Stem Cell Research and Therapeutics

Yanhong Shi • Dennis O. Clegg
Editors

Stem Cell Research and Therapeutics

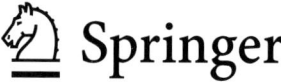 Springer

Editors
Yanhong Shi
Beckman Research Intitute of City of Hope
Duarte, CA
USA

Dennis O. Clegg
University of California
Santa Barbara, CA
USA

ISBN: 978-1-4020-8501-7   e-ISBN: 978-1-4020-8502-4

Library of Congress Control Number: 2008927237

Printed on acid-free paper

9 8 7 6 5 4 3 2 1

springer.com

Preface

This book is an updated reference for one of the most exciting field of biomedical researches- Stem Cell Research and its therapeutic applications. Stem cell research holds great promise for the treatment of many human diseases that currently lack effective therapies. The set of chapters in this book provide insights into both basic stem cell biology and clinical applications of stem cell-based cell replacement therapies for a variety of human diseases, including cardiovascular diseases, neurological disorders, and liver degeneration. It also covers novel technologies for the culture and differentiation of both human embryonic stem cells and adult tissue stem cells. This book summarizes our current state of knowledge in stem cell research and integrates basic stem cell biology with regenerative medicine in an overall context. It is an essential reference for students, postdoctoral fellows, academic and industrial scientists, and clinicians.

Acknowledgements

The editors would like to thank Ms. Jill Brantley, Rose Chavarin, Alina Haas, and Emily Sun for their administrative assistance and proof-reading of this book. We would also like to thank all the authors for their contributions.

The editors wish to dedicate this book to our mentors Ron Evans, Fred Gage, and, in memory of Daniel E. Koshland, Jr.

Contents

Contributors

Timothy Allsopp
Stem Cell Sciences UK Ltd, Minerva Building 250, Babraham Research Campus,
Cambridge, UK CB22 3AT

Basam Z. Barkho
Department of Neurosciences and University of New Mexico, School of
Medicine, Albuquerque, NM 87131, USA

Ronnda Bartel
Aastrom Biosciences, Inc., P.O. Box 376, Ann Arbor, MI 48106, USA

Crestina L. Beites
Department of Anatomy & Neurobiology, 264 Med Surge II,
University of California, Irvine College of Medicine, Irvine, CA 92697-1275,
USA

Paul Bello
Stem Cell Sciences Pty Ltd., Melbourne, Australia

Federico Benetti
Benetti Foundation, Rosario, Argentina

Alexandre Bonnin
Department of Pharmacology, and the Kennedy Center for Research on
Human Development Vanderbilt University, 465 – 21st Avenue,
South Nashville, TN 37232, USA

Daniel Brusich
Cardiac Surgical and Heart Failure Department, Asociacion Espanola,
Montevideo, Uruguay

David Buchholz
Center for Stem Cell Biology and Engineering, Neuroscience Research Institute,
University of California, Santa Barbara, CA 93106, USA

Anne L. Calof
Departments of Anatomy and Neurobiology, Developmental and Cell
Biology, and Ophthalmology, 264 Med Surge II, University of California,
Irvine College of Medicine, Irvine, CA 92697-1275, USA

Yen Choo
Plasticell Ltd., Imperial Bioincubator, Bessemer Building (RSM), Prince Consort
Road, South Kensington, London SW7 2BP, UK

Dennis O. Clegg
Center for Stem Cell Biology and Engineering and Neuroscience Research
Institute, University of California, Santa Barbara, CA 93106, USA

Wangde Dai
The Heart Institute and Good Samaritan Hospital, Division of Cardiovascular
Medicine of the Keck School of Medicine at University of Southern California,
Los Angeles, CA 90017-2395, USA

James Dennis
Department of Orthopaedics, Case Western Reserve University, Cleveland, OH
44106, USA

Agustin Fronzutti
Cardiac Surgical and Heart Failure Department, Asociacion Espanola,
Montevideo, Uruguay

Norma Fulton
Stem Cell Sciences UK Ltd., Roger Land Building, Kings Buildings, West Mains
Road, Edinburgh, UK EH9 3JQ

Luis Geffner
Stem Cell Program, Junta de Beneficencia, Guayaquil, Ecuador

Loyal A. Goff
W. M. Keck Center for Collaborative Neuroscience, and Rutgers Stem Cell
Research Center, Rutgers University, Piscataway, NJ 08854, USA

Kimberly K. Gokoffski
Department of Developmental and Cell Biology,
264 Med Surge II, University of California, Irvine College of Medicine,
Irvine, CA 92697-1275, USA

Kristin L. Goltry
Aastrom Biosciences, Inc.,24 Frank Lloyd Wright Drive, Lobby K Ann Arbor,
MI 48105, USA

Michelle Greene
Bioscience Division, Millipore Corporation, 28820 Single Oak Drive, Temecula,
CA 92590, USA

Nagy Habib
Department of Surgery, Hammersmith Campus, Imperial College, London, UK

Jason A. Hamilton
Department of Anatomy and Neurobiology, 264 Med Surge II, University of California, Irvine College of Medicine, Irvine, CA 92697-1275, USA

Ronald P. Hart
W. M. Keck Center for Collaborative Neuroscience, and Rutgers Stem Cell Research Center, Rutgers University, 604 Allison Road, Room D251, Piscataway, NJ 08854, USA

Sherry Hikita
Center for Stem Cell Biology and Engineering, Neuroscience Research Institute, University of California, Santa Barbara, CA 93106, USA

Robert M. Hoffman
AntiCancer, Inc., 7917 Ostrow Street, San Diego, CA 92111, USA

Piper L. W. Hollenbeck
Graduate Student, Department of Anatomy and Neurobiology, 264 Med Surge II, University of California, Irvine College of Medicine, Irvine, CA 92697-1275, USA

Lilian Hook
Stem Cell Sciences UK Ltd., Roger Land Building, Kings Buildings, West Mains Road, Edinburgh, UK EH9 3JQ

Qirui Hu
Center for Stem Cell Biology and Engineering, Neuroscience Research Institute, University of California, Santa Barbara, CA 93106, USA

Jacqui Johnson
Stem Cell Sciences Pty Ltd., Melbourne, Australia

Lincoln V. Johnson
Center for Stem Cell Biology and Engineering, Neuroscience Research Institute, University of California, Santa Barbara, CA 93106, USA

Shimako Kawauchi
Department of Anatomy and Neurobiology, 264 Med Surge II, University of California, Irvine College of Medicine, Irvine, CA 92697-1275, USA

Joon Kim
Department of Neurosciences, University of California at San Diego, Leichtag 332, 9500 Gilman Drive, La Jolla, CA 92093, USA

Henry J. Klassen
Stem Cell and Retinal Regeneration Program, Department of Ophthalmology, School of Medicine, University of California, Irvine, 101 The City Drive, Bldg. 55, Room 204, Orange, CA 92868-4380, USA

Robert A. Kloner
The Heart Institute, Good Samaritan Hospital, 1225 Wilshire Boulevard, Los
Angeles, CA 90017, USA

Robert Kovelman
Bioscience Division, Millipore Corporation, 28820 Single Oak Drive, Temecula,
CA 92590, USA

Uma Lakshmipathy
Regenerative Medicine, Invitrogen, Inc., P.O. Box 6482, Carlsbad, CA 92008, USA

Nataša Levičar
Department of Surgery, Hammersmith Campus, Imperial College, London, UK

Xuekun Li
Department of Neurosciences, University of New Mexico, School of Medicine,
Albuquerque, NM 87131, USA

Juan Paganini
Cardiac Surgical and Heart Failure Department, Asociacion Espanola,
Montevideo, Uruguay

Roberto Paganini
Cardiac Surgical and Heart Failure Department, Asociacion Espanola,
Montevideo, Uruguay

Madhava Pai
Department of Surgery, Hammersmith Campus, Imperial College, London, UK

Amit Patel
University of Pittsburgh, McGowan Institute for Regenerative Medicine,
Pittsburgh, PA

Kenneth Pollock
ReNeuron Ltd., 10 Nugent Road, Surrey Research Park, Guildford, GU2 7AF, UK

Teisha Rowland
Center for Stem Cell Biology and Engineering, Neuroscience Research Institute,
University of California, Santa Barbara, CA 93106, USA

Jon Rowley
Aastrom Biosciences, Inc., P.O. Box 376, Ann Arbor, MI 48106, USA

Gregor Russell
Stem Cell Sciences UK Ltd., Roger Land Building, Kings Buildings, West Mains
Road, Edinburgh, UK EH9 3JQ

Rosaseyla Santos
Department of Anatomy and Neurobiology, 264 Med Surge II, University of
California, Irvine College of Medicine, Irvine, CA 92697-1275, USA

Yanhong Shi
Division of Neurosciences, and Center for Gene Expression and Drug Discovery,
Beckman Research Institute of City of Hope, 1500 E. Duarte Road, Duarte, CA
91010, USA

John D. Sinden
ReNeuron Ltd., 10 Nugent Road, Surrey Research Park, Guildford, GU2 7AF, UK

Matthew A. Singer
Bioscience Division, Millipore Corporation, 28820 Single Oak Drive, Temecula,
CA 92590, USA

Douglas Smith
Aastrom Biosciences, Inc., P.O. Box 376, Ann Arbor, MI 48106, USA

GuoQiang Sun
Division of Neurosciences, and Center for Gene Expression and Drug Discovery,
Beckman Research Institute of City of Hope, 1500 E. Duarte Road, Duarte, CA
91010, USA

Hsiao-Huei Wu
Research Instructor, Department of Biochemistry, Vanderbilt University Medical
School, Nashville, TN 37232, USA

Chunnian Zhao
Division of Neurosciences, and Center for Gene Expression and Drug Discovery,
Beckman Research Institute of City of Hope, 1500 E. Duarte Road, Duarte, CA
91010, USA

Xinyu Zhao
Department of Neurosciences, University of New Mexico, School of Medicine,
MSC 08 4740, 915 Camino de Salud NE, Albuquerque, NM 87131-0001, USA

Chapter 1
Retinal Pigment Epithelial Cells: Development *In Vivo* and Derivation from Human Embryonic Stem Cells *In Vitro* for Treatment of Age-Related Macular Degeneration

Dennis O. Clegg*, David Buchholz, Sherry Hikita, Teisha Rowland, Qirui Hu, and Lincoln V. Johnson

Abstract The retinal pigment epithelium (RPE) plays a key role in supporting photoreceptor survival and function, and RPE loss and dysfunction in age-related macular degeneration (AMD) leads to photoreceptor death. AMD is one of the leading causes of blindness, yet there is neither a cure nor a way to prevent it. In this chapter, we discuss recent progress in the study of AMD, summarize what is known about RPE development, and review recent progress in deriving RPE from human embryonic stem cells (hESC). The RPE is derived from the optic vesicle, which in turn is derived from the eye field of the anterior neural plate. Multiple extracellular signaling factors and transcriptional regulators have been identified that are crucial to RPE development. Knowledge of these events is guiding efforts to understand how hESC differentiate into RPE cells that might be used therapeutically for AMD. RPE derived from hESC are remarkably similar to fetal RPE with respect to gene expression and cellular function. Future research on these cells will lead to a better understanding of RPE development and the advancement of cellular therapy for AMD.

Keywords Age-related macular degeneration, human embryonic stem cells, ocular development, retinal cells, retinal pigment epithelium

---

Center for Stem Cell Biology and Engineering, Neuroscience Research Institute, University of California, Santa Barbara, CA 93106, USA

*Corresponding Author:
e-mail: clegg@lifesci.ucsb.edu

Abbreviations AMD Age-related macular degeneration; hESC Human embryonic stem cells; hESC-RPE RPE-like cells derived from human embryonic stem cells; PEDF Pigment epithelium-derived factor; RPE Retinal pigment epithelium; VEGF Vascular endothelial growth factor

1.1   Introduction

Most diseases that result in loss of vision are not lethal, but are certainly some of the most insidious because of their horrible influence on the quality of life. AMD is the leading cause of blindness in elderly people of the western world. AMD is a daunting public health problem; an estimated 10–30% of people over 75 years of age are afflicted, totaling 30 million people, and the incidence of AMD is predicted to double over the next 25 years [117]. There is no effective treatment or cure for the disease, and the molecular mechanisms are not completely understood.

1.2   Molecular, Cellular and Genetic Studies of AMD

Loss of vision in AMD is a result of degeneration of rod and cone photoreceptors in the macular region of the central retina, which is responsible for high acuity vision [37, 104]. Death of the photoreceptors appears to be a consequence of degeneration and apoptosis of neighboring RPE cells [28, 32, 115]. In ~10% of cases, further disease progression leads to exudative or wet AMD, which is characterized by neovascularization of the retina. AMD is a heterogeneous, multifactorial disease with both environmental and genetic factors contributing to the disease [116, 134]. Epidemiological studies link the disease to four risk factors: age, obesity, cigarette smoking and inheritance. (See Gehrs et al. [41] for a recent comprehensive review of AMD.)

The formation of drusen, abnormal deposits in Bruch's membrane underlying the RPE, is an important hallmark of AMD [1, 47]. Significant drusen formation appears to precede the occurrence of visual symptoms in AMD. Many investigators hypothesize that drusen are a cause of AMD, although the possibility that they are simply a consequence of the disease cannot be ruled out. Typically, drusen lie between the RPE basement membrane and the inner collagenous layer of Bruch's membrane and contain a variety of ECM molecules, such as collagens, laminin, fibronectin, vitronectin and heparan sulfate. Other reported drusen components include integrins, β-amyloid, amyloid P component, ubiquitin, apolipoprotein E, α1-antitrypsin, IgG, complement factors C5 and C5b-9, TIMP-3, and advanced glycation end products [5, 16, 23, 29, 38, 47, 58–60, 81, 82, 95, 97, 102]. Proteomic analysis has identified 126 proteins in drusen, many of which contain carboxyethyl pyrrole modifications derived from docosahexaenoate-containing lipids [54].

This growing list of drusen components includes acute phase reactant plasma proteins that are up-regulated during immune responses. This led some investigators to propose that drusen may result from an inflammatory immune reaction against RPE cells [4, 47, 58, 104]. In support of this idea, Ig-G, C5b-9 – positive "compromised" RPE cells were identified, and macrophage cell processes have been imaged that pass from the choroid through Bruch's membrane to the core of drusen particles [26, 58, 62, 103]. It is not understood why the drusen particles are not cleared by immune cells. One idea is that the RPE monolayer attempts to repair Bruch's membrane, and as a result shuts out immune cells and precludes clearance [47].

A major breakthrough in our understanding of AMD has come from genetic studies, which have implicated multiple genes encoding proteins important in immune function. As many as 75% of AMD cases can be explained by polymorphisms in two genes encoding regulatory factors in the alternative complement pathway: Factor H and Factor B [2, 34, 44, 48, 49, 65, 112]. In addition, smaller percentages of AMD, are linked to mutations in ABCA4, which encodes a transporter [3], fibulin-5, encoding a matrix protein in Bruch's membrane [121], and CX3CR1, a chemokine receptor important in leukocyte function [129]. These findings confirm earlier suspicions that immune function is involved, and also point the crucial functions of the extracellular matrix in AMD.

One hypothesis to explain the progression of some forms of AMD may be as follows: (1) RPE cells may die via complement attack due to improper regulation of the alternative complement pathway, or via loss of attachment to Bruch's membrane, or via accumulation of nondegradable retinoid-phosopholipid adducts such as A2E in lipofuscin [118]. (2) An inflammatory immune reaction and wound repair response occurs in an attempt to clear RPE debris. (3) Leftover debris accumulates in the form of drusen deposits, and (4) The presence of drusen may lead to further disruption of RPE attachment and RPE death [4, 22, 41, 47].

1.2.1 Cellular Therapy for AMD

Therapeutic options for the treatment of AMD are limited. While some recent progress has been made in treating the wet form of AMD, using Veg-F inhibitors such as Avastin and Leucentis, and with surgical intervention, treatments for the majority of cases are lacking [24, 41]. Since loss of RPE cells is thought to give rise to AMD, then one treatment option might be to replace RPE cells in the macula via cellular transplantation. If RPE could be replenished before the demise of macular photoreceptors, and at the same time genetic defects could be addressed, it might be possible to prevent vision loss. Proof of principal for such an approach has already been demonstrated by transplantation in animal models and by trials in humans where autologous transplantation of RPE/choroid from peripheral eye has been carried out (see review by da Cruz et al. [24]).

Our laboratory and others have recently shown that RPE-like cells can be derived from mouse, primate and human embryonic stem cells (hESC) [53, 61, 66, 101, 131]. Others have reported that bone marrow-derived stem cells can differentiate into RPE-like cells [11, 78]. These stem cell-derived RPE may provide a source of cells for transplantation therapy. In addition, human embryonic stem cell-derived RPE provide an invaluable model for studying human RPE development and differentiation. Below, we describe RPE cell structure, function, and development, as well as recent studies of RPE-like cells derived from hESC.

1.3   The Retinal Pigment Epithelium

The RPE is a highly polarized monolayer of cuboidal cells intimately associated with the rod and cone photoreceptors of the adult retina. A comprehensive review of RPE function in the visual system has recently been published [122]. Situated behind the neural retina, the RPE is a typical polarized epithelium, with the basal side attached to a basal lamina that is part of Bruch's membrane. Apical microvilli interdigitate between the outer segments of rods and cones. Many roles are fulfilled by the RPE that are necessary for proper visual function. As pigmented cells, the RPE absorbs stray light to increase visual sensitivity and protect against photo-oxidation. As an epithelium with tight junctions, the RPE forms part of the blood/retina barrier, transporting nutrients and ions between the photoreceptors at its apical surface and the choriocapillaris at its basal surface. The RPE secretes two important factors in the healthy eye: the neuroprotective/antiangiogenic pigment epithelium-derived factor (PEDF) to the neural retina, and the vasoprotective/angiogenic vascular endothelial growth factor (VEGF) to the choroid. In the visual cycle, the RPE takes up all-*trans*-retinal from the photoreceptors and reisomerizes it to 11-*cis*-retinal, returning the functional chromophore to the photoreceptors. In addition to recycling 11-*cis*-retinal for the photoreceptors, the RPE also phagocytoses photoreceptor outer segments, according to a daily circadian cycle, to relieve the photoreceptors of light-induced free radicals. Together the RPE and photoreceptors form a functional unit where degeneration of one leads to degeneration of the other. With its many critical roles, it is no surprise that several diseases are associated with RPE dysfunction or degeneration. In addition to AMD, some forms of retinitis pigmentosa and Stargardt's disease have also been traced to RPE dysfunction [41, 51, 69].

1.3.1   RPE Development

Ocular development has been studied in many model organisms, most extensively in *Drosophila*, *Xenopus*, zebrafish, chick and mouse. Despite major advances in elucidating transcription factor and signaling networks specifying the eye field and its subsequent cell types, there remain many key questions regarding how these networks are integrated to direct differentiation. Knowledge of human ocular development is restricted to analysis of naturally occurring mutations. hESCs provide a human system to test and expand upon networks defined in other model organisms.

The developmental journey that culminates in RPE differentiation involves neural induction, followed by eye field specification, bisection of the eye field, and then differentiation of the optic cup to become RPE. The following is a brief review of what is known of RPE development with the intent of highlighting key extracellular signaling factors that may be used to direct hESC differentiation as well as intracellular regulatory factors that may be used as markers of progenitor and mature states.

1.3.1.1 Neural Induction and Eye Field Specification in the Anterior Neural Plate

The RPE is derived from cells of the optic vesicle which itself arises from a subset of cells in the anterior neural plate known as the eye field [21, 142]. It has been demonstrated in *Xenopus* that the eye field is partially specified prior to gastrulation, although the mechanism remains unclear [139]. Neural induction arises through the combined activities of: (1) FGF and Notch signaling; (2) Time-dependent canonical Wnt activation and inhibition; and (3) Inhibition of BMP signaling by Noggin, Chordin and Follistatin. The result is the generation of the definitive neural plate [120]. The neural plate then develops anterior characteristics during early gastrulation via inhibition or exclusion of caudalizing factors [132]. The secreted proteins Cerberus and Insulin-like Growth Factor (IGF) combine to inhibit many of these caudalizing pathways and to induce expression of anterior transcription factors such as *Otx2* [19, 45, 107].

Next, the anterior neural plate is patterned into the telencephalon, eye field and diencephalon by many extracellular signaling pathways (Fig. 1.1). The anterior neural border expresses *Fgf3*, *Fgf8* and *tiarin*, which specify the telencephalon. Telencephalic expression of the Wnt inhibitor *Tlc*, a secreted Frizzled Related Protein (sFRP), is also required for development of the telencephalon [33, 132]. Diencephalic characteristics are specified by canonical *Wnt8b/Wnt1* signaling as well as retinoic acid [36, 50].

Eye field specification relies on many extracellular factors including Wnts, sFRPs, ephrins, Notch and IGF. Like the telencephalon, the eye field requires inhibition of canonical Wnt signaling. This is achieved through expression of the Wnt/β-catenin inhibitors *sFRP1* and *sFRP5* (activated by *Lhx5*), and direct transcriptional repression of Wnt/β-catenin by the transcription factor *Six3* [20, 63, 73, 91, 105]. Non-canonical Wnt signaling through *Wnt11/Wnt4*, similar to the *Drosophila* planar cell polarity pathway, also serves many functions to specify the early eye field. Through *Wnt11/Wnt4* and their receptors *Fz5/Fz3*, non-canonical Wnt signaling inhibits canonical Wnt/β-catenin signaling and induces expression of the eye field marker *Rx*. In addition, these Wnts induce *ephrinB1* signaling, which promotes cell migration into the eye field [20, 76, 91]. Following these morphogenetic movements, Notch signaling appears to be necessary for expression of the transcription factors that mark the early eye field [72, 76, 100, 139].

IGF signals through two major pathways: the MAP Kinase pathway (MAPK) and the PI3-Kinase/Akt pathway (PI3K/Akt) [99]. *Igf1* utilizes both pathways in early

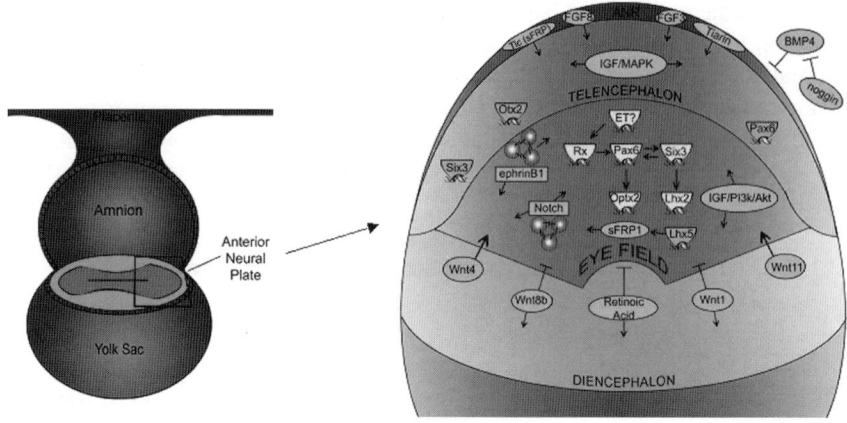

Fig. 1.1 Patterning of the eye field and anterior neural plate. The eye field is found within the anterior neural plate and bordered by the telencephalon rostrally and the diencephalon caudally. The anterior neural plate develops in a BMP-negative environment through the inhibitory action of noggin. The telencephalon and eye field are induced by suppression of the caudalizing retinoic acid and canonical Wnt/β-catenin signals whereas the diencephalon is specified by these signals (through Wnt8b/Wnt1 and RA). Wnt non-canonical signaling on the other hand specifies the eye field (through Wnt4/Wnt11). Signaling from the anterior neural ridge (ANR) specifies the telencephalon. IGF appears to activate the telencephalon and eye field through different pathways, MAPK for the telencephalon and PI3K/Akt for the eye field. Notch and ephrin cell-cell signaling guides and specifies cells to the eye field. The eye field is characterized by the overlapping expression patterns of several transcription factors, highlighted in yellow. Other important transcription factors are indicated in orange. Signaling molecules are indicated in blue (*See Color Plates*)

neural development. The IGF-MAPK pathway induces forebrain markers such as *Otx2* and *Sox3* [106, 107]. The IGF/PI3k/Akt pathway regulates expression of several eye field transcription factors including *Rx, Lhx2, Pax6* and *Six3* [114, 135].

1.3.1.2   Eye Field Transcription Factors

The eye field is designated by the overlapping expression patterns of the transcription factors *ET, Rx1, Pax6, Six3, Lhx2* and *Optx2* in *Xenopus* (similarly in other vertebrates and even *Drosophila*) and arises from a *noggin/Otx2/Hesx1* positive environment in the anterior neural plate [7, 71, 139, 142]. These eye field transcription factors partially regulate each other, as loss or overexpression of one often affects the others in a similar way [142]. An overview of this hierarchical system is shown in Fig. 1.1 and examined in more detail below.

   ET(Tbx3) is a T-box transcription factor (Tbx) of the *Tbx2* family that appears to be at the head of eye field specification hierarchy, at least in *Xenopus*. *Tbx2* and *Tbx3* may be functionally redundant in *Xenopus*, while *Tbx2* may be the functional equivalent in zebrafish [30, 123]. It is unclear which Tbx gene, if any, is the functional human homolog of *Xenopus ET* [142]. It is also unclear how *ET* expression is directly induced. However, noggin overexpression can inhibit expression of *ET* and this inhibition can be rescued by Otx2 overexpression [142]. None of the other eye field transcription factors can induce *ET* expression while *ET* can drive *Rx1*, *Lhx2* and *tll* expression [77, 142]. Overexpression of *ET* results in ventral optic cup malformations including a loss of ventral RPE [123, 133].

The retinal homeobox transcription factor (*Rx/Rax*) is necessary for eye formation in all vertebrates studied, but does not appear to play a direct role in *Drosophila* eye development [12]. *Rx* expression is positively regulated, either directly or indirectly, by *chordin, noggin, Igf1, Wnt-4, Wnt-11, notch, hedgehog* and *Six3* [9, 20, 43, 73, 91, 100, 135, 142]. In turn, *Rx* positively regulates *Pax6, Lhx2, tll, Optx2, BF-1, Zic2, Hairy2* and *Hmgb3* and negatively regulates *Otx2, Ngnr-1, Delta-1, p27Kip1* and *N-tubulin* in the early eye field [8, 9, 127, 142]. Loss of *Rx* results in loss of optic vesicle evagination from the forebrain and a thinning of the ventral forebrain [12]. Overexpression of *Rx* results in over-proliferation of both the neural retina and the RPE [12]. The roles of *Rx* at the neural plate stage appear to be specification of the eye field, promotion of cell proliferation, and inhibition of neurulation/maintenance of a progenitor state [9, 12, 127, 140].

The paired box and paired-like homeobox transcription factor *Pax6* has been touted as a master regulator of eye development because ectopic expression can induce eye formation in flies, and because of its high degree of conservation throughout evolution [70]. Although it is now clear that there is no single "master regulator" of eye development, *Pax6* is clearly one of the major players [21]. Null mutants lack a fully developed optic cup, never develop differentiated neural retina or RPE, and die at birth [52]. Heterozygotes develop a range of phenotypes including aniridia and microphthalmia [52]. Interestingly, overexpression also results in microphthalmia, indicating a critical role for *Pax6* gene dosage [52]. *Pax6* is positively regulated by *noggin, Six3, Rx, Lhx2, tll, Wnt-4, Igf1* and *notch* [91, 100, 135, 142]. *Pax6* enhances expression of *Six3, Lhx2, tll*, and *Optx2* and inhibits the forebrain gene *Hesx1* in the early eye field [119, 142].

Six3 is a Six domain/homeodomain containing transcription factor necessary for proper forebrain and eye development [21]. Loss of *Six3* results in loss of forebrain and posteriorization of the remaining forebrain tissue, while overexpression leads to enlargement of the eye and forebrain expansion [73, 83]. Many roles for *Six3* have been identified during patterning of the anterior neural plate. These include: direct transcriptional inhibition of *Wnt1* and *Bmp4*, mutual repression against *Irx3* forming an anterior/posterior forebrain boundary, enhancement of proliferation/maintenance of a progenitor state through transcriptional regulation of *cyclinD1, p27, Zic2, Hairy2* and direct binding to Geminin, and positive regulation of the eye field transcription factors *Pax6, Lhx2* [27, 43, 68, 73, 142]. Transcriptional repression by *Six3* is modulated by interactions with the *groucho* family genes *Tle1* and *Aes* [83]. *Six3* is positively regulated by *Igf1, notch, noggin, Pax6* and *tll* [100, 135, 142].

Lhx2 is a LIM-homeodomain containing transcription factor required for eye and forebrain development [110]. Overexpression or knockdown of *Lhx2* shows similar phenotypes to *Six3* overexpression or knockdown [6]. Indeed, *Lhx2* appears to function downstream of *Six3* to regulate proliferation in the anterior neural plate

[6]. *Lhx2* is positively regulated by *noggin, ET, Pax6, Six3, Rx* and *tll* [142]. Little is known of the downstream effectors of *Lhx2*. *Pax6* is upregulated by overexpression of *Lhx2* and based on its ability to rescue *Six3* mutants, *Lhx2* may regulate cell cycle genes such as *cyclinD1* and *p27* [6, 142].

Optx2 (also known as *Six6* or *Six9*) is another *Six*-homeodomain containing transcription factor related to *Six3* [21]. Expression of *Optx2* begins later than *Six3* and the other eye field transcription factors and *Optx2* cannot regulate the others [142]. Consistent with its later role in the eye field, mutations result in anophthalmia rather than larger scale forebrain malformations [40]. *Optx2* requires *Rx/Rax* for expression and is also positively regulated by *noggin* and *Pax6* [127, 142]. Like *Six3*, *Optx2* can interact with the *groucho* homologues *Tle1* and *Aes* and causes over-proliferation when overexpressed [83].

1.3.1.3   Bisection of the Eye Field and Patterning of the Optic Vesicle into RPE, Neural Retina and Optic Stalk

The formation of two symmetric optic vesicles results from *Sonic Hedgehog (shh)* signaling, which arises from the prechordal plate [136] (Fig. 1.2A). An elegant demonstration of *shh* function is found in nature, where sheep that eat corn lilies have lambs with a single eye, due to lack of eye field bisection. Corn lilies contain the alkaloid cyclopamine, which inhibits the *shh* signaling pathway [64]. In *Xenopus* and chick, *shh* represses eye field transcription factors in the midline, while in zebrafish eye field separation is accompanied by cell migration away from the midline [35, 77]. The result is two symmetric eye fields that begin to evaginate from the forebrain towards the surface ectoderm as optic vesicles (at ~4 weeks in human, ~E8.5 in mouse) [14]. As previously mentioned, *Rx* is necessary for this optic vesicle evagination [12]. *Shh* not only suppresses the eye field in the midline, it also sets up early polarity in the optic vesicle, specifying the proximal/ventral region that will become the optic stalk and ventral neuroretina (characterized *Vax1* and *Vax2* expression) [21]. At this early optic vesicle stage, many genes are co-expressed throughout the optic vesicle including: *Pax6, Pax2, Six3, Rx, Otx1/2* [13, 88] (Fig. 1.2B).

Otx1/2 is one of the two master transcription factors in RPE differentiation [87]. Little is known about the direct activation of *Otx1/2* in the optic vesicle as it appears to be repressed in the early eye field [142], but *Rx* may play a role. In zebrafish there are three *Rx* genes (*Rx1–3*). Zebrafish *Rx3* has been implicated in specification of RPE, where it lies upstream of both *Otx2* and the other master RPE transcription factor, *Micropthalmia-associated Transcription Factor (Mitf)* [113]. Similarly, overexpression of *Rx* in *Xenopus* generates both ectopic RPE and neural retina [89]. Interestingly, in the anterior neural plate, *Rx* may be one of the factors that represses *Otx2* [142]. Stage-specific cofactors may be required to direct the function of *Rx*. It is worthwhile to note that the RPE may arise from the *Otx2* positive periphery of the eye field and never experience an *Otx2* negative environment [12, 88].

As the optic vesicle makes contact with the surface ectoderm, extracellular signals begin to resolve the vesicle into the three regions of the initially tri-potent optic vesicle: the presumptive optic stalk, presumptive neural retina and presumptive RPE [88] (Fig. 1.2B). At this time, the master pigment gene *Mitf*, is activated. In mouse, *Mitf* is initially expressed throughout the optic vesicle while in chick initial expression is localized to the distal optic vesicle [13, 94]. BMP signaling from the surface ectoderm induces *Mitf* expression in the distal optic vesicle in chick [94]. Also in chick, the BMP related molecule Activin A has been shown to suffice for the extraocular mesenchyme in the specification of RPE although this may represent a maintenance effect rather than specification [39, 94]. In mouse, alterations in the levels of *Bmp4* signaling have also been shown to affect RPE development, implicating the morphogen activity of BMPs in the regionalization of the optic vesicle [14]. *Pax6* and *Pax2* appear to act redundantly in the activation of at least one isoform of *Mitf*, which exists in nine isoforms, although *Pax2* may only act in the absence of *Pax6* [13, 88].

Following *Mitf* induction, FGF signaling, again from the surface ectoderm, induces *Chx10* expression in the presumptive neural retina, which subsequently downregulates neural retina expression of *Mitf* [55, 94]. *Otx1/2* is also downregulated in the presumptive neural retina although it is unclear if this is a direct effect of *Chx10*. *Otx1/2* and *Mitf* are both necessary for the maintained expression of each other and the downregulation of *Otx1/2* may be the result of the direct inhibition of *Mitf* by *Chx10* [15]. *Otx1/2* and *Mitf* are thus relegated to the dorsal optic vesicle, where their expression is maintained by extraocular mesenchyme, which expresses BMPs (possibly including Activin A) [39, 94]. As previously mentioned, ventrally expressed *shh* induces expression of *Vax1/2* in the presumptive optic stalk, forming a distinct boundary with *Mitf* expression where the two may mutually repress each other [15]. The presumptive RPE is now bounded dorsal/distally by the neural retina and ventral/proximally by the optic stalk.

Interestingly, as *Otx1/2* and *Mitf* expression becomes isolated to the presumptive RPE, the expression of *Rx*, *Pax6* and *Pax2*, transcription factors thought to activate these genes, is reduced there (along with the other early eye field transcription factors) [88]. *Rx* and *Pax6* segregate to the neural retina and *Pax2* to the optic stalk [88]. *Pax6* may be downregulated by direct protein-protein interaction with Mitf, which leads to mutual inhibition in vitro [109].

1.3.1.4 Optic Cup Formation and RPE Pigmentation

After reaching the surface ectoderm, both the optic vesicle and ectoderm invaginate to form the optic cup [21] (Fig. 1.2C). Both *Pax6* and *Lhx2* are independently required for the morphogenetic transition from optic vesicle to optic cup [21]. During this time the RPE spreads ventrally to envelop the neural retina at the back of the optic cup [15].

At this stage hedgehog signaling appears to play a role in RPE maintenance. Inhibition of *shh* in chick during the optic vesicle/optic cup transition or afterwards

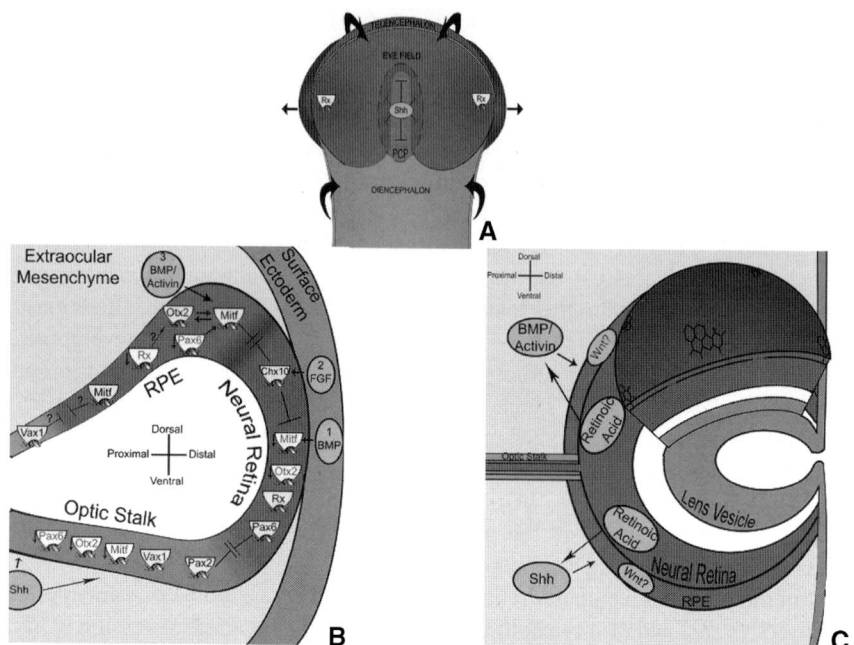

Fig. 1.2 From optic vesicle to optic cup. (**A**) *Sonic Hedgehog* (Shh) arising from the ventrally located prechordal plate (PCP) divides the eye field by down-regulating eye field transcription factors in the midline. *Rx* signaling is necessary for optic vesicle evagination towards the surface ectoderm as the neural tube folds. Arrows show morphogenetic movements. (**B**) As the optic vesicle reaches the surface ectoderm, the presumptive RPE, neural retina and optic stalk begin to differentiate. BMP signaling from the surface ectoderm induces *Mitf* expression (1). This is followed by a wave of FGF signaling from the surface ectoderm which induces *Chx10* expression (2). *Chx10* down regulates *Mitf* within the presumptive neural retina. *Mitf* is maintained/specified in the dorsal/distal optic vesicle by BMP/Activin signaling (3). Transcription factors in gray are initially expressed but eventually down-regulated. (**C**) Both the optic vesicle and the surface ectoderm invaginate to form the optic cup and lens vesicle. The RPE spreads ventrally to surround the neural retina. Many signaling molecules are thought to act at this stage, although their exact mechanisms and functions remain to be elucidated (*See Color Plates*)

results in a loss of ventral RPE [141]. Similarly in *Xenopus*, cyclopamine treatment after eye field separation leads to a reduction in peripheral RPE pigmentation [108]. Additionally, the RPE itself becomes a source of hedgehog proteins, with strong expression centrally located and hedgehog receptors located peripherally [108]. A short time later retinal ganglion cell axons entering the optic stalk secrete *shh*, loss of which results in a conversion of optic stalk to RPE [25]. The cell cycle inhibitor *Gas1* can interact positively or negatively with *shh*. In *Gas1* mutants, the ventral RPE transdifferentiates to neural retina, showing a gradual loss of *Mitf* [75].

Wnt signaling may also play a role at this stage in RPE development. *Wnt/β-catenin* signaling can directly regulate the melanocyte specific isoform of *Mitf* (*Mitf-M*) [125]. Additionally, *Wnt* signaling can synergize with *Mitf-M* to activate melanin synthesis proteins in melanocytes [137]. Although it is unclear whether the *Mitf* isoforms in RPE respond in the same way, a GFP-Wnt/β-catenin reporter construct shows that the RPE is Wnt responsive in zebrafish at the optic cup stage [31]. Finally, several Wnts, Frizzleds and SFRPs are expressed by the RPE in the optic cup stage [57, 80].

Retinoic acid is synthesized in the optic vesicle and its target is the extraocular mesenchyme [90, 93]. Although RA does not directly signal back onto the optic vesicle, it likely regulates *Bmp*, *Fgf* and *Shh* signaling coming from the extraocular mesenchyme [50, 111]. Studies in *retinaldehyde dehydrogenase* mutant mice and the vitamin A deficient (VAD) quail model, as well as studies of mice with mutations in the RA inducible *AP-2α* gene, show retinoic acid plays a role in proper morphogenesis and maintenance, if not specification, of the optic vesicle and RPE [50, 85, 90, 93].

Pigmentation and the final differentiation of RPE to a cuboidal epithelial monolayer with tight junctions occurs during the optic cup stage, accompanying neural retina differentiation[122]. *Otx2* and *Mitf* synergize to activate the melanin pigment synthesis genes *Tyrosinase*, *Trp1* and *Trp2 (Dct)* and the melanosomal glycoprotein *QNR71* [87, 126]. Additional signaling molecules such as hedgehogs and Wnts likely play a role in activating transcription of melanin synthesis genes [88]. In humans, pigmentation is first observed after 5.5 weeks in utero [98].

Proliferation of RPE cells occurs in two phases in rodents (Stroeva and Mitashov, 1983), and the second phase of mitosis does not always include cytokinesis, resulting in some binucleate cells [131]. *Mitf* expression is associated with a reduction in cell proliferation and exit from the cell cycle [15]. In melanocytes this is achieved by activation of the cell cycle inhibitor p21Cip1[18]. It is unclear whether or not a similar pathway exists in RPE, but *Mitf* loss-of-function mutations lead to increased proliferation in the presumptive RPE [15].

The role for *Mitf* in specification and differentiation of RPE may be transient as *Mitf* is not detected in the RPE after birth in mouse or chick [92, 96]. *Otx2* expression on the other hand is maintained in the mature adult RPE [88]. Other markers of mature RPE include: integrin $\alpha_v\beta_5$ (binds photoreceptor outer segments [79]); the apical proteins EMMPRIN, Ezrin and N-CAM-140; *melanosomal matrix protein 115 (MMP115)*; *CRBP*, *CRALBP* and *RPE-65* (visual cycle components); and the tight junction components *ZO-1* and *occluding* [86, 122]. Final differentiation of the RPE occurs in association with photoreceptor outer segment extension; the RPE envelop the outer segments with long and short microvilli, thus beginning their lifelong partnership [122].

1.4 Differentiation of hESC into RPE-Like Cells

If a stem cell is to assume the RPE fate, presumably it must undergo a developmental progression similar to the complex pathway described above. As mentioned earlier, embryonic stem cells from mouse, monkey and human have been reported to differentiate into RPE-like cells [53, 61, 66, 101, 131]. This can occur spontaneously in a small percentage of cells, after simply removing bFGF to allow widespread differentiation of hESC [66, 67]. Others have used methods to induce ocular and RPE fate, for example, using co-culture with PA-6 cells, a bone marrow stromal cell line with neuralizing activity [61], or using matrix from human amniotic membrane [130].

Ideally, a protocol with defined factors to induce large scale ocular differentiation would be desirable. Wnt2B may be useful in that regard, as it has been reported to increase ocular differentiation of mouse ES cells [10]. In another report, this same group used serum-free embryoid body culture, followed by treatment with the canonical Wnt antagonist Dkk-1, nodal antagonist lefty-A, fetal calf serum, and activin to induce retinal progenitors [56]. This protocol increased Mit-F-positive RPE-like cells from 2% to 17%. More recently, Reh and coworkers described methods for differentiation of ocular precursors from hESC [74]. They treat dispersed embryoid bodies with IgF-1, Dkk-1 and noggin and obtain neural retinal cell phenotypes, mostly retinal ganglion and amacrine cells. Co-culture with developing mouse neural retinal cells has been utilized to induce photoreceptor development [56, 74].

Even though only a small percentage of hESC spontaneously differentiate into RPE-like cells, they are easily identified by their pigmentation and cuboidal morphology (Fig. 1.3). Following the protocols pioneered by Klimanskaya et al. [66, 67], we have isolated a number of RPE-like cell lines by manually picking pigmented hESC derivatives. While these cells have potential for the treatment of AMD, many questions remain. Can efficiency of hESC differentiation into RPE be improved? Can they be isolated/sorted/cloned? Do they express the same mRNAs and proteins as native RPE? Can they fulfill all the functions of native RPE? How stable are they? Is the mechanism of differentiation of hESC into RPE the same at that documented in vivo in other species? Below, we summarize recent studies aimed at answering these questions.

1.4.1 Efficiency of Derivation

hESC will spontaneously differentiate to RPE-like cells under a variety of conditions in monolayer culture and in embryoid bodies, and this may reflect the fact that neural differentiation seems to be the default pathway followed by hESC. It has been noted that these pigmented clusters appear in close proximity to cells with neural phenotypes (J. Thomson, personal communication, 2006) [66, 67], and cell-cell signaling in the hESC culture may be similar to in vivo interactions. Interestingly, differentiation in vitro is on the same time scale as in vivo. But the percentage of cells that become pigmented is small, and it would be advantageous to improve the efficiency of conversion, since it may not be possible to passage and expand the hESC-RPE indefinitely. Furthermore, mechanical picking of colonies is not ideal, since contaminating cells might have the potential to form tumors or differentiate into other cells types.

While co-culture with PA6 cells was reported to help induce ocular cells in mouse ES (see above), in our hands this does not speed RPE differentiation of hESC. We might be able to improve efficiency by imitating the normal embryonic

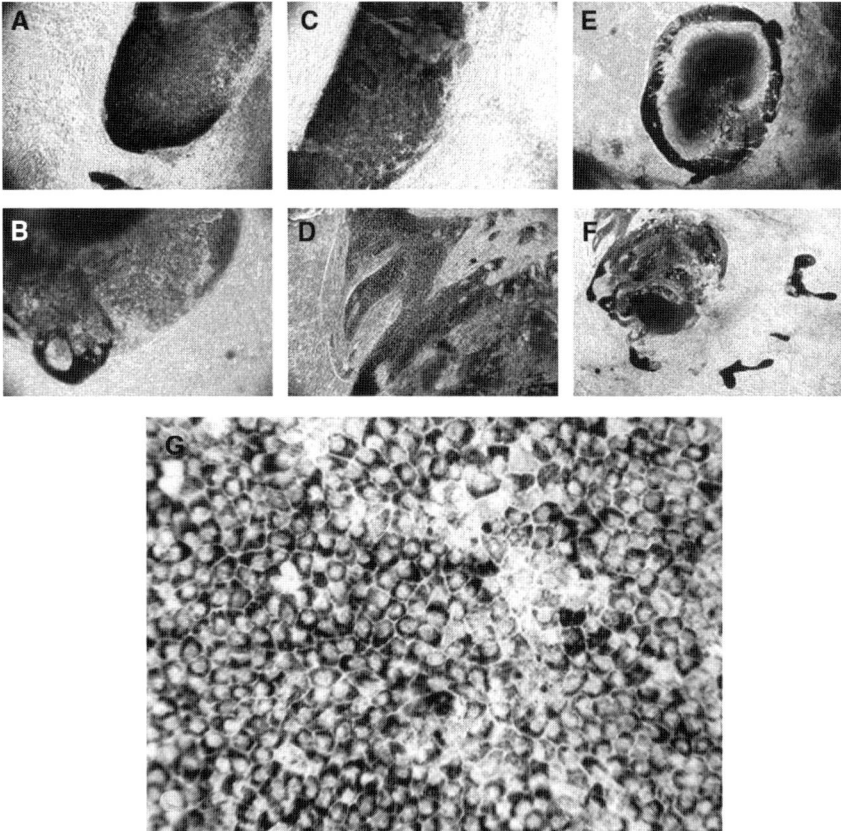

Fig. 1.3 RPE-like colonies in differentiating hESC. (**A–F**) Examples of pigmented colonies after 40 days of culture in media without bFGF are shown. (**G**) Higher magnification view of pigmented RPE-like cells (passage 1) expanded onto a 6 well plate (*See Color Plates*)

program of RPE differentiation. In vivo, a number of factors have been identified that regulate the developmental progression of undifferentiated cells to neural cells, anterior neural plate, eye field, optic cup, and then RPE (see above). For example, a temporal protocol similar to that used by Ikeda et al. [56], which mimics the in vivo process, might be applied to hESC.

It may be possible to improve isolation of RPE cells using cell sorting methods. We have been able to enrich for pigmented cells by sorting on the basis of light scattering (Fig. 1.4). Using a conventional cell sorter, we have been able to achieve a threefold increase in purity of darkly pigmented cells, with 90% of cells containing high concentrations of melanin granules. Such methods may alleviate the tedious manual picking of colonies and decrease the possibility of contaminating cells.

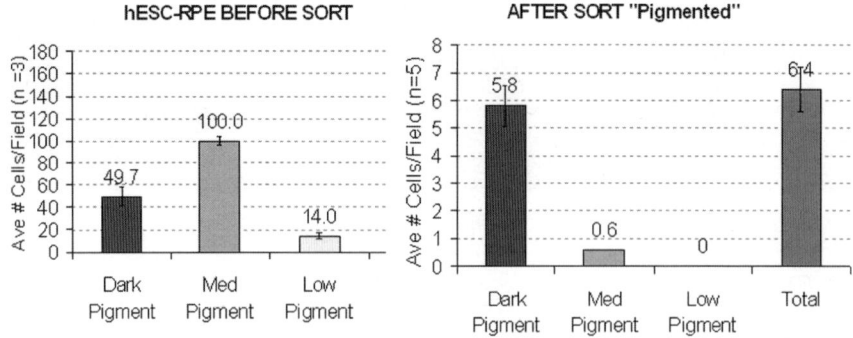

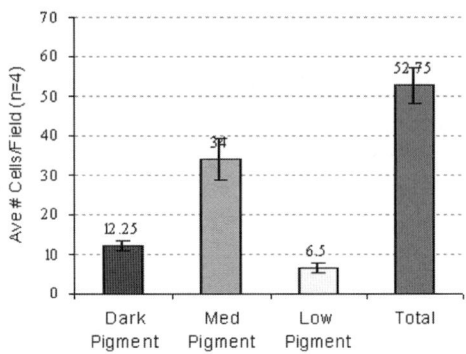

Fig. 1.4 Sorting of hESC-RPE. Shown are results of a FACS Aria sort based on light scattering. The mixed cell population contained 30.4% darkly pigmented cells before the sort and 90.6% darkly pigmented cells after the sort (*See Color Plates*)

1.4.2 Characterization of hESC-RPE

Earlier reports have shown that hESC-RPE express many of the markers present in native RPE, more similar than RPE cell lines [66]. We have extended these studies and investigated expression profiles of hESC-RPE after continued passage. We have also used immunohistology to examine protein expression and localization. Results thus far indicate that hESC-RPE are strikingly similar but not identical to native RPE. Surprisingly, levels of RPE markers are in some instances higher than native fetal RPE. In addition, hESC-RPE express some markers of RPE precursor cells, including Pax6. These results may be explained by the presence of a subpopulation of precursors, or by precursor genes whose expression has persisted.

Immunofluoresence studies show that hESC-RPE are properly polarized and express markers in an appropriately polarized fashion. For example, EMMPRIN is expressed in a basolateral pattern in vivo, and the same distribution is seen in vitro (Fig. 1.5). EM images indicate that hESC have elaborate apical microvilli and contain

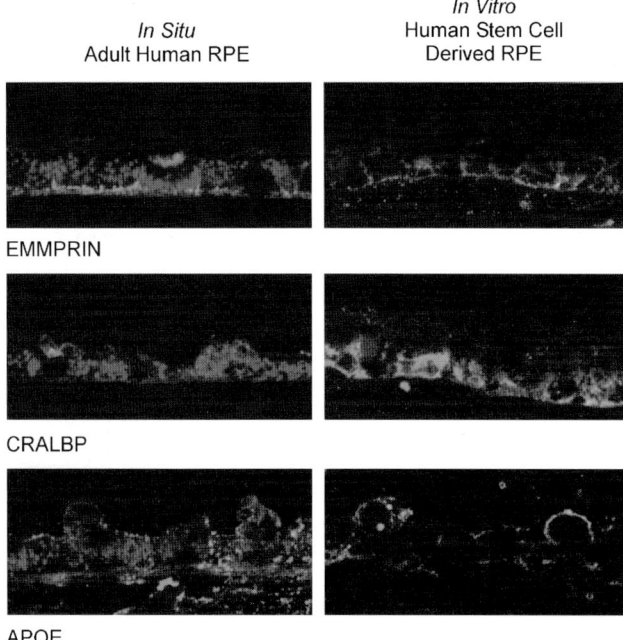

Fig. 1.5 Expression of RPE markers in hESC-RPE. The panel on the left show sections of adult human donor RPE/Choroid with staining of the marker EMPRIN indicated in green, and autofluorescent lipofuscin shown in red. The panel on the right shows a similar aspect of confluent hESC-RPE cultures (*See Color Plates*)

abundant melanin granules. hESC-RPE differ from native RPE with regard to their content of autofluorescent lipofuscin in the lysosomes. Lipofuscin is "molecular garbage" consisting of oxidatively modified proteins and lipids that accumulate after phagocytosis of rod outer segments [128]. Some of the lipid adducts found here have been shown to have toxic qualities, and lipofuscin load correlates with poor cellular function, so the fact that hESC-RPE lack this substance is likely a good thing.

Functionally, hESC-RPE are likewise similar to native RPE in vitro. They form tight junctions, transport ions to the basal side and generate "domes" in culture (Fig. 1.6). These structures are easily seen in confluent cultures and are a simple indicator of proper polarization and formation of tight junctions [17]. Klimanskaya et al. reported that these cells are capable of phagocytosis when presented with latex beads [66]. We have extended these results to show that similar to RPE cell lines, hESC phagocytose purified bovine photoreceptor outer segments and they use the same molecular mechanism, since antibodies to integrin alpha-v/beta-5 block outer segment binding [79].

Transplantation of hESC-RPE into animal models of RPE dysfunction is just beginning. Lund et al. [84] showed that they could preserve vision in the RCS rat model, where photoreceptors perish due to lack of phagocytosis by RPE. The hESC-RPE were as efficient as the ARPE-19 cell line in rescuing photoreceptors. While

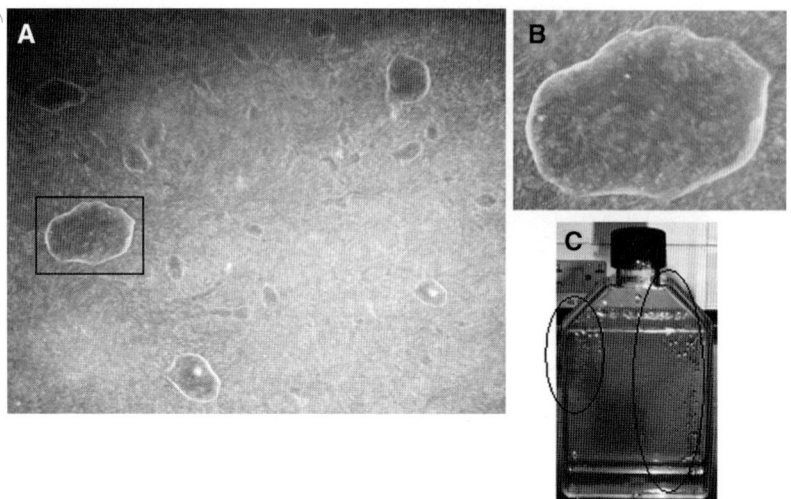

Fig. 1.6 Domes in hESC-RPE cultures. (**A**) Low magnification view of hESC-RPE after three passages. Boxed area is magnified in (**B**), showing dome. (**C**) Domes are visible to the naked eye in culture flasks (*See Color Plates*)

these results demonstrate RPE function in vivo, it should be noted that the RCS rat is not a model for AMD and that many cell types can achieve the same level of rescue, including non-ocular cells. Further studies will be necessary to more thoroughly investigate function of hESC-RPE.

Investigators have cultured native RPE from adult and fetal sources for many years, and a great deal of literature indicates that they lose some functionality and can take on mesenchymal morphology or transdifferentiate after repeated passage [17, 42, 46]. We have found that hESC can grow as monolayers for prolonged periods (up to 11 months) without any obvious changes in morphology. However, after five passages, a subset of hESC-RPE take on a fibroblastic appearance and tend to overgrow the monolayer. This can be taken as evidence that they behave much like native RPE, but it could be problematic in achieving the necessary expansion for generating cells for therapy.

1.5 Future Directions

Our knowledge of the molecular mechanism underlying differentiation of hESC into RPE are very rudimentary at best. As mentioned earlier, this new culture system provides for the first time an opportunity to investigate human RPE differentiation. Information learned form such studies will likely have relevance to improving conditions for generation and maintenance of hESC-RPE.

Recently, reprogramming of human fibroblasts into pluripotent stem cells has been reported by the Yamanaka and Thomson groups [124, 138]. By expressing a specific set of transcription factors (Oct-4, Sox-2, Klf-4, and c-Myc [124]; or Oct-4, Sox-2, Lin-28, and nanog [138]), fibroblasts were converted to a pluripotent cell that resembled human embryonic stem cells (called iPS for induced pluripotent stem cells). If these cells can differentiate into RPE cells, which seems likely, then autologous, patient-specific RPE-like cells can be generated for therapeutic use. This approach has great appeal, since immune rejection of transplanted cells could occur using heterologous cells. However, if the patient's own cells have some sort of genetic defect, the problem might persist, so this approach would have to include steps to repair the original defect (for example by supplying beneficial alternative complement proteins in the blood). Future studies are likely to generate new RPE-like cells from a variety of sources; time will tell which ones are best for therapies.

There are many challenges that lie ahead in developing cellular therapies in the eye. Diseased or damaged tissue is obviously a very different environment than that of an embryo or culture dish. Timing of treatment for AMD with RPE cells will be crucial, so that photoreceptors can be rescued before they perish. Once disease has progressed, the environment can be severely modified in ways that make the tissue inhospitable for transplanted cells (see Vugler et al. [131] for an extensive discussion). Muller cell hypertrophy and gliosis, changes in downstream neural pathways, complications due to angiogenesis, inflammation, and alteration in growth factors released are examples. However, experiments in animal models give reasons to believe that in the future, stem cell-based cellular therapies will be a reality.

Acknowledgements We wish to acknowledge the intellectual contributions of our colleagues and collaborators, especially Don Anderson, Craig Hawker, Ken Kosik, Erkki Ruoslahti, Mike West, Jamie Thomson, Pete Coffey, Anthony Vugler, Jun Parsons, Evan Snyder, and Dean Bok. This work was made possible by funding from California Institute for Regenerative Medicine, Institute for Collaborative Biotechnologies, Army Research Office, Fight for Sight, TriCounties Blood Bank, Chemicon/Millipore, Sigma Xi, Advanced Cell Technology, Primegen Biotech, Santa Barbara Cottage Hospital, and Private Donors.

References

1. Abdelsalam, A., L. Del Priore, and M.A. Zarbin, *Drusen in age-related macular degeneration: pathogenesis, natural course, and laser photocoagulation-induced regression.* Surv Ophthalmol, 1999. **44**(1): 1–29.
2. Abrera-Abeleda, M.A., C. Nishimura, J.L. Smith, S. Sethi, J.L. McRae, B.F. Murphy, G. Silvestri, C. Skerka, M. Jozsi, P.F. Zipfel, G.S. Hageman, and R.J. Smith, *Variations in the complement regulatory genes factor H (CFH) and factor H related 5 (CFHR5) are associated with membranoproliferative glomerulonephritis type II (dense deposit disease).* J Med Genet, 2006. **43**(7): 582–9.
3. Allikmets, R., N.F. Shroyer, N. Singh, J.M. Seddon, R.A. Lewis, P.S. Bernstein, A. Peiffer, N.A. Zabriskie, Y. Li, A. Hutchinson, M. Dean, J.R. Lupski, and M. Leppert, *Mutation of the Stargardt disease gene (ABCR) in age-related macular degeneration.* Science, 1997. **277**(5333): 1805–7.

4. Anderson, D.H., R.F. Mullins, G.S. Hageman, and L.V. Johnson, *A role for local inflammation in the formation of drusen in the aging eye.* Am J Ophthalmol, 2002. **134**(3): 411–31.

5. Anderson, D.H., K.C. Talaga, A.J. Rivest, E. Barron, G.S. Hageman, and L.V. Johnson, *Characterization of beta amyloid assemblies in drusen: the deposits associated with aging and age-related macular degeneration.* Exp Eye Res, 2004. **78**(2): 243–56.

6. Ando, H., M. Kobayashi, T. Tsubokawa, K. Uyemura, T. Furuta, and H. Okamoto, *Lhx2 mediates the activity of Six3 in zebrafish forebrain growth.* Dev Biol, 2005. **287**(2): 456–68.

7. Andoniadou, C.L., M. Signore, E. Sajedi, C. Gaston-Massuet, D. Kelberman, A.J. Burns, N. Itasaki, M. Dattani, and J.P. Martinez-Barbera, *Lack of the murine homeobox gene Hesx1 leads to a posterior transformation of the anterior forebrain.* Development, 2007. **134**(8): 1499–508.

8. Andreazzoli, M., G. Gestri, D. Angeloni, E. Menna, and G. Barsacchi, *Role of Xrx1 in Xenopus eye and anterior brain development.* Development, 1999. **126**(11): 2451–60.

9. Andreazzoli, M., G. Gestri, F. Cremisi, S. Casarosa, I.B. Dawid, and G. Barsacchi, *Xrx1 controls proliferation and neurogenesis in Xenopus anterior neural plate.* Development, 2003. **130**(21): 5143–54.

10. Aoki, H., A. Hara, S. Nakagawa, T. Motohashi, M. Hirano, Y. Takahashi, and T. Kunisada, *Embryonic stem cells that differentiate into RPE cell precursors in vitro develop into RPE cell monolayers in vivo.* Exp Eye Res, 2006. **82**(2): 265–74.

11. Arnhold, S., P. Heiduschka, H. Klein, Y. Absenger, S. Basnaoglu, F. Kreppel, S. Henke-Fahle, S. Kochanek, K.U. Bartz-Schmidt, K. Addicks, and U. Schraermeyer, *Adenovirally transduced bone marrow stromal cells differentiate into pigment epithelial cells and induce rescue effects in RCS rats.* Invest Ophthalmol Vis Sci, 2006. **47**(9): 4121–9.

12. Bailey, T.J., H. El-Hodiri, L. Zhang, R. Shah, P.H. Mathers, and M. Jamrich, *Regulation of vertebrate eye development by Rx genes.* Int J Dev Biol, 2004. **48**(8–9): 761–70.

13. Baumer, N., T. Marquardt, A. Stoykova, D. Spieler, D. Treichel, R. Ashery-Padan, and P. Gruss, *Retinal pigmented epithelium determination requires the redundant activities of Pax2 and Pax6.* Development, 2003. **130**(13): 2903–15.

14. Behesti, H., J.K. Holt, and J.C. Sowden, *The level of BMP4 signaling is critical for the regulation of distinct T-box gene expression domains and growth along the dorso-ventral axis of the optic cup.* BMC Dev Biol, 2006. **6**: 62.

15. Bharti, K., M.T. Nguyen, S. Skuntz, S. Bertuzzi, and H. Arnheiter, *The other pigment cell: specification and development of the pigmented epithelium of the vertebrate eye.* Pigment Cell Res, 2006. **19**(5): 380–94.

16. Brem, R.B., S.G. Robbins, D.J. Wilson, L.M. O'Rourke, R.N. Mixon, J.E. Robertson, S.R. Planck, and J.T. Rosenbaum, *Immunolocalization of integrins in the human retina.* Invest Ophthalmol Vis Sci, 1994. **35**(9): 3466–74.

17. Burke, J.M., C.M. Skumatz, P.E. Irving, and B.S. McKay, *Phenotypic heterogeneity of retinal pigment epithelial cells in vitro and in situ.* Exp Eye Res, 1996. **62**(1): 63–73.

18. Carreira, S., J. Goodall, I. Aksan, S.A. La Rocca, M.D. Galibert, L. Denat, L. Larue, and C.R. Goding, *Mitf cooperates with Rb1 and activates p21Cip1 expression to regulate cell cycle progression.* Nature, 2005. **433**(7027): 764–9.

19. Carron, C., A. Bourdelas, H.Y. Li, J.C. Boucaut, and D.L. Shi, *Antagonistic interaction between IGF and Wnt/JNK signaling in convergent extension in Xenopus embryo.* Mech Dev, 2005. **122**(11): 1234–47.

20. Cavodeassi, F., F. Carreira-Barbosa, R.M. Young, M.L. Concha, M.L. Allende, C. Houart, M. Tada, and S.W. Wilson, *Early stages of zebrafish eye formation require the coordinated activity of Wnt11, Fz5, and the Wnt/beta-catenin pathway.* Neuron, 2005. **47**(1): 43–56.

21. Chow, R.L. and R.A. Lang, *Early eye development in vertebrates.* Annu Rev Cell Dev Biol, 2001. **17**: 255–96.

22. Coffey, P.J., C. Gias, C.J. McDermott, P. Lundh, M.C. Pickering, C. Sethi, A. Bird, F.W. Fitzke, A. Maass, L.L. Chen, G.E. Holder, P.J. Luthert, T.E. Salt, S.E. Moss, and J. Greenwood, *Complement factor H deficiency in aged mice causes retinal abnormalities and visual dysfunction.* Proc Natl Acad Sci U S A, 2007. **104**(42): 16651–6.

23. Crabb, J.W., M. Miyagi, X. Gu, K. Shadrach, K.A. West, H. Sakaguchi, M. Kamei, A. Hasan, L. Yan, M.E. Rayborn, R.G. Salomon, and J.G. Hollyfield, *Drusen proteome analysis: an approach to the etiology of age-related macular degeneration*. Proc Natl Acad Sci U S A, 2002. **99**(23): 14682–7.

24. da Cruz, L., F.K. Chen, A. Ahmado, J. Greenwood, and P. Coffey, *RPE transplantation and its role in retinal disease*. Prog Retin Eye Res, 2007. **26**(6): 598–635.

25. Dakubo, G.D., Y.P. Wang, C. Mazerolle, K. Campsall, A.P. McMahon, and V.A. Wallace, *Retinal ganglion cell-derived sonic hedgehog signaling is required for optic disc and stalk neuroepithelial cell development*. Development, 2003. **130**(13): 2967–80.

26. Dastgheib, K. and W.R. Green, *Granulomatous reaction to Bruch's membrane in age-related macular degeneration*. Arch Ophthalmol, 1994. **112**(6): 813–8.

27. Del Bene, F., K. Tessmar-Raible, and J. Wittbrodt, *Direct interaction of geminin and Six3 in eye development*. Nature, 2004. **427**(6976): 745–9.

28. Del Priore, L.V., Y.H. Kuo, and T.H. Tezel, *Age-related changes in human RPE cell density and apoptosis proportion in situ*. Invest Ophthalmol Vis Sci, 2002. **43**(10): 3312–8.

29. Dentchev, T., A.H. Milam, V.M. Lee, J.Q. Trojanowski, and J.L. Dunaief, *Amyloid-beta is found in drusen from some age-related macular degeneration retinas, but not in drusen from normal retinas*. Mol Vis, 2003. **9**: 184–90.

30. Dheen, T., I. Sleptsova-Friedrich, Y. Xu, M. Clark, H. Lehrach, Z. Gong, and V. Korzh, *Zebrafish tbx-c functions during formation of midline structures*. Development, 1999. **126**(12): 2703–13.

31. Dorsky, R.I., L.C. Sheldahl, and R.T. Moon, *A transgenic Lef1/beta-catenin-dependent reporter is expressed in spatially restricted domains throughout zebrafish development*. Dev Biol, 2002. **241**(2): 229–37.

32. Dunaief, J.L., T. Dentchev, G.S. Ying, and A.H. Milam, *The role of apoptosis in age-related macular degeneration*. Arch Ophthalmol, 2002. **120**(11): 1435–42.

33. Eagleson, G.W. and R.D. Dempewolf, *The role of the anterior neural ridge and Fgf-8 in early forebrain patterning and regionalization in Xenopus laevis*. Comp Biochem Physiol B Biochem Mol Biol, 2002. **132**(1): 179–89.

34. Edwards, A.O., R. Ritter, 3rd, K.J. Abel, A. Manning, C. Panhuysen, and L.A. Farrer, *Complement factor H polymorphism and age-related macular degeneration*. Science, 2005. **308**(5720): 421–4.

35. England, S.J., G.B. Blanchard, L. Mahadevan, and R.J. Adams, *A dynamic fate map of the forebrain shows how vertebrate eyes form and explains two causes of cyclopia*. Development, 2006. **133**(23): 4613–7.

36. Esteve, P. and P. Bovolenta, *Secreted inducers in vertebrate eye development: more functions for old morphogens*. Curr Opin Neurobiol, 2006. **16**(1): 13–9.

37. Evans, J.R., *Risk factors for age-related macular degeneration*. Prog Retin Eye Res, 2001. **20**(2): 227–53.

38. Fariss, R.N., S.S. Apte, B.R. Olsen, K. Iwata, and A.H. Milam, *Tissue inhibitor of metalloproteinases-3 is a component of Bruch's membrane of the eye*. Am J Pathol, 1997. **150**(1): 323–8.

39. Fuhrmann, S., E.M. Levine, and T.A. Reh, *Extraocular mesenchyme patterns the optic vesicle during early eye development in the embryonic chick*. Development, 2000. **127**(21): 4599–609.

40. Gallardo, M.E., J. Lopez-Rios, I. Fernaud-Espinosa, B. Granadino, R. Sanz, C. Ramos, C. Ayuso, M.J. Seller, H.G. Brunner, P. Bovolenta, and S. Rodriguez de Cordoba, *Genomic cloning and characterization of the human homeobox gene SIX6 reveals a cluster of SIX genes in chromosome 14 and associates SIX6 hemizygosity with bilateral anophthalmia and pituitary anomalies*. Genomics, 1999. **61**(1): 82–91.

41. Gehrs, K.M., D.H. Anderson, L.V. Johnson, and G.S. Hageman, *Age-related macular degeneration–emerging pathogenetic and therapeutic concepts*. Ann Med, 2006. **38**(7): 450–71.

42. Geisen, P., J.R. McColm, B.M. King, and M.E. Hartnett, *Characterization of barrier properties and inducible VEGF expression of several types of retinal pigment epithelium in medium-term culture*. Curr Eye Res, 2006. **31**(9): 739–48.

43. Gestri, G., M. Carl, I. Appolloni, S.W. Wilson, G. Barsacchi, and M. Andreazzoli, *Six3 functions in anterior neural plate specification by promoting cell proliferation and inhibiting Bmp4 expression.* Development, 2005. **132**(10): 2401–13.
44. Gold, B., J.E. Merriam, J. Zernant, L.S. Hancox, A.J. Taiber, K. Gehrs, K. Cramer, J. Neel, J. Bergeron, G.R. Barile, R.T. Smith, G.S. Hageman, M. Dean, and R. Allikmets, *Variation in factor B (BF) and complement component 2 (C2) genes is associated with age-related macular degeneration.* Nat Genet, 2006. **38**(4): 458–62.
45. Gould, S.E. and R.M. Grainger, *Neural induction and antero-posterior patterning in the amphibian embryo: past, present and future.* Cell Mol Life Sci, 1997. **53**(4): 319–38.
46. Grisanti, S. and C. Guidry, *Transdifferentiation of retinal pigment epithelial cells from epithelial to mesenchymal phenotype.* Invest Ophthalmol Vis Sci, 1995. **36**(2): 391–405.
47. Hageman, G.S., P.J. Luthert, N.H. Victor Chong, L.V. Johnson, D.H. Anderson, and R.F. Mullins, *An integrated hypothesis that considers drusen as biomarkers of immune-mediated processes at the RPE-Bruch's membrane interface in aging and age-related macular degeneration.* Prog Retin Eye Res, 2001. **20**(6): 705–32.
48. Hageman, G.S., D.H. Anderson, L.V. Johnson, L.S. Hancox, A.J. Taiber, L.I. Hardisty, J.L. Hageman, H.A. Stockman, J.D. Borchardt, K.M. Gehrs, R.J. Smith, G. Silvestri, S.R. Russell, C.C. Klaver, I. Barbazetto, S. Chang, L.A. Yannuzzi, G.R. Barile, J.C. Merriam, R.T. Smith, A.K. Olsh, J. Bergeron, J. Zernant, J.E. Merriam, B. Gold, M. Dean, and R. Allikmets, *A common haplotype in the complement regulatory gene factor H (HF1/CFH) predisposes individuals to age-related macular degeneration.* Proc Natl Acad Sci U S A, 2005. **102**(20): 7227–32.
49. Haines, J.L., M.A. Hauser, S. Schmidt, W.K. Scott, L.M. Olson, P. Gallins, K.L. Spencer, S.Y. Kwan, M. Noureddine, J.R. Gilbert, N. Schnetz-Boutaud, A. Agarwal, E.A. Postel, and M.A. Pericak-Vance, *Complement factor H variant increases the risk of age-related macular degeneration.* Science, 2005. **308**(5720): 419–21.
50. Halilagic, A., V. Ribes, N.B. Ghyselinck, M.H. Zile, P. Dolle, and M. Studer, *Retinoids control anterior and dorsal properties in the developing forebrain.* Dev Biol, 2007. **303**(1): 362–75.
51. Hartong, D.T., E.L. Berson, and T.P. Dryja, *Retinitis pigmentosa.* Lancet, 2006. **368**(9549): 1795–809.
52. Hever, A.M., K.A. Williamson, and V. van Heyningen, *Developmental malformations of the eye: the role of PAX6, SOX2 and OTX2.* Clin Genet, 2006. **69**(6): 459–70.
53. Hirano, M., A. Yamamoto, N. Yoshimura, T. Tokunaga, T. Motohashi, K. Ishizaki, H. Yoshida, K. Okazaki, H. Yamazaki, S. Hayashi, and T. Kunisada, *Generation of structures formed by lens and retinal cells differentiating from embryonic stem cells.* Dev Dyn, 2003. **228**(4): 664–71.
54. Hollyfield, J.G., R.G. Salomon, and J.W. Crabb, *Proteomic approaches to understanding age-related macular degeneration.* Adv Exp Med Biol, 2003. **533**: 83–9.
55. Horsford, D.J., M.T. Nguyen, G.C. Sellar, R. Kothary, H. Arnheiter, and R.R. McInnes, *Chx10 repression of Mitf is required for the maintenance of mammalian neuroretinal identity.* Development, 2005. **132**(1): 177–87.
56. Ikeda, H., F. Osakada, K. Watanabe, K. Mizuseki, T. Haraguchi, H. Miyoshi, D. Kamiya, Y. Honda, N. Sasai, N. Yoshimura, M. Takahashi, and Y. Sasai, *Generation of Rx⁺ /Pax6⁺ neural retinal precursors from embryonic stem cells.* Proc Natl Acad Sci U S A, 2005. **102**(32): 11331–6.
57. Jin, E.J., L.W. Burrus, and C.A. Erickson, *The expression patterns of Wnts and their antagonists during avian eye development.* Mech Dev, 2002. **116**(1–2): 173–6.
58. Johnson, L.V., S. Ozaki, M.K. Staples, P.A. Erickson, and D.H. Anderson, *A potential role for immune complex pathogenesis in drusen formation.* Exp Eye Res, 2000. **70**(4): 441–9.
59. Johnson, L.V., W.P. Leitner, M.K. Staples, and D.H. Anderson, *Complement activation and inflammatory processes in Drusen formation and age related macular degeneration.* Exp Eye Res, 2001. **73**(6): 887–96.
60. Johnson, P.T., G.P. Lewis, K.C. Talaga, M.N. Brown, P.J. Kappel, S.K. Fisher, D.H. Anderson, and L.V. Johnson, *Drusen-associated degeneration in the retina.* Invest Ophthalmol Vis Sci, 2003. **44**(10): 4481–8.

61. Kawasaki, H., H. Suemori, K. Mizuseki, K. Watanabe, F. Urano, H. Ichinose, M. Haruta, M. Takahashi, K. Yoshikawa, S. Nishikawa, N. Nakatsuji, and Y. Sasai, *Generation of dopaminergic neurons and pigmented epithelia from primate ES cells by stromal cell-derived inducing activity.* Proc Natl Acad Sci U S A, 2002. **99**(3): 1580–5.

62. Killingsworth, M.C., J.P. Sarks, and S.H. Sarks, *Macrophages related to Bruch's membrane in age-related macular degeneration.* Eye, 1990. **4 (Pt 4)**: 613–21.

63. Kim, H.S., J. Shin, S.H. Kim, H.S. Chun, J.D. Kim, Y.S. Kim, M.J. Kim, M. Rhee, S.Y. Yeo, and T.L. Huh, *Eye field requires the function of Sfrp1 as a Wnt antagonist.* Neurosci Lett, 2007. **414**(1): 26–9.

64. Kiselyov, A.S., *Targeting the hedgehog signaling pathway with small molecules.* Anticancer Agents Med Chem, 2006. **6**(5): 445–9.

65. Klein, R.J., C. Zeiss, E.Y. Chew, J.Y. Tsai, R.S. Sackler, C. Haynes, A.K. Henning, J.P. SanGiovanni, S.M. Mane, S.T. Mayne, M.B. Bracken, F.L. Ferris, J. Ott, C. Barnstable, and J. Hoh, *Complement factor H polymorphism in age-related macular degeneration.* Science, 2005. **308**(5720): 385–9.

66. Klimanskaya, I., J. Hipp, K.A. Rezai, M. West, A. Atala, and R. Lanza, *Derivation and comparative assessment of retinal pigment epithelium from human embryonic stem cells using transcriptomics.* Cloning Stem Cells, 2004. **6**(3): 217–45.

67. Klimanskaya, I., *Retinal pigment epithelium.* Methods Enzymol, 2006. **418**: 169–94.

68. Kobayashi, D., M. Kobayashi, K. Matsumoto, T. Ogura, M. Nakafuku, and K. Shimamura, *Early subdivisions in the neural plate define distinct competence for inductive signals.* Development, 2002. **129**(1): 83–93.

69. Koenekoop, R.K., *The gene for Stargardt disease, ABCA4, is a major retinal gene: a mini-review.* Ophthalmic Genet, 2003. **24**(2): 75–80.

70. Kozmik, Z., *Pax genes in eye development and evolution.* Curr Opin Genet Dev, 2005. **15**(4): 430–8.

71. Kumar, J.P. and K. Moses, *Eye specification in Drosophila: perspectives and implications.* Semin Cell Dev Biol, 2001. **12**(6): 469–74.

72. Kumar, J.P. and K. Moses, *EGF receptor and Notch signaling act upstream of Eyeless/Pax6 to control eye specification.* Cell, 2001. **104**(5): 687–97.

73. Lagutin, O.V., C.C. Zhu, D. Kobayashi, J. Topczewski, K. Shimamura, L. Puelles, H.R. Russell, P.J. McKinnon, L. Solnica-Krezel, and G. Oliver, *Six3 repression of Wnt signaling in the anterior neuroectoderm is essential for vertebrate forebrain development.* Genes Dev, 2003. **17**(3): 368–79.

74. Lamba, D.A., M.O. Karl, C.B. Ware, and T.A. Reh, *Efficient generation of retinal progenitor cells from human embryonic stem cells.* Proc Natl Acad Sci U S A, 2006. **103**(34): 12769–74.

75. Lee, C.S., N.R. May, and C.M. Fan, *Transdifferentiation of the ventral retinal pigmented epithelium to neural retina in the growth arrest specific gene 1 mutant.* Dev Biol, 2001. **236**(1): 17–29.

76. Lee, H.S., Y.S. Bong, K.B. Moore, K. Soria, S.A. Moody, and I.O. Daar, *Dishevelled mediates ephrinB1 signalling in the eye field through the planar cell polarity pathway.* Nat Cell Biol, 2006. **8**(1): 55–63.

77. Li, H., C. Tierney, L. Wen, J.Y. Wu, and Y. Rao, *A single morphogenetic field gives rise to two retina primordia under the influence of the prechordal plate.* Development, 1997. **124**(3): 603–15.

78. Li, Y., P. Atmaca-Sonmez, C.L. Schanie, S.T. Ildstad, H.J. Kaplan, and V. Enzmann, *Endogenous bone marrow derived cells express retinal pigment epithelium cell markers and migrate to focal areas of RPE damage.* Invest Ophthalmol Vis Sci, 2007. **48**(9): 4321–7.

79. Lin, H. and D.O. Clegg, *Integrin alphavbeta5 participates in the binding of photoreceptor rod outer segments during phagocytosis by cultured human retinal pigment epithelium.* Invest Ophthalmol Vis Sci, 1998. **39**(9): 1703–12.

80. Liu, H., O. Mohamed, D. Dufort, and V.A. Wallace, *Characterization of Wnt signaling components and activation of the Wnt canonical pathway in the murine retina.* Dev Dyn, 2003. **227**(3): 323–34.

81. Loeffler, K.U. and N.J. Mangini, *Immunolocalization of ubiquitin and related enzymes in human retina and retinal pigment epithelium.* Graefes Arch Clin Exp Ophthalmol, 1997. **235**(4): 248–54.

82. Loffler, K.U., D.P. Edward, and M.O. Tso, *Immunoreactivity against tau, amyloid precursor protein, and beta-amyloid in the human retina.* Invest Ophthalmol Vis Sci, 1995. **36**(1): 24–31.

83. Lopez-Rios, J., K. Tessmar, F. Loosli, J. Wittbrodt, and P. Bovolenta, *Six3 and Six6 activity is modulated by members of the groucho family.* Development, 2003. **130**(1): 185–95.

84. Lund, R.D., S. Wang, I. Klimanskaya, T. Holmes, R. Ramos-Kelsey, B. Lu, S. Girman, N. Bischoff, Y. Sauve, and R. Lanza, *Human embryonic stem cell-derived cells rescue visual function in dystrophic RCS rats.* Cloning Stem Cells, 2006. **8**(3): 189–99.

85. Maden, M., A. Blentic, S. Reijntjes, S. Seguin, E. Gale, and A. Graham, *Retinoic acid is required for specification of the ventral eye field and for Rathke's pouch in the avian embryo.* Int J Dev Biol, 2007. **51**(3): 191–200.

86. Marmorstein, A.D., S.C. Finnemann, V.L. Bonilha, and E. Rodriguez-Boulan, *Morphogenesis of the retinal pigment epithelium: toward understanding retinal degenerative diseases.* Ann N Y Acad Sci, 1998. **857**: 1–12.

87. Martinez-Morales, J.R., V. Dolez, I. Rodrigo, R. Zaccarini, L. Leconte, P. Bovolenta, and S. Saule, *OTX2 activates the molecular network underlying retina pigment epithelium differentiation.* J Biol Chem, 2003. **278**(24): 21721–31.

88. Martinez-Morales, J.R., I. Rodrigo, and P. Bovolenta, *Eye development: a view from the retina pigmented epithelium.* Bioessays, 2004. **26**(7): 766–77.

89. Mathers, P.H., A. Grinberg, K.A. Mahon, and M. Jamrich, *The Rx homeobox gene is essential for vertebrate eye development.* Nature, 1997. **387**(6633): 603–7.

90. Matt, N., V. Dupe, J.M. Garnier, C. Dennefeld, P. Chambon, M. Mark, and N.B. Ghyselinck, *Retinoic acid-dependent eye morphogenesis is orchestrated by neural crest cells.* Development, 2005. **132**(21): 4789–800.

91. Maurus, D., C. Heligon, A. Burger-Schwarzler, A.W. Brandli, and M. Kuhl, *Noncanonical Wnt-4 signaling and EAF2 are required for eye development in Xenopus laevis.* Embo J, 2005. **24**(6): 1181–91.

92. Mochii, M., Y. Mazaki, N. Mizuno, H. Hayashi, and G. Eguchi, *Role of Mitf in differentiation and transdifferentiation of chicken pigmented epithelial cell.* Dev Biol, 1998. **193**(1): 47–62.

93. Molotkov, A., N. Molotkova, and G. Duester, *Retinoic acid guides eye morphogenetic movements via paracrine signaling but is unnecessary for retinal dorsoventral patterning.* Development, 2006. **133**(10): 1901–10.

94. Muller, F., H. Rohrer, and A. Vogel-Hopker, *Bone morphogenetic proteins specify the retinal pigment epithelium in the chick embryo.* Development, 2007. **134**(19): 3483–93.

95. Mullins, R.F., L.V. Johnson, D.H. Anderson, and G.S. Hageman, *Characterization of drusen-associated glycoconjugates.* Ophthalmology, 1997. **104**(2): 288–94.

96. Nakayama, A., M.T. Nguyen, C.C. Chen, K. Opdecamp, C.A. Hodgkinson, and H. Arnheiter, *Mutations in microphthalmia, the mouse homolog of the human deafness gene MITF, affect neuroepithelial and neural crest-derived melanocytes differently.* Mech Dev, 1998. **70**(1–2): 155–66.

97. Newsome, D.A., A.T. Hewitt, W. Huh, P.G. Robey, and J.R. Hassell, *Detection of specific extracellular matrix molecules in drusen, Bruch's membrane, and ciliary body.* Am J Ophthalmol, 1987. **104**(4): 373–81.

98. O'Rahilly, R., *The prenatal development of the human eye.* Exp Eye Res, 1975. **21**(2): 93–112.

99. Oldham, S. and E. Hafen, *Insulin/IGF and target of rapamycin signaling: a TOR de force in growth control.* Trends Cell Biol, 2003. **13**(2): 79–85.

100. Onuma, Y., S. Takahashi, M. Asashima, S. Kurata, and W.J. Gehring, *Conservation of Pax 6 function and upstream activation by Notch signaling in eye development of frogs and flies.* Proc Natl Acad Sci U S A, 2002. **99**(4): 2020–5.

101. Ooto, S., M. Haruta, Y. Honda, H. Kawasaki, Y. Sasai, and M. Takahashi, *Induction of the differentiation of lentoids from primate embryonic stem cells.* Invest Ophthalmol Vis Sci, 2003. **44**(6): 2689–93.

102. Pauleikhoff, D., S. Zuels, G.S. Sheraidah, J. Marshall, A. Wessing, and A.C. Bird, *Correlation between biochemical composition and fluorescein binding of deposits in Bruch's membrane.* Ophthalmology, 1992. **99**(10): 1548–53.

103. Penfold, P.L., M.C. Killingsworth, and S.H. Sarks, *Senile macular degeneration: the involvement of immunocompetent cells.* Graefes Arch Clin Exp Ophthalmol, 1985. **223**(2): 69–76.

104. Penfold, P.L., M.C. Madigan, M.C. Gillies, and J.M. Provis, *Immunological and aetiological aspects of macular degeneration.* Prog Retin Eye Res, 2001. **20**(3): 385–414.

105. Peng, G. and M. Westerfield, *Lhx5 promotes forebrain development and activates transcription of secreted Wnt antagonists.* Development, 2006. **133**(16): 3191–200.

106. Pera, E.M., O. Wessely, S.Y. Li, and E.M. De Robertis, *Neural and head induction by insulin-like growth factor signals.* Dev Cell, 2001. **1**(5): 655–65.

107. Pera, E.M., A. Ikeda, E. Eivers, and E.M. De Robertis, *Integration of IGF, FGF, and anti-BMP signals via Smad1 phosphorylation in neural induction.* Genes Dev, 2003. **17**(24): 3023–8.

108. Perron, M., S. Boy, M.A. Amato, A. Viczian, K. Koebernick, T. Pieler, and W.A. Harris, *A novel function for Hedgehog signalling in retinal pigment epithelium differentiation.* Development, 2003. **130**(8): 1565–77.

109. Planque, N., L. Leconte, F.M. Coquelle, P. Martin, and S. Saule, *Specific Pax-6/microphthalmia transcription factor interactions involve their DNA-binding domains and inhibit transcriptional properties of both proteins.* J Biol Chem, 2001. **276**(31): 29330–7.

110. Porter, F.D., J. Drago, Y. Xu, S.S. Cheema, C. Wassif, S.P. Huang, E. Lee, A. Grinberg, J.S. Massalas, D. Bodine, F. Alt, and H. Westphal, *Lhx2, a LIM homeobox gene, is required for eye, forebrain, and definitive erythrocyte development.* Development, 1997. **124**(15): 2935–44.

111. Ribes, V., Z. Wang, P. Dolle, and K. Niederreither, *Retinaldehyde dehydrogenase 2 (RALDH2)-mediated retinoic acid synthesis regulates early mouse embryonic forebrain development by controlling FGF and sonic hedgehog signaling.* Development, 2006. **133**(2): 351–61.

112. Rodrigues, E.B., *Inflammation in dry age-related macular degeneration.* Ophthalmologica, 2007. **221**(3): 143–52.

113. Rojas-Munoz, A., R. Dahm, and C. Nusslein-Volhard, *chokh/rx3 specifies the retinal pigment epithelium fate independently of eye morphogenesis.* Dev Biol, 2005. **288**(2): 348–62.

114. Rorick, A.M., W. Mei, N.L. Liette, C. Phiel, H.M. El-Hodiri, and J. Yang, *PP2A:B56epsilon is required for eye induction and eye field separation.* Dev Biol, 2007. **302**(2): 477–93.

115. Sarks, J.P., S.H. Sarks, and M.C. Killingsworth, *Evolution of geographic atrophy of the retinal pigment epithelium.* Eye, 1988. **2 (Pt 5)**: 552–77.

116. Seddon, J.M., U.A. Ajani, and B.D. Mitchell, *Familial aggregation of age-related maculopathy.* Am J Ophthalmol, 1997. **123**(2): 199–206.

117. Smith, W., J. Assink, R. Klein, P. Mitchell, C.C. Klaver, B.E. Klein, A. Hofman, S. Jensen, J.J. Wang, and P.T. de Jong, *Risk factors for age-related macular degeneration: pooled findings from three continents.* Ophthalmology, 2001. **108**(4): 697–704.

118. Sparrow, J.R., B. Cai, N. Fishkin, Y.P. Jang, S. Krane, H.R. Vollmer, J. Zhou, and K. Nakanishi, *A2E, a fluorophore of RPE lipofuscin: can it cause RPE degeneration?* Adv Exp Med Biol, 2003. **533**: 205–11.

119. Spieler, D., N. Baumer, J. Stebler, M. Koprunner, M. Reichman-Fried, U. Teichmann, E. Raz, M. Kessel, and L. Wittler, *Involvement of Pax6 and Otx2 in the forebrain-specific regulation of the vertebrate homeobox gene ANF/Hesx1.* Dev Biol, 2004. **269**(2): 567–79.

120. Stern, C.D., *Neural induction: 10 years on since the 'default model'.* Curr Opin Cell Biol, 2006. **18**(6): 692–7.

121. Stone, E.M., T.A. Braun, S.R. Russell, M.H. Kuehn, A.J. Lotery, P.A. Moore, C.G. Eastman, T.L. Casavant, and V.C. Sheffield, *Missense variations in the fibulin 5 gene and age-related macular degeneration.* N Engl J Med, 2004. **351**(4): 346–53.

122. Strauss, O., *The retinal pigment epithelium in visual function.* Physiol Rev, 2005. **85**(3): 845–81.

123. Takabatake, Y., T. Takabatake, S. Sasagawa, and K. Takeshima, *Conserved expression control and shared activity between cognate T-box genes Tbx2 and Tbx3 in connection with Sonic hedgehog signaling during Xenopus eye development.* Dev Growth Differ, 2002. **44**(4): 257–71.

124. Takahashi, K., K. Tanabe, M. Ohnuki, M. Narita, T. Ichisaka, K. Tomoda, and S. Yamanaka, *Induction of pluripotent stem cells from adult human fibroblasts by defined factors.* Cell, 2007. **131**(5): 861–72.

125. Takeda, K., K. Yasumoto, R. Takada, S. Takada, K. Watanabe, T. Udono, H. Saito, K. Takahashi, and S. Shibahara, *Induction of melanocyte-specific microphthalmia-associated transcription factor by Wnt-3a.* J Biol Chem, 2000. **275**(19): 14013–6.

126. Takeda, K., S. Yokoyama, K. Yasumoto, H. Saito, T. Udono, K. Takahashi, and S. Shibahara, *OTX2 regulates expression of DOPAchrome tautomerase in human retinal pigment epithelium.* Biochem Biophys Res Commun, 2003. **300**(4): 908–14.

127. Terada, K., A. Kitayama, T. Kanamoto, N. Ueno, and T. Furukawa, *Nucleosome regulator Xhmgb3 is required for cell proliferation of the eye and brain as a downstream target of Xenopus rax/Rx1.* Dev Biol, 2006. **291**(2): 398–412.

128. Terman, A., B. Gustafsson, and U.T. Brunk, *Autophagy, organelles and ageing.* J Pathol, 2007. **211**(2): 134–43.

129. Tuo, J., C.M. Bojanowski, and C.C. Chan, *Genetic factors of age-related macular degeneration.* Prog Retin Eye Res, 2004. **23**(2): 229–49.

130. Ueno, M., M. Matsumura, K. Watanabe, T. Nakamura, F. Osakada, M. Takahashi, H. Kawasaki, S. Kinoshita, and Y. Sasai, *Neural conversion of ES cells by an inductive activity on human amniotic membrane matrix.* Proc Natl Acad Sci U S A, 2006. **103**(25): 9554–9.

131. Vugler, A., J. Lawrence, J. Walsh, A. Carr, C. Gias, M. Semo, A. Ahmado, L. da Cruz, P. Andrews, and P. Coffey, *Embryonic stem cells and retinal repair.* Mech Dev, 2007. **124**(11–12): 807–29.

132. Wilson, S.W. and C. Houart, *Early steps in the development of the forebrain.* Dev Cell, 2004. **6**(2): 167–81.

133. Wong, K., Y. Peng, H.F. Kung, and M.L. He, *Retina dorsal/ventral patterning by Xenopus TBX3.* Biochem Biophys Res Commun, 2002. **290**(2): 737–42.

134. Wright, A., B. Charlesworth, I. Rudan, A. Carothers, and H. Campbell, *A polygenic basis for late-onset disease.* Trends Genet, 2003. **19**(2): 97–106.

135. Wu, J., M. O'Donnell, A.D. Gitler, and P.S. Klein, *Kermit 2/XGIPC, an IGF1 receptor interacting protein, is required for IGF signaling in Xenopus eye development.* Development, 2006. **133**(18): 3651–60.

136. Yang, X.J., *Roles of cell-extrinsic growth factors in vertebrate eye pattern formation and retinogenesis.* Semin Cell Dev Biol, 2004. **15**(1): 91–103.

137. Yasumoto, K., K. Takeda, H. Saito, K. Watanabe, K. Takahashi, and S. Shibahara, *Microphthalmia-associated transcription factor interacts with LEF-1, a mediator of Wnt signaling.* Embo J, 2002. **21**(11): 2703–14.

138. Yu, J., M.A. Vodyanik, K. Smuga-Otto, J. Antosiewicz-Bourget, J.L. Frane, S. Tian, J. Nie, G.A. Jonsdottir, V. Ruotti, R. Stewart, Slukvin, II, and J.A. Thomson, *Induced pluripotent stem cell lines derived from human somatic cells.* Science, 2007. **318**(5858): 1917–20.

139. Zaghloul, N.A., B. Yan, and S.A. Moody, *Step-wise specification of retinal stem cells during normal embryogenesis.* Biol Cell, 2005. **97**(5): 321–37.

140. Zaghloul, N.A. and S.A. Moody, *Alterations of rx1 and pax6 expression levels at neural plate stages differentially affect the production of retinal cell types and maintenance of retinal stem cell qualities.* Dev Biol, 2007. **306**(1): 222–40.

141. Zhang, X.M. and X.J. Yang, *Temporal and spatial effects of Sonic hedgehog signaling in chick eye morphogenesis.* Dev Biol, 2001. **233**(2): 271–90.

142. Zuber, M.E., G. Gestri, A.S. Viczian, G. Barsacchi, and W.A. Harris, *Specification of the vertebrate eye by a network of eye field transcription factors.* Development, 2003. **130**(21): 5155–67.

143. Stroeva, O.G. and V.I. Mitashov, *Retinal pigment epithelium: proliferation and differentiation during development and regeneration.* Int Rev Cytol, 1983. **83**: p. 221–93.

Chapter 2
Progenitor Cell Transplantation for Retinal Disease

Henry J. Klassen

Abstract Diseases of the retina frequently result in permanent visual impairment. One strategy for recovering lost function is to replace retinal neurons lost to the disease process, while another is to protect these neurons from dying in the first place. Retinal progenitor cell transplantation is an experimental approach that has relevance to both strategies and holds promise as a potential therapeutic intervention. Work to date has shown that retinal progenitor cells can be cultured from the neural retina in a range of mammalian species, from mouse to human. These cells proliferate in response to exogenous mitogens and express primitive neuroepithelial genes. Unlike many other cell types, they express retinal-specific markers under conditions favoring differentiation, particularly transplantation to the subretinal space. The cells integrate into the retina, exhibit morphologies appropriate to their location, and have been associated with photoreceptor phenotype and preservation of photosensitivity. In mouse and pig allograft models, retinal progenitor cells survive transplantation to the retina for extended periods without exogenous immune suppression. Research areas of ongoing interest include detailed examination of marker expression, alternate potential cell types, optimization of proliferation and differentiation, genetic modification of donor cells, elucidation of the role of stem cells in cancer, assuring cessation of proliferation following transplantation, and the use of biodegradable materials as a substrate for cell delivery. Attention to these issues should hasten the advent of regenerative therapies for retinal diseases.

Keywords Neural stem cells, transplantation, neuroprotection, cell replacement

Assistant Professor, Director, Stem Cell and Retinal Regeneration Program, Department of Ophthalmology, School of Medicine, University of California, Irvine, 101 The City Drive, Bldg. 55, Room 204, Orange, CA 92868-4380, USA
e-mail: hklassen@uci.edu

Y. Shi, D.O. Clegg (eds.) *Stem Cell Research and Therapeutics*,

2.1   Neural Repair

In lower vertebrates, both the retina and the brain show considerable regenerative ability throughout the life of the animal. In mammals, unfortunately, such is not the case. While the loss of neurons in the central nervous system (CNS) can be compensated for, up to a point, adult neurogenesis is quite limited and CNS lesions in mammalian species tend to have long-lasting and often debilitating consequences. In the human retina, a wide range of diseases lead to the loss of neurons and permanent visual deficits. These include hereditary degenerations of photoreceptors and the optic nerve, as well as more widespread conditions such as macular degeneration, retinal detachment, and glaucoma. Because lost retinal neurons are not spontaneously replaced in humans, there is a pressing need for novel therapeutic approaches to retinal regeneration.

The inability of the human central nervous system to effectively regenerate has been known for centuries, but it was the pioneering work of Cajal that clearly demonstrated the histopathological consequences of CNS injuries at the microscopic level [1]. His work revealed the immense complexity of the mammalian nervous system and the relatively miniscule amount of regeneration that typically follows a lesion. Basically, he showed the CNS to be a single integrated organ system organized at the level of neurons and their processes. He surmised the presence of synaptic connections, although it was not until the advent of the electron microscope that his hypothesis could be confirmed. These data gave rise to a view of the adult CNS as a vast, hard-wired loom of intricate connections that are permanently specified and essentially irreplaceable. The most realistic conclusion that one could gather from his data was that notions of clinical CNS repair should be relegated to the realm of fanciful thinking.

While the view outlined above continues to serve as a practical guide, a wealth of new information has come forward during the latter part of the 20th century indicating that a considerable degree of functional reorganization is possible in the CNS. For example, dramatic plasticity in ocular dominance columns of the cerebral cortex have been documented [2–4], and synapses can change dynamically within structures such as the hippocampus [5]. A surprising degree of regenerative capacity can be elicited following experimental manipulations, such as the transplantation of embryonic CNS tissue [6] or manipulation of the local microenvironment in ways that favor regeneration [7–9]. Similar breakthroughs were also reported from work in the visual system, including embryonic retinal tissue transplantation [10, 11] and through manipulation of the local microenvironment [12–14]. Results such as these provide evidence that neuronal reconstruction and neuroprotection are indeed possible, and collectively redefine what is achievable in terms of mammalian CNS repair.

2.2   Retinal Repair

The neural retina arises from an out-pouching of the brain early in development, and differentiates into a layered structure that has been well characterized anatomically and functionally. Light-sensing photoreceptors are in the back of the retina, where they are interdigitated with apical processes of the retinal pigment epithelium (RPE), which supports and nourishes the photoreceptors (see Chapter 1). The potential space between the photoreceptors and RPE is known as the subretinal space. Stimulated photoreceptors signal via several interneurons (bipolar, horizontal and amacrine cells) to the retinal ganglion cells (RGCs), which extend axons along the inner (vitreal) surface of the retina, down the optic nerve, to the brain. Muller glial cells and microglia are the resident supporting cells within the neural retina.

As with other compartments of the CNS, the human retina is subject to a wide range of diseases. Those involving the loss of photoreceptors and other neurons result in permanent visual deficits. Examples include hereditary degenerations of the photoreceptors such as the rod-cone dystrophies, as well as more common conditions such as macular degeneration, retinal detachment, diabetic maculopathy, vascular occlusions and inflammatory conditions. The increasing prevalence of these conditions relates to current demographic factors such as increases in longevity and average age of the population, as well as increasing rates of myopia, eye surgery, and diabetes throughout much of the world. Because of the lack of effective self-repair in the human retina, there is a pressing need for novel approaches to retinal regeneration that are clinically applicable. One proposed treatment is retinal replacement through the use of an in-dwelling photosensitive electronic prosthesis [15, 16]. This strategy has a distinct technological appeal to it, yet has thus far proven unpractical, partly because of power supply issues, but largely because of fundamental problems with information transfer at the bioelectronic interface. Hopefully, attention to this problem will yield results soon. An alternate approach to the retinal "chip," as it is known, is biologically grounded and involves cellular reconstruction of the neural retina.

The goal of replacing the photoreceptors and neurons of the mammalian retina was all but unthinkable a quarter century ago, yet since that time there have been many astonishing advances in the field of neural regeneration and quite a few of these have specifically involved the retina. Work in retinal transplantation has shown that not only can a grafted embryonic retina survive ectopically within the host nervous system without immune suppression, but it can also develop a normal-appearing laminar organization and establish specific projections to the appropriate host nuclei. Furthermore, these graft-host connections are capable of generating a range of appropriate responses in the host, including electrophysiological, reflex, and behavioral activities [10, 11, 17–19]. Analogous experiments in which fetal retinas were transplanted orthotopically, i.e., to the subretinal space, has demonstrated that such grafts can also survive for extended periods and develop normal laminar organization, however, there was a failure to reliably establish connections with the host retina. This appears to be due to hypertrophic glial changes at the level of the outer limiting membrane (OLM) that present a barrier cell migration and neurite extension. The use of embryonic and fetal transplants for retinal repair has therefore been limited by both the availability of donor tissue and the problem of functional connectivity with the host visual system [20–22]. Recently, results obtained from the transplantation of cultured stem cells have indicated that the barriers to graft-host integration in the retina are not insurmountable.

2.3 Transplantation of Neural Progenitor Cells to the Retina

Transplantation studies in the rat eye first revealed the ability of cultured neural progenitor cells, in this case derived from the adult rat hippocampus, to migrate from the vitreous cavity into the immature retina. Within this ectopic microenvironment, the cells adopted a range of morphologies, many of which were strikingly similar to those of resident neurons [23]. Additional work demonstrated that a similar effect could be reproduced when grafting brain-derived progenitors across species, in this case from mouse to the very immature eyes of the Brazilian opossum [24]. In sharp contrast, allogeneic neural progenitor cells did not migrate into the normal mature retina when transplanted to the vitreous cavity [25]. In this same study we did, however, show that neural progenitor cells (NPCs) would selectively integrate into the adult retina in the setting of retinal dystrophy or mechanical injury. This directed response to injury, or "wound tropism," represents a highly desirable feature for a grafted cell type. Also of interest, and potential clinical significance, was the fact that donor NPCs survived in unrelated allorecipients without immune suppression. In mice, this cellular form of immune privilege even protected NPCs transplanted to non-privileged sites [26]. A significant limitation that emerged from transplantation studies using NPCs was restricted expression of mature markers appropriate to cells at the recipient site. The paucity of retinal-specific markers suggests a limited ability of brain-derived donor cells to fully differentiate into cells of retinal lineage, despite the striking morphological similarities that were seen. This issue was particularly problematic when considering expression of photoreceptor markers, since opsins and many others are essential for normal functioning of these highly specialized cells. Our solution to this problem involved the derivation of immature cells that are inherently predisposed towards a retinal cell fate as part of normal development. These are the progenitor cells of the developing neural retina.

2.4 Retinal Progenitor Cells

In the last several years, we and others have cultured retinal progenitor cells (RPCs) from the neural retina in a range of mammalian species, including mouse [27, 28], rat [29–31], pig [32], and human [33–35]. Work in the mouse has shown that RPCs can be propagated continuously for over a year, expanded in great numbers, and banked and re-cultured after extended periods in liquid nitrogen. Expanded RPC cultures continue to exhibit widespread expression of immature markers and, importantly, express mature retinal markers following transplantation to the subretinal space of diseased or injured allorecipients [27]. Specifically, RPCs express photoreceptor-associated markers, integrate into host cellular layers including the ONL, developed local neuronal and photoreceptor-like morphologies, and have been associated with local neuroprotection [27] and behavioral benefits in retinal dystrophic recipients [27, 28]. As with NPCs, donor RPCs also survive in unrelated murine allorecipients without immune suppression.

Overall, these results have been very encouraging with respect to the application of RPCs to retinal regeneration, however, the ultimate implications of these results must be viewed with caution due to the biological and physical constraints of the rodent models used. While there is much research yet to do, including in rodents, validation of key findings in a large animal allograft model, together with proof-of-principle data obtained using human cells in the laboratory and in animal models, would together provide considerable reassurance prior to the translation of this approach into clinical trials.

In ongoing work, we have extended this work to a pig allograft model in which we have thus far been able to replicate many of the findings seen in mice [32]. Evidence of extended survival post-transplantation without immune suppression, morphological integration of donor cells into the host neural retina and RPE, as well as widespread differentiation into cells expressing multiple photoreceptor markers has been obtained [32]. Furthermore, progenitor cells have been cultured from the immature human neural retina [33, 34]. These cells expand in culture and exhibit many of the progenitor markers anticipated from work in animal models. We have previously shown that human retinal progenitor cells (hRPCs), obtained from post-mortem infants born prematurely at mid-gestation, express a number of potentially important surface markers [34]. In addition, distinct subpopulations of hRPCs express various mature markers, and this expression increases under differentiation conditions. Examination of the capacity of these cells to express a range of rod- and cone-associated photoreceptor markers has begun, as has initial studies involving the transplantation of labeled hRPCs to the subretinal space in animal models.

In summary, research over the past several decades has demonstrated the potential utility of cell and tissue transplantation as a means of diminishing retinal cell loss and even restoring retinal cell types and function. Despite all these advances, it is not yet known whether such strategies will result in clinically significant visual benefits in patients. Only clinical trials can answer that question. In the following sections, I will address the progress made and some of the potential problems that need to be considered if stem cell-related therapies are to be successful in the setting of retinal disease.

2.5   Marker Expression

The identification and analysis of phenotype-associated molecular markers is crucial to the stem cell field because this is the most important method for identifying the cells present in a given culture, including the immature and more differentiated types, and also for establishing the fate of cells following transplantation. In addition, marker expression can be used to sort stem cells from other cell types within a mixed population, as is now common practice in clinical hematology for the isolation of CD34-positive hematopoietic progenitor cells from blood or bone marrow [36].

Cytoplasmic markers are central to studies of CNS progenitors and the most important of these relate to the cytoskeleton. This makes some sense intuitively in that the cytoskeleton is an important determinant of cellular morphology and probably plasticity as well. The intermediate filament nestin is heavily expressed by the majority of cells in neural progenitor cultures and the related marker vimentin often shows a similar expression pattern in retinal cultures, as has been shown for both human [34] and pig [32] (Fig. 2.1). The intermediate filament GFAP is associated with the astroglial lineage, although expression within progenitor populations is a recurring observation [37, 38] and, in the eye, GFAP can be up-regulated in Mueller glia following a variety of perturbations [39]. Other cytoskeletal markers are associated with cells of neuronal lineage, including doublecortin (DCX), β-III tubulin, MAPs, and neurofilaments which have been associated with migratory neuroblasts, immature neurons, neurons, and projection neurons respectively. An added benefit of using anti-cytoskeletal antibodies is that the target antigens label robustly and nicely showcase the morphology of the cells.

Nuclear markers are also important for assessing progenitor cells, both in terms of genetic regulation and cell cycle activity. Among the former, nuclear transcription factors (NTFs) are widely used in the investigation of cellular identity. Because these factors are intimately involved in the epigenetic regulation of cell fate, they are a

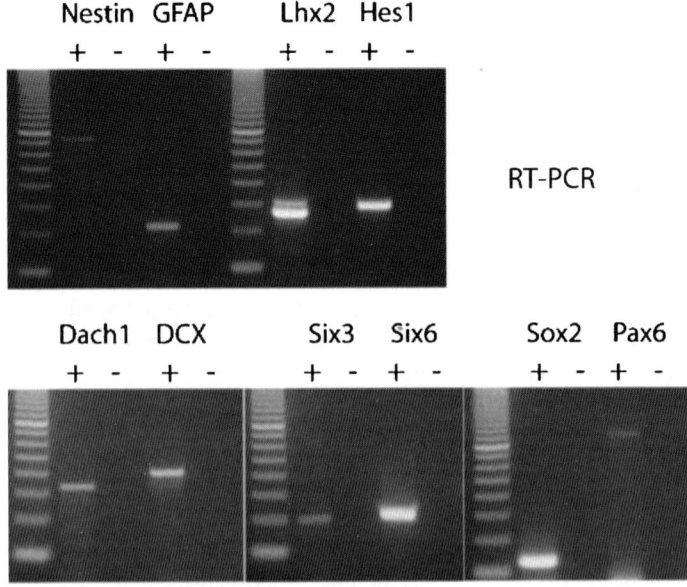

Fig. 2.1 RT-PCR analysis of porcine retinal progenitor cells. Primers designed for human genes were used to probe RNA extracted from cultured porcine retinal progenitor cells. Evidence was found for expression of nestin (faint), GFAP, Lhx2, Hes1, Dach1, DCX, Six3, Six6, Sox2, and Pax6 (faint). Alternating lanes contain sample with (+) and without (−) reverse transcriptase, the latter serving as negative control. 100-bp ladders provided for reference (From [32]; reprinted courtesy of Stem Cells)

natural choice when looking for markers closely associated with ontogenetic status. The functional role of NTFs suggests that expression of these genes might be more tightly correlated with changes in developmental stage than cytoskeletal proteins. Generally, NTFs are not uniquely related to a particular cellular phenotype, however, they can be illuminating when viewed in a defined context. For instance, the pattern of expression can define cell types if analyzed in the setting of cellular populations derived from a particular tissue at a distinct developmental time point, and in concert with other markers, including other NTFs [37]. In this way, Sox2, which is expressed in a variety of cell types, is nevertheless frequently co-expressed with nestin within cell populations derived from the CNS during mid-development. Sox2 is thus an important marker for progenitor cells throughout the CNS, even if it is not entirely specific to these cell types. Other NTFs of particular interest for CNS progenitor cells are Hes1 and Hes5 which are downstream effectors of the notch signaling pathway and also associated with a primitive, progenitor-like state. There are additional NTFs associated with retinal development and these include Pax6, Six3, Six6, Lhx2, Dach1, and Chx10, as well as the photoreceptor precursor markers Crx and Nrl. Antibodies against most of these markers are gradually becoming available.

In contrast to NTFs, cell cycle-associated markers are much less cell type-specific, yet provide very useful information regarding the proportion of cells in a population that are actively proliferating. This is particularly true after transplantation since the failure of donor cells to cease proliferative activity could presage serious local, and even systemic, complications. Widely used markers of this type include Ki-67, PCNA, and BrdU, the last following administration and uptake of that particular compound. Cyclins and other cell cycle proteins can also be examined [38].

Surface epitopes represent another important class of markers, both because they are frequently associated with developmental stages and because they can be used to sort living cells from a mixed population. One example is CD133 (prominin-1), which is seen on hematopoietic progenitors and cells from the developing human brain [40, 41]. Interestingly, some of the more attractive surface markers from a developmental standpoint relate to carbohydrate modifications of underlying proteins or non-protein membrane components such as PSA-NCAM [42], CD15 [43, 44], and selected gangliosides [44–46].

The preceding discussion of markers represents a basic starting point rather than a comprehensive list for neural progenitor markers. As gene expression profiling becomes increasingly practical, we may soon approach the point of knowing and evaluating all relevant genes simultaneously. Dealing with changes in the many possible combinations and quantitative levels of gene expression will then present a significant challenge, as will simultaneous assessment of the different profiles likely to be present within a given sample at a given point in time. Even then, genome-wide genetic analysis is not likely to be sufficient for an understanding of cultured stem cells. For instance, it would not directly address the proteome, epigenetic tags such as DNA and histone modifications, metabolic status, or developmentally regulated glycosylation. Furthermore, mapping out the developmental potential of such cells under many relevant possible culture conditions represents a task of daunting scope. Fortunately, it appears that much can be achieved without the necessity of completing a body of knowledge at the detailed level just described.

2.6   Immunology of CNS Progenitor Cells

Any cell-based therapy must take into consideration the immunological response of the host to the grafted cells and any associated materials. In this regard, the retina represents an inviting target because of the immune privilege attributed to this location, similar to the phenomenon seen in the cornea [47]. In addition, neural progenitors themselves appear to be an immune privileged cell type, at least in the mouse [26], thereby doubly predisposing them to survival when grafted to the vitreous or subretinal space of allorecipients. Indeed, many studies have replicated this finding in the mouse, showing that immunosuppressive agents need not be administered in these types of experiments. What has been less clear is whether the findings in the mouse would apply to larger mammals that more accurately reflect the situation in humans. This is significant from a clinical standpoint because the use of immune suppression introduces the known risk of serious systemic complications, including death, making clinical trials for a non-lethal medical condition such as retinal degeneration much less palatable.

Examination of the immune-related markers of the major histocompatibility complex (MHC) expressed by neural progenitor cells from mouse, rat, and human has shown that none of these cells express class II MHC antigens at a level detectable by flow cytometry, whereas the levels of class I MHC antigens vary considerably between species [48]. Specifically, mouse neural progenitors do not express any detectable MHC class I [26, 44], while rat cells express low levels [49], and human cells express high levels of these molecules [34, 44]. The absence of MHC class II expression across species bodes well for survival of this cell type in allorecipients, particularly when grafting to the subretinal space. However, such survival is far from assured as there are many other potential determinants of immune rejection, MHC class I being just one of them. In terms of immunological considerations, studies in the mouse represents an important but limited step and translation of the results obtained to animals with a more sophisticated immune system is prudent before generalizing to humans.

Work in the pig has been instructive as to how the limits of immune tolerance can more easily be exceeded in a large adult mammal as opposed to a mouse or immature marsupial. The same sort of murine progenitor cells that express no detectable MHC molecules and are well tolerated in allorecipients, even in non-privileged sites [26], and also survive transplantation to the xenogeneic eye of the Brazilian opossum [24], elicit a vigorous choroidal immune response when grafted to the subretinal space of juvenile porcine xenorecipients where they are completely rejected within 5 weeks [50, 51]. In contrast, work with porcine retinal progenitor cells has shown that these allogeneic cells survive in the pig eye for the same period without signs of immunological reaction [32]. Furthermore, in ongoing work we have extended that time point considerably.

So how well would allogeneic CNS progenitor cells be tolerated in non-immune suppressed humans? Without specific data, it is too early to say, but my guess is that results in the pig will prove fairly predictive. Indeed, in somewhat related trials of fetal retinal tissue transplantation in patients, immunological reactions have not been reported [52–54]. I remain optimistic that immune suppression will not be necessary for CNS progenitor transplantation to the retina anymore than is the case for corneal transplantation. The absence of a requirement for routine immune suppression would eliminate one significant barrier to the initiation of clinical safety trials involving the application of progenitor cells for retinal disease. On the other hand, use of porcine xenografts is contraindicated at this time. In my opinion, any potential donor cells would require extensive modifications to render them immune-compatible before such an approach would be worth revisiting.

2.7 Proliferation

Control of cellular proliferation is important from two very different standpoints. First, the availability of immature human tissue is limited relative to the potential clinical need for donor cells. Second, it is clinically imperative that grafted cells not continue to proliferate for extended periods following transplantation because of the risk of tumor formation.

Unless the donor cells can be induced to proliferate sufficiently to generate an adequate supply, it will not be feasible to rely on human retinal progenitor cells for therapeutic application, even if these cells show promise in limited clinical trials. This point is all the more critical for any contemplated use of post-mitotic cells, such as Nrl-positive rod photoreceptor precursor cells [28], which by definition are not self-renewing. These would have to be generated anew for each recipient, presumably from a population of retinal progenitor cells, the latter perhaps derived from a population of human ES cells [55]. Traditionally, cultured neural progenitors require exogenous mitotic stimulation to proliferate and abruptly cease proliferation and differentiate upon mitogen withdrawal. Unlike ES cells, however, human CNS progenitor cells tend to senesce with repeated passaging in culture. In fact, finding the optimal culture conditions for sustained proliferation of human retinal progenitor cells has proven especially difficult, particularly given the challenge of obtaining sufficient donor material [34]. One method that has been used to overcome this problem is immortalization of the cells, for instance by introducing variants of the proliferation-associated myc gene [56–58]. This strategy has proven successful in experimental applications, however, continued over-expression of myc is known to interfere with differentiation and frequently results in tumor formation [59–61]. Conditional expression of the immortalizing transgene is one strategy for circumventing this problem, at least until alternate methods such as optimal culture conditions can be identified.

As pointed out above, cessation of proliferation is another major aspect of stem cell research. In general, tumor formation is more often seen with immortal cell types, such as ES cells [62], or with constitutively immortalized progenitor cells. The tendency of human CNS progenitors to senesce, on the other hand, provides something of a safety factor. Indeed, the primary role of senescence in human cells may be to protect against tumor formation. That being said, extended passaging of cells in culture with prolonged exposure to high levels of mitogens could result in transformational events. The process of clonal selection also potentially favors cells that have undergone transformation since they survive the isolation process more readily than normal progenitors, particularly with reference to human cells. Clinical application will require special attention to the possibility of tumor formation, regardless of the safety record in animals. In terms of patient safety, it certainly makes sense to first test prospective cells in a non-seeing eye where they can be directly observed and, in the worst case, removed along with the sequestering globe. This contrasts sharply with the options available following transplantation of cells to a vital structure such as the brain.

Interestingly, another proposed role for neural progenitor cells is the targeting of malignant brain lesions. Both grafted [63] and endogenous [64] neural progenitor cells show a pronounced tropism for tumor cells implanted at a distance within the forebrain. Therefore, exogenous neural progenitor grafts represent one potential method for delivery of anti-oncogenic genes to tumors in a directed manner. Similarly, retinal progenitor cells might be used to treat retinal tumors such as retinoblastoma. As I have cautioned previously, this intriguing strategy could backfire if the grafted cells are activated by mitogens secreted by the tumor [65]. It is known that CNS tumor cells can secrete growth factors such as bFGF that induce neural progenitor proliferation [66–68]. If tumors both attract and stimulate exogenous progenitors, this could result in recruitment of the grafted cells into the malignant process. The reason I bring up this potentially grim scenario is to emphasize the more general need for adequate measures to insure that grafted cells will not be induced to proliferate by the local microenvironment following implantation. Whether post-mitotic precursors maintain their competency for migration and tropism for tumors is, I believe, a very pertinent question. On this point I again remain optimistic. Studies of migratory neuroblasts, as well as recent work in the retina [28], suggest that such might be the case. As an aside, I believe it is worth considering whether recruitment of endogenous progenitor cells contributes to the rapid progression of childhood CNS malignancies such as brainstem tumors and retinoblastoma [65].

2.8 Differentiation

The advantage of grafting immature cells is that they retain the capacity for injury-directed migration, as well as morphological integration in to the mature retina. In order to induce neuroprotection, perfect differentiation might not always be necessary. However, for integration to be significant at the level of cell replacement, the donor cells must exhibit the appropriate functional characteristics associated with the local cellular phenotype in question. In the case of photoreceptors, this means light sensitivity and implies the successful expression of all genes necessary for the successful transduction of photic stimuli, including those mediating the phototransduction cascade.

As mentioned earlier, studies of brain-derived progenitors grafted to the retina have shown that these cells do not typically express phototransduction proteins, even if they can exhibit photoreceptor-like morphology [23, 25]. Therefore, one of the distinct advantages of using progenitor cells derived from the developing neural retina is their inherent propensity for differentiating into photoreceptor cells. We and others have shown that retinal progenitor and precursor cells can express photoreceptor markers both before (Fig. 2.2), and particularly after, transplantation to the retina [27, 28, 32, 34] (Fig. 2.3). In the allogeneic pig model, cells in the vicinity of the ONL and subretinal space expressed multiple photoreceptor markers in abundance [32]. In addition, there is evidence for improvement in light perception [27, 28], however,

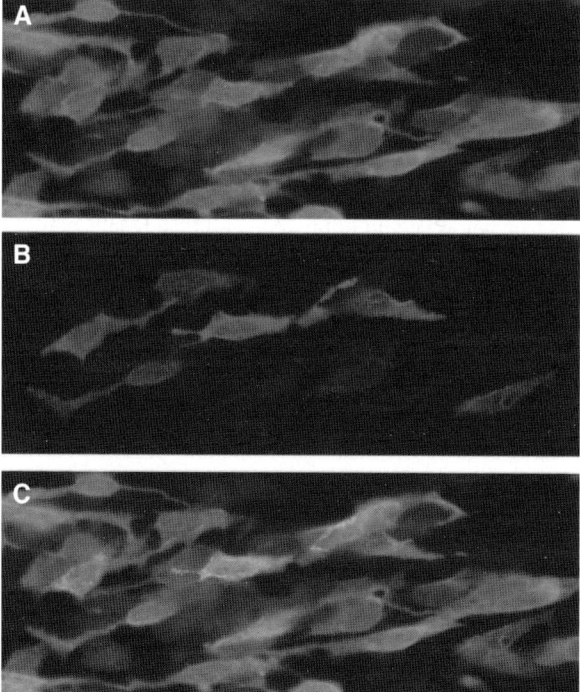

Fig. 2.2 Expression of photoreceptor markers in culture. Under differentiation conditions, porcine retinal progenitor cells expressed the photoreceptor markers recoverin (green) (**A**) and rhodopsin (red) (**B**), with co-expression of both markers in a subset of cells (**C**). Cells co-expressing rhodopsin and recoverin frequently exhibited morphologies suggestive of rod photoreceptors (From [32]; reprinted courtesy of Stem Cells) (*See Color Plates*)

Fig. 2.3 Subretinal transplantation in allogeneic recipients. Cultured porcine retinal progenitor cells were prelabeled with DAPI (blue) prior to transplantation. Following transplantation, many donor cells exhibited rod-like morphologies and co-expressed the photoreceptor marker rhodopsin (red). DAPI-labeled donor cells formed characteristic rosettes (arrows), suggestive of an advanced level of photoreceptor differentiation. Rhodopsin was also expressed by the DAPI-negative rods of the host (red, below) (Detail from [32]; reprinted courtesy of Stem Cells) (*See Color Plates*)

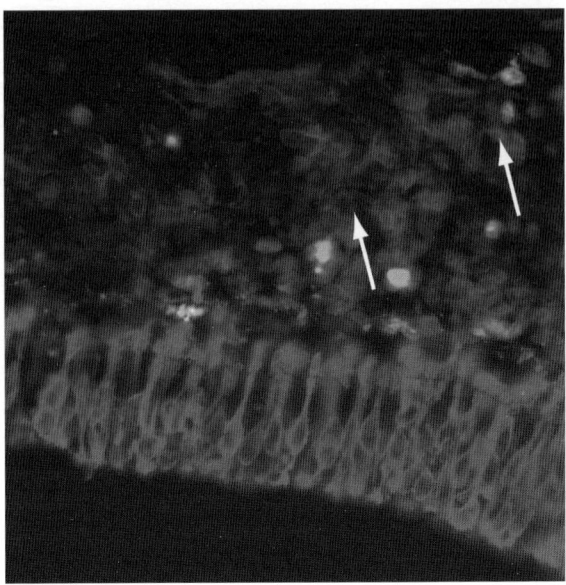

truly understanding the functional capabilities of progenitor cells following integration is a subject for detailed further investigation. Noticeable improvements in patterned vision as a result of cell replacement are unlikely at present, although this goal should be achievable in the case of neuroprotection. Ongoing improvements in cell delivery methods (see below) could improve anatomical results across larger areas of the retina and thereby enhance functional outcome by virtue of cell replacement.

Potential donor cell types other than retinal progenitor and precursor cells present greater difficulties when it comes to differentiating into retinal cell types such as photoreceptors. Pluripotent stem cells, such as ES cells, are theoretically capable of generating any somatic cell type, yet coaxing them to do so predictably and in significant numbers is not necessarily straightforward. Another challenge is the extended time frame required for the differentiation process. Nevertheless, recent progress in a number of laboratories suggests that this approach will become increasingly feasible in the future [55, 69, 70].

2.9   Cell Delivery

As mentioned above, deliver of donor cells to the subretinal space is an area where there is considerable room for improvement. Bolus injections of cells, as are currently used in animal experiments, are relatively simple to perform and allow for informative initial investigations of progenitor cell behavior within the host retina, as well as the immunological response of the host to the donor cells. On the other hand, when functional evaluations and clinical applications are being contemplated, it is desirable to achieve a more widespread and uniform result. In addition, donor cell attrition following grafting can be a major problem, necessitating the injection of large quantities of cells to ensure adequate graft survival. When cell survival is high, such boluses can easily overshoot the intended goal and result in substantial retention of donor cells beneath the retina. The cells in these grafts often adhere to each other, rather than integrating into the retina, and the resulting mass can significantly distort the overlying retina. Fortunately, there is an emerging technology that represents a potential solution to these problems, namely tissue engineering.

A number of biodegradable polymers are currently available and each of these can be tested as a means of delivering cells. Examples include polylactic acid (PLA), polylactic-co-glycolic acid (PLGA), polycaprolactone (PCL), and polyglycerol sebacate (PGS), to name a few [71]. Each differs in chemical composition, method and rate of degradation, as well as the nature of the degradation products. They also vary in terms of transparency, flexibility, permeability, and strength. The materials can be fashioned into sheets of varying thickness and texture, depending upon the distinctive physical characteristics of the polymer used. Importantly, there can be significant differences in biocompatibility, and this aspect is particularly important for any material that is being placed in contact with the delicate photoreceptor and RPE layers of the eye.

Characterization of the biocompatibility of various polymer formulations in the subretinal space is now underway. In addition, evaluation of the ability of progenitor cells to adhere to these constructs, as well as the influence that adherence to the polymer has on gene expression are current areas of interest. Work to date shows that retinal progenitor cells adhere avidly to porous PLGA scaffolds [72], resulting in radial organization of the grafted cells following transplantation to the subretinal space [50]. A regular, radial organization is certainly more desirable for ONL replacement than the relatively

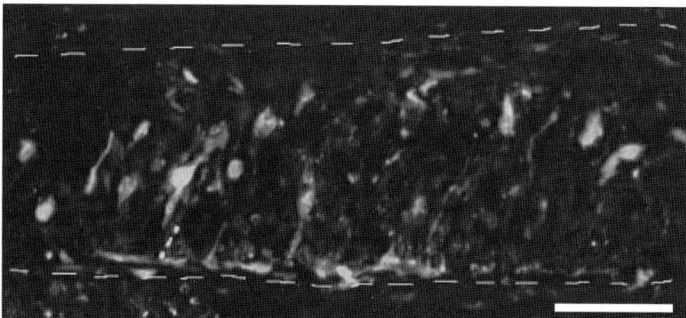

Fig. 2.4 Polymer-progenitor composite graft in the eye. GFP-transgenic mouse retinal progenitor cells were co-cultured on a sheet of PLGA followed by transplantation to the subretinal space of a pig. Note that the cells have conformed to the porous structure of the polymer by extending processes with a radial orientation. Dashed lines indicate the border of the polymer scaffold. The host RPE lies above the graft, while the host retina lies below. Scale bar 90 um. (From [50] reprinted courtesy Archives of Ophthalmology) (*See Color Plates*)

disorganized mass resulting from bolus injection (Fig. 2.4), however, increasing the cell density within the polymer scaffold is also import. PLA/PLGA blends appear to exert a differentiating effect on mouse CNS progenitor cells in vitro [72] and in vivo and promote survival after transplantation [73]. The presence of a giant cell reaction, however, represents a disadvantage when using this polymer in the subretinal space.

Exploration of the uses for progenitor cell/polymer composite grafts is in the early stages and the many available polymers and many possible ways in which they can be configured, together with the possibility of functionalizing the polymers to deliver pharmacological agents, suggests that this approach will play a significant role in any future clinical application of the type being considered here.

2.10   Gene Delivery

Gene delivery is another potential role for grafted progenitor cells. For instance, by delivering neuroprotective cyokines, CNS progenitors might favorably influence visual performance in a degenerative eye without the added requirements for differentiation into photoreceptors and integration into the host retina. This approach would also circumvent the need for direct delivery of viral-based vectors to patients, a strategy that has been associated with a number of fatalities. Neuroprotection studies in the rodent retina have been quite successful, however the size of the human eye and the extended course of the degenerative process make direct translation of rodent methodologies to humans untenable. Challenges to a cell-based approach to clinical neuroprotection include regulation of transgene expression, choice of neuroprotective agent and disease entity, how, where, and when to deliver the cells for optimal effect, and how best to monitor functional outcome in a long term neuroprotection study. In my opinion, the development of an appropriate non-rodent model that provides a more human-like eye and allows for more detailed visual assessment would be very helpful in terms of moving this promising strategy forward.

2.11   Alternate Cell Types

One of the uncertainties facing the field of regenerative medicine as a whole, including retinal transplantation, relates to the question of which donor cell type will be the most efficacious. While I have focused the present discussion on the use of retinal progenitor cells, these are by no means the only candidates worthy of attention.

Post-mitotic rod precursor cells have recently been implicated as the cells most capable of morphological integration into the retinal ONL [28]. There is at present no way to source these cells from humans, however the introduction of a GFP-reporter gene on an Nrl promoter into ES or progenitor cells could make this feasible. In any event, the available evidence indicates that retinal progenitor cells yield results similar to rod precursors. Furthermore, it might be possible to induce progenitors to become Nrl-positive rod precursors immediately prior to transplantation, should that turn out to be important.

Ciliary epithelial cells have been reported to contain a small subpopulation of stem cells predisposed toward a retinal fate [74]. It is evident that these cells can express a number of retina-specific genes [75, 76]. The degree to which they are suitable for cell replacement in the retina remains unclear. Certainly the transformation from a pigmented epithelial cell to a retinal neuron represents a significant degree of transdifferentiation [77], arguably more than is usually seen in mammals. These cells could be obtained autologously from patients, although this would add another surgery and would presumably not be efficacious in patients whose retinas were degenerating secondary to a genetic condition, since autologous ciliary cells would carry the same mutant genes.

The quintessential stem cell is arguably the embryonic stem cell (ES cell). These cells can multiply for indefinite periods of time and expand in vast numbers, making them attractive from an industrial standpoint. In addition to a lack of senescence, another strong point for these cells is pluripotentiality which means they are relatively unrestricted in terms of what phenotypes they can adopt. As noted above, these strong points of ES cells both have a downside. The capacity for unrelenting proliferation is likely related to the known tendency towards tumor formation [62], while the immature, pluripotent state is likely responsible for the challenges faced when trying to achieve complete differentiation and formation of photoreceptor cells. Once a way can be found to select for a population of post-mitotic progeny, or render the entire grafted population post-mitotic following transplantation, it will be quite helpful to the field of ES cell transplantation. Likewise, a deeper understanding of the means by which these cells can be directed down specific phenotypic pathways to complete differentiation should prove to be valuable.

Another class of potential donor cells are bone marrow-derived, particularly the non-hematopoietic bone marrow progenitor population. Cells of this general type have been thought to evidence considerable degrees of plasticity [78, 79] and therefore might also be useful for retinal cell replacement. In addition, mouse data suggests that bone marrow-derived endothelial precursors are capable of integrating into the retinal vasculature following intravitreal injection and in some way secondarily rescuing retinal photoreceptors in a model of retinal dystrophy [80]. On the plus side, bone marrow cells can be derived autologously, thereby eliminating any genetic incompatibility. However, not all patients will be eager to have their bone marrow harvested, in addition to eye surgery, especially prior to definitive clinical substantiation of the utility of this approach. In the setting of genetically based retinal disease, it is very unclear whether a patient's own cells would be of benefit since they carry the same disease-causing mutation. Furthermore, these cells are not necessarily an immune privileged cell type, at least not in the manner of neural progenitor cells [81, 82], and further research is needed to determine whether they are suitable for human allografting in the absence of immune suppression.

In summary, every candidate cell type has apparent advantages and disadvantages. It could be that one particular type comes to dominate the field clinically although, even if this were the case, such a cell type is likely to be displaced from its preeminence as technology advances. For example, the recent finding that mouse dermal fibroblasts can be genetically reprogrammed to a pluripotent, ES cell-like state shows how dramatically the available options can change in a relatively short period of time [83, 84]. It is my belief that any immunologically compatible cell that confers a reliable and clinically significant level of neuroprotection, without a corresponding tumor forming risk to the patient, represents a good candidate for initial studies. For cell replacement, it seems to me that the retinal progenitor cell is the best candidate we have at present and it has potential for neuroprotection as well. Whether retinal progenitor cells can be generated from human ES cells on an industrial scale is certainly an interesting question.

2.12   Conclusion

Experimental evidence of functional recovery from a variety of disease states following transplantation of stem cells has generated considerable optimism within the biomedical community regarding the prospects for developing restorative treatments for many currently incurable diseases. Included on this list are a variety of blinding conditions of the retina. While such optimism must inevitably be tempered by recognition of the complexity of human biology, as well as the many significant hurdles yet to be dealt with, it nevertheless appears to be justified. That being the case, there is a growing appreciation of the need to study stem, progenitor, and precursor cells in considerably greater detail that has so far been the case. In the preceding discussion I have attempted to highlight some important areas in which further efforts should be directed.

Acknowledgements I would particularly like to acknowledge all the many collaborators and colleagues who worked on the research described here. I am also grateful for past and present research support from Sigma Xi, the NSF, NIH, Foundation Fighting Blindness, Discovery Eye Foundation, Lincy Foundation, Siegal Foundation, Larry Hoag Foundation, CHOC Foundation, and the BMRC of Singapore.

References

1. Ramon y Cajal S (1995) Histology of the Nervous System. Oxford University Press, New York
2. Wiesel TN, Hubel DH (1965) Extent of recovery from the effects of visual deprivation in kittens. J Neurophysiol 28:1060–1072
3. Blakemore C, Van Sluyters RC (1974) Reversal of the physiological effects of monocular deprivation in kittens: further evidence for a sensitive period. J Physiol 237:195–216

4. Allard T, Clark SA, Jenkins WM, Merzenich MM (1991) Reorganization of somatosensory area 3b representations in adult owl monkeys after digital syndactyly. J Neurophysiol 66:1048–1058
5. Fagan AM, Gage FH (1994) Mechanisms of sprouting in the adult central nervous system: cellular responses in areas of terminal degeneration and reinnervation in the rat hippocampus. Neuroscience 58:705–725
6. Bjorklund A, Stenevi U, Dunnett SB, Iversen SD (1981) Functional reactivation of the deafferented neostriatum by nigral transplants. Nature 289:497–499
7. Bray GM, Vidal-Sanz M, Aguayo AJ (1987) Regeneration of axons from the central nervous system of adult rats. Prog Brain Res 71:373–379
8. Schnell L, Schwab ME (1990) Axonal regeneration in the rat spinal cord produced by an antibody against myelin-associated neurite growth inhibitors. Nature 343:269–272
9. Nakahara Y, Gage FH, Tuszynski MH (1996) Grafts of fibroblasts genetically modified to secrete NGF, BDNF, NT-3, or basic FGF elicit differential responses in the adult spinal cord. Cell Transplant 5:191–204
10. Klassen H, Lund RD (1987) Retinal transplants can drive a pupillary reflex in host rat brains. Proc Natl Acad Sci USA 84:6958–6960
11. Klassen H, Lund RD (1990a) Retinal graft-mediated pupillary responses in rats: restoration of a reflex function in the mature mammalian brain. J Neurosci 10:578–587
12. Cho EY, So KF (1989) Regrowth of retinal ganglion cell axons into a peripheral nerve graft in the adult hamster is enhanced by a concurrent optic nerve crush. Exp Brain Res 78:567–574
13. Weibel D, Cadelli D, Schwab ME (1994) Regeneration of lesioned rat optic nerve fibers is improved after neutralization of myelin-associated neurite growth inhibitors. Brain Res 642:259–266
14. Faktorovich EG, Steinberg RH, Yasumura D, Matthes MT, LaVail MM (1990) Photoreceptor degeneration in inherited retinal dystrophy delayed by basic fibroblast growth factor. Nature 347:83–86
15. Colodetti L, Weiland JD, Colodetti S, Ray A, Seiler MJ, Hinton DR, Humayun MS (2007) Pathology of damaging electrical stimulation in the retina. Exp Eye Res 85:23–33
16. Schanze T, Hesse L, Lau C, Greve N, Haberer W, Kammer S, Doerge T, Rentzos A, Stieglitz T (2007) An optically powered single-channel stimulation implant as test system for chronic biocompatibility and biostability of miniaturized retinal vision prostheses. IEEE Trans Biomed Eng 54:983–992
17. Young MJ, Rao K, Lund RD (1989) Integrity of the blood-brain barrier in retinal xenografts is correlated with the immunological status of the host. J Comp Neurol 283:107–117
18. Coffey PJ, Lund RD, Rawlins JN (1989) Retinal transplant-mediated learning in a conditioned suppression task in rats. Proc Natl Acad Sci USA 86:7248–7249
19. Klassen H, Lund RD (1990b) Parameters of retinal graft-mediated responses are related to underlying target innervation. Brain Res 533:181–191
20. Turner JE, Seiler M, Aramant R, Blair JR (1988) Embryonic retinal grafts transplanted into the lesioned adult rat retina. Prog Brain Res 78:131–139
21. Silverman MS, Hughes SE (1989) Transplantation of photoreceptors to light- damaged retina. Invest Ophthalmol Vis Sci 30:1684–1690
22. Gouras P, Tanabe T (2003) Survival and integration of neural retinal transplants in rd mice. Graefes Arch Clin Exp Ophthalmol 241:403–409
23. Takahashi M, Palmer TD, Takahashi J, Gage FH (1998) Widespread integration and survival of adult-derived neural progenitor cells in the developing optic retina. Mol Cell Neurosci 12:340–348
24. Van Hoffelen SJ, Young MJ, Shatos MA, Sakaguchi DS (2003) Incorporation of murine brain progenitor cells into the developing mammalian retina. Invest Ophthalmol Vis Sci 44:426–434
25. Young MJ, Ray J, Whiteley SJ, Klassen H, Gage FH (2000) Neuronal differentiation and morphological integration of hippocampal progenitor cells transplanted to the retina of immature and mature dystrophic rats. Mol Cell Neurosci 16:197–205

26. Hori J, Ng TF, Shatos M, Klassen H, Streilein JW, Young MJ (2003) Neural progenitor cells lack immunogenicity and resist destruction as allografts. Stem Cells 21:405–416

27. Klassen HJ, Ng TF, Kurimoto Y, Kirov I, Shatos M, Coffey P, Young MJ (2004) Multipotent retinal progenitors express developmental markers, differentiate into retinal neurons, and preserve light-mediated behavior. Invest Ophthalmol Vis Sci 45:4167–4173

28. MacLaren RE, Pearson RA, MacNeil A, Douglas RH, Salt TE, Akimoto M, Swaroop A, Sowden JC, Ali RR (2006) Retinal repair by transplantation of photoreceptor precursors. Nature 444:203–207

29. Chacko DM, Rogers JA, Turner JE, Ahmad I (2000) Survival and differentiation of cultured retinal progenitors transplanted in the subretinal space of the rat. Biochem Biophys Res Commun 268:842–846

30. Yang P, Seiler MJ, Aramant RB, Whittemore SR (2002) Differential lineage restriction of rat retinal progenitor cells in vitro and in vivo. J Neurosci Res 69:466–476

31. Yang J, Klassen H, Pries M, Wang W, Nissen MH (2006) Aqueous humor enhances the proliferation of rat retinal precursor cells in culture, and this effect is partially reproduced by ascorbic acid. Stem Cells 24:2766–2775

32. Klassen H, Kiilgaard JF, Zahir T, Ziaeian B, Kirov I, Scherfig E, Warfvinge K, Young MJ (2007) Progenitor cells from the porcine neural retina express photoreceptor markers after transplantation to the subretinal space of allorecipients. Stem Cells 25:1222–1230

33. Kelley MW, Turner JK, Reh TA (1995) Regulation of proliferation and photoreceptor differentiation in fetal human retinal cell cultures. Invest Ophthalmol Vis Sci 36:1280–1289

34. Klassen H, Ziaeian B, Kirov II, Young MJ, Schwartz PH (2004) Isolation of retinal progenitor cells from post-mortem human tissue and comparison with autologous brain progenitors. J Neurosci Res 77:334–343

35. Carter DA, Mayer EJ, Dick AD (2007) The effect of postmortem time, donor age and sex on the generation of neurospheres from adult human retina. Br J Ophthalmol 91: 1216–1218

36. Baum CM, Weissman IL, Tsukamoto AS, Buckle AM, Peault B (1992) Isolation of a candidate human hematopoietic stem-cell population. Proc Natl Acad Sci USA 89:2804–2808

37. Klassen H, Sakaguchi DS, Young MJ (2004) Stem cells and retinal repair. Prog Retin Eye Res 23:149–181

38. Schwartz PH, Nethercott H, Kirov II, Ziaeian B, Young MJ, Klassen H (2005) Expression of neurodevelopmental markers by cultured porcine neural precursor cells. Stem Cells 23:1286–1294

39. Klassen H, Schwartz P, Nethercott H, Ziaeian B, Young M, Narfstrom K (2007) Neural precursors isolated from the developing cat brain show retinal integration following transplantation to the retina of the dystrophic cat. Vet Ophthalmol 10:245–253

40. Uchida N, Buck DW, He D, Reitsma MJ, Masek M, Phan TV, Tsukamoto AS, Gage FH, Weissman IL (2000) Direct isolation of human central nervous system stem cells. Proc Natl Acad Sci USA 97:14720–14725

41. Schwartz P, Bryant P, Fuja T, Su H, O'Dowd D, Klassen H (2003) Isolation and characterization of neural progenitor cells from post-mortem human cortex. J Neurosci Res 74: 838–851

42. Szele FG, Chesselet MF (1996) Cortical lesions induce an increase in cell number and PSA-NCAM expression in the subventricular zone of adult rats. J Comp Neurol 368:439–454

43. Allendoerfer KL, Durairaj A, Matthews GA, Patterson PH (1999) Morphological domains of Lewis-X/FORSE-1 immunolabeling in the embryonic neural tube are due to developmental regulation of cell surface carbohydrate expression. Dev Biol 211:208–219

44. Klassen H, Schwartz MR, Bailey AH, Young MJ (2001) Surface markers expressed by multipotent human and mouse neural progenitor cells include tetraspanins and non-protein epitopes. Neurosci Lett 312:180–182

45. Sparrow JR, Barnstable CJ (1988) A gradient molecule in developing rat retina: expression of 9-O-acetyl GD3 in relation to cell type, developmental age, and GD3 ganglioside. J Neurosci Res 21:398–409

46. Yanagisawa M, Nakamura K, Taga T (2005) Glycosphingolipid synthesis inhibitor represses cytokine-induced activation of the Ras-MAPK pathway in embryonic neural precursor cells. J Biochem 138:285–291

47. Williamson JS, Streilein JW (1989) Induction of delayed hypersensitivity to alloantigens coinjected with Langerhans cells into the anterior chamber of the eye. Abrogation of anterior chamber-associated immune deviation. Transplantation 47:519–524

48. Klassen H (2006) Transplantation of cultured progenitor cells to the mammalian retina. Expert Opin Biol Ther 6:443–451

49. Klassen H, Imfeld KL, Ray J, Young MJ, Gage FH, Berman MA (2003) The immunological properties of adult hippocampal progenitor cells. Vision Res 43:947–956

50. Warfvinge K, Kiilgaard JF, Lavik EB, Scherfig E, Langer R, Klassen HJ, Young MJ (2005) Retinal progenitor cell xenografts to the pig retina: morphologic integration and cytochemical differentiation. Arch Ophthalmol 123:1385–1393

51. Warfvinge K, Kiilgaard J, Klassen H, Zamiri P, Scherfig E, Streilein JW, Prause J, Young M (2006) Retinal progenitor cell xenografts to the pig retina: immunological reactions. Cell Transplant 15:603–612

52. Humayun MS, de Juan E Jr, del Cerro M, Dagnelie G, Radner W, Sadda SR, del Cerro C (2000) Human neural retinal transplantation. Invest Ophthalmol Vis Sci 41:3100–3106

53. Berger AS, Tezel TH, Del Priore LV, Kaplan HJ (2003) Photoreceptor transplantation in retinitis pigmentosa: short-term follow-up. Ophthalmology 110:383–391

54. Radtke ND, Aramant RB, Seiler MJ, Petry HM, Pidwell D (2004) Vision change after sheet transplant of fetal retina with retinal pigment epithelium to a patient with retinitis pigmentosa. Arch Ophthalmol 122:1159–1165

55. Lamba DA, Karl MO, Ware CB, Reh TA (2006) Efficient generation of retinal progenitor cells from human embryonic stem cells. Proc Natl Acad Sci USA 103:12769–12774

56. Snyder EY, Deitcher DL, Walsh C, Arnold-Aldea S, Hartwieg EA, Cepko CL (1992) Multipotent neural cell lines can engraft and participate in development of mouse cerebellum. Cell 68:33–51

57. Rashid-Doubell F, Kershaw TR, Sinden JD (1994) Effects of basic fibroblast growth factor and gamma interferon on hippocampal progenitor cells derived from the H-2Kb-tsA58 transgenic mouse. Gene Ther 1 Suppl 1:S63

58. Cacci E, Villa A, Parmar M, Cavallaro M, Mandahl N, Lindvall O, Martinez- Serrano A, Kokaia Z (2007) Generation of human cortical neurons from a new immortal fetal neural stem cell line. Exp Cell Res 313:588–601

59. Kitchens DL, Snyder EY, Gottlieb DI (1994) FGF and EGF are mitogens for immortalized neural progenitors. J Neurobiol 25:797–807

60. Fults D, Pedone C, Dai C, Holland EC (2002) MYC expression promotes the proliferation of neural progenitor cells in culture and in vivo. Neoplasia 4:32–39

61. Su X, Gopalakrishnan V, Stearns D, Aldape K, Lang FF, Fuller G, Snyder E, Eberhart CG, Majumder S (2006) Abnormal expression of REST/NRSF and Myc in neural stem/progenitor cells causes cerebellar tumors by blocking neuronal differentiation. Mol Cell Biol 26:1666–1678

62. Arnhold S, Klein H, Semkova I, Addicks K, Schraermeyer U (2004) Neurally selected embryonic stem cells induce tumor formation after long-term survival following engraftment into the subretinal space. Invest Ophthalmol Vis Sci 45:4251–4255

63. Aboody KS, Brown A, Rainov NG, Bower KA, Liu S, Yang W, Small JE, Herrlinger U, Ourednik V, Black PM, Breakefield XO, Snyder EY (2000) Neural stem cells display extensive tropism for pathology in adult brain: evidence from intracranial gliomas. Proc Natl Acad Sci USA 97:12846–12851

64. Glass R, Synowitz M, Kronenberg G, Walzlein JH, Markovic DS, Wang LP, Gast D, Kiwit J, Kempermann G, Kettenmann H (2005) Glioblastoma-induced attraction of endogenous neural precursor cells is associated with improved survival. J Neurosci 25:2637–2646

65. Klassen H (2007) Recruitment of endogenous neural progenitor cells by malignant neoplasms of the central nervous system. Curr Stem Cell Res Ther 2:113–119

66. Takahashi JA, Mori H, Fukumoto M, Igarashi K, Jaye M, Oda Y, Kikuchi H, Hatanaka M (1990) Gene expression of fibroblast growth factors in human gliomas and meningiomas: demonstration of cellular source of basic fibroblast growth factor mRNA and peptide in tumor tissues. Proc Natl Acad Sci USA 87:5710–5714

67. Paulus W, Sage EH, Jellinger K, Roggendorf W (1990) Localization of basic fibroblast growth factor, a mitogen and angiogenic factor, in human brain tumors. Acta Neuropathol (Berl) 79:418–423

68. Behl C, Winkler J, Bogdahn U, Meixensberger J, Schligensiepen KH, Brysch W (1993) Autocrine growth regulation in neuroectodermal tumors as detected with oligodeoxynucleotide antisense molecules. Neurosurgery 33:679–684

69. Ikeda H, Osakada F, Watanabe K, Mizuseki K, Haraguchi T, Miyoshi H, Kamiya D, Honda Y, Sasai N, Yoshimura N, Takahashi M, Sasai Y (2005) Generation of Rx$^+$/Pax6$^+$ neural retinal precursors from embryonic stem cells. Proc Natl Acad Sci USA 102:11331–11336

70. Zhao X, Liu J, Ahmad I (2006) Differentiation of embryonic stem cells to retinal cells in vitro. Methods Mol Biol 330:401–416

71. Gunatillake PA, Adhikari R (2003) Biodegradable synthetic polymers for tissue engineering. Eur Cell Mater 5:1–16

72. Lavik EB, Klassen H, Warfvinge K, Langer R, Young MJ (2005) Fabrication of degradable polymer scaffolds to direct the integration and differentiation of retinal progenitors. Biomaterials 26:3187–3196

73. Tomita M, Lavik E, Klassen H, Zahir T, Langer R, Young MJ (2005) Biodegradable polymer composite grafts promote the survival and differentiation of retinal progenitor cells. Stem Cells 23:1579–1588

74. Tropepe V, Coles BL, Chiasson BJ, Horsford DJ, Elia AJ, McInnes RR, van der Kooy D (2000) Retinal stem cells in the adult mammalian eye. Science 287:2032–2036

75. Bertazolli-Filho R, Ghosh S, Huang W, Wollmann G, Coca-Prados M (2001) Molecular evidence that human ocular ciliary epithelium expresses components involved in phototransduction. Biochem Biophys Res Commun 8, 284:317–325

76. Haruta M, Kosaka M, Kanegae Y, Saito I, Inoue T, Kageyama R, Nishida A, Honda Y, Takahashi M (2001) Induction of photoreceptor-specific phenotypes in adult mammalian iris tissue. Nat Neurosci 4:1163–1164

77. Sakaguchi DS, Janick LM, Reh TA (1997) Basic fibroblast growth factor (FGF-2) induced transdifferentiation of retinal pigment epithelium: generation of retinal neurons and glia. Dev Dyn 209:387–398

78. Mezey E, Key S, Vogelsang G, Szalayova I, Lange GD, Crain B (2003) Transplanted bone marrow generates new neurons in human brains. Proc Natl Acad Sci USA 100:1364–1369

79. Castro RF, Jackson KA, Goodell MA, Robertson CS, Liu H, Shine HD (2002) Failure of bone marrow cells to transdifferentiate into neural cells in vivo. Science 297:1299

80. Otani A, Dorrell MI, Kinder K, Moreno SK, Nusinowitz S, Banin E, Heckenlively J, Friedlander M (2004) Rescue of retinal degeneration by intravitreally injected adult bone marrow-derived lineage-negative hematopoietic stem cells. J Clin Invest 114:765–774

81. Klyushnenkova E, Mosca JD, Zernetkina V, Majumdar MK, Beggs KJ, Simonetti DW, Deans RJ, McIntosh KR (2005) T cell responses to allogeneic human mesenchymal stem cells: immunogenicity, tolerance, and suppression. J Biomed Sci 12:47–57

82. Poncelet AJ, Vercruysse J, Saliez A, Gianello P (2007) Although pig allogeneic mesenchymal stem cells are not immunogenic in vitro, intracardiac injection elicits an immune response in vivo. Transplantation 83:783–790

83. Okita K, Ichisaka T, Yamanaka S (2007) Generation of germline-competent induced pluripotent stem cells. Nature 448:313–317

84. Wernig M, Meissner A, Foreman R, Brambrink T, Ku M, Hochedlinger K, Bernstein BE, Jaenisch R (2007) In vitro reprogramming of fibroblasts into a pluripotent ES-cell-like state. Nature 448:318–324

Chapter 3
Negative Regulation of Endogenous Stem Cells in Sensory Neuroepithelia: Implications for Neurotherapeutics

Jason A. Hamilton[1], Crestina L. Beites[1], Kimberly K. Gokoffski[2], Piper L. W. Hollenbeck[1], Shimako Kawauchi[1], Rosaseyla Santos[1], Alexandre Bonnin[3], Hsiao-Huei Wu[4], Joon Kim[5], and Anne L. Calof[1*]

Abstract Stem cell therapies to treat central nervous system (CNS) injuries and diseases face many obstacles, one of which is the fact that the adult CNS often presents an environment hostile to the development and differentiation of neural stem and progenitor cells. Close examination of two regions of the nervous system – the olfactory epithelium (OE), which regenerates, and the neural retina, which does not – have helped identify endogenous signals, made by differentiated neurons, which act to inhibit neurogenesis by stem/progenitor cells within these tissues. In this chapter, we provide background information on these systems and their neurogenic signaling systems, with the goal of providing insight into how manipulation of endogenous signaling molecules may enhance the efficacy of stem cell neurotherapeutics.

Keywords BMP, FGF, follistatin, GDF11, proneural genes, regeneration, Sox2

[1]Department of Anatomy and Neurobiology, 264 Med Surge II, University of California, Irvine College of Medicine, Irvine, CA 92697-1275, USA

[2]Department of Developmental and Cell Biology, 264 Med Surge II, University of California, Irvine College of Medicine, Irvine, CA 92697-1275, USA

[3]Department of Pharmacology, and the Kennedy Center for Research on Human Development, Vanderbilt University, 465 – 21st Avenue, South Nashville, TN 37232, USA

[4]Department of Biochemistry, Vanderbilt University Medical School, Nashville, TN 37232, USA

[5]Department of Neurosciences, University of California at San Diego, Leichtag 332, 9500, Gilman Drive, La Jolla, CA 92093, USA

*Corresponding Author:
Departments of Anatomy and Neurobiology, Developmental and Cell Biology, and Ophthalmology.
e-mail: alcalof@uci.edu

Y. Shi, D.O. Clegg (eds.) *Stem Cell Research and Therapeutics*,
© Springer Science + Business Media B.V. 2008

3.1 Introduction

Stem cells are increasingly viewed as viable sources of treatment for injured or diseased nervous system tissues, in which the mammalian capacity for regeneration of damaged tissue is severely limited. Great efforts have been made to understand the molecular signals regulating the growth and differentiation of neural stem cells during normal development in many model systems. Understanding the molecular signals that regulate endogenous stem cell populations will provide information that should eventually permit us to harness these signals and stimulate growth and regeneration of neural tissues from endogenous stem cell pools. In addition, such information will permit us to utilize appropriate molecular tools for production of specialized neural cell types in vitro for use in transplantation-based therapies.

3.2 Olfactory Epithelium as a Model System for Understanding Molecular Regulation of Endogenous Neural Stem Cells

The adult mammalian central nervous system (CNS), relative to other tissues, possesses a severely limited cohort of stem cells. Following development, basal stem cell activity is low, suggesting that stem cells are under tight negative regulation. This regulation, which likely keeps stem cells in a "locked" or dormant state, is in part responsible for the poor regeneration seen in injured or diseased CNS. Currently, only three mammalian CNS stem cell niches are known to persist into adulthood: the subventricular zone (SVZ) of the lateral ventricle, the subgranular layer (SGL) of the dentate gyrus, and the olfactory epithelium (OE) [reviewed in 1, 2].

The OE is unique amongst mammalian neurogenic tissues: it continually generates neurons throughout life, making it an attractive model system for studying not only neurogenesis, but neural regeneration as well. OE neurogenesis is tightly regulated to allow for regeneration when many or most neurons are lost, but also to prevent abnormal overgrowth. It is possible that a similar regulatory mechanism may repress neurogenesis within non-regenerative neural tissues. An understanding of the molecular signals that permit ongoing OE neurogenesis and regulate regeneration should provide insight into how these same signals could be harnessed to promote regeneration of other brain regions following disease or injury.

3.2.1 Structure and Development of the Olfactory Epithelium

The posterodorsal region of the nasal cavity in mammals (Fig. 3.1A) is lined with an olfactory mucosa consisting of the olfactory epithelium (OE) and its underlying lamina propria [3–5]. OE development begins around gestational day 9 (E9) in mice, at which time bilateral thickenings of the surface ectoderm, called the olfactory placodes (OPs), are first evident. The OP invaginates to form the olfactory pit, and over time the epithelium thickens and comes to consist of three major cellular compartments: (1) apical, (2) basal, and (3) intermediate or middle (Fig. 3.1B). The apical layer is adjacent to the nasal cavity, and is comprised of a single layer of supporting or sustentacular (SUS) cells. These cells extend their endfeet to the basal lamina (BL) and, like glia of the CNS, provide architectural support to growing neurons [6, 7]. Atop the BL lies the basal compartment, which contains a single layer of horizontal basal cells (HBCs) and one to two layers of globose basal cells (GBCs). HBCs are situated closest to the BL and express keratin intermediate filaments [8]. Although HBCs do not appear to be part of the OE neuronal lineage during development, severe induced damage to the OE has been shown to stimulate this population to repopulate the OE, at least partially [9–11]. GBCs lie directly above the HBCs. GBCs are actually a mixed cell population, which has been shown to contain the stem/progenitor cell types that give rise to olfactory receptor neurons (ORNs) in vivo [12–15]. Between sustentacular and progenitor cells sit four to five layers of ORNs, the sensory neurons of the OE. The axons of ORNs project subjacent to the epithelium into the lamina propria, through the cribriform plate of the ethmoid bone, directly into the CNS, where they synapse on neurons of the main olfactory bulb (Fig. 3.1A). An additional olfactory sensory epithelium, the vomeronasal organ (VNO), lies within the septum ventral to main OE (Fig. 3.1A). The VNO detects pheromonal chemical signals that influence mating and social behavior. Afferent axons of vomeronasal neurons connect to the accessory olfactory bulb.

Studies by us and others have shown that ORNs are generated via a lineage consisting of three distinct proliferating cell types identified by specific markers (Fig. 3.1C). (1) The *neural stem cell*, which expresses *Sox2*, a SRY-family transcription factor expressed by many stem cells including embryonic stem cells and many neuroepithelial cells, is the first cell in the lineage [1, 16–21]. *Sox2*-expressing stem cells give rise to (2) *committed progenitor cells* that express *Mash1* (*Ascl1*), a proneural gene that encodes a basic helix-loop-helix transcription factor required for ORN development [22–24]. *Mash1*-expressing neuronal progenitors give rise to (3) *immediate neuronal precursors* (INPs), which expresses the proneural gene *Neurogenin1* (*Ngn1*) and give rise to daughter cells that undergo terminal differentiation into ORNs (Fig. 3.1C) [1, 8]. ORNs, which are the odor signal-transducing neurons of the OE, reside within the middle compartment, sandwiched between the apical and basal cell layers. ORNs extend cilia into the nasal cavity and axons into the CNS (Fig. 3.1). All postmitotic ORNs can be identified by their expression of the neural cell adhesion molecule, NCAM [8].

3.2.2   FGF8 Expression Defines Primordial Neural Stem Cells During Early OE Development

These three cell types are evident from the earliest stages of OE development [22, 25]. Expression patterns from in situ hybridization studies indicate that, at the

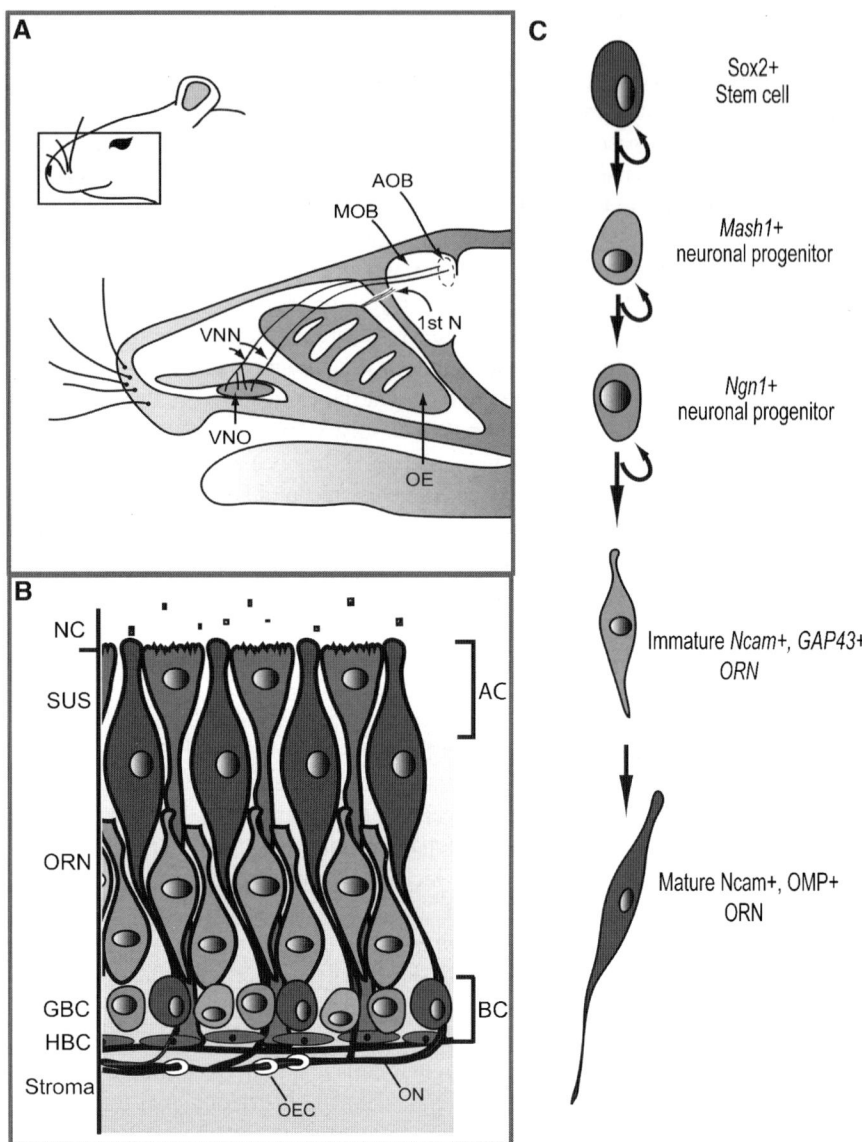

Fig. 3.1 Schematic drawings of olfactory structures and relevant developmental cell types. (**A**) Sagittal view of the nasal cavity and rostral forebrain of a mouse. The olfactory epithelium (OE) lines the nasal cavity and contains olfactory receptor neurons (ORNs), which project through the cribriform plate to glomeruli in the main olfactory bulb (MOB) within the central nervous system. Pheromone-detecting vomeronasal neurons (VNN) of the vomeronasal organ (VNO) project to the accessory olfactory bulb (AOB). (**B**) Diagram of the OE showing relative positions of cell types. From apical to basal, these include sustentacular cells (SUS; green), ORNs, and globose and horizontal basal cells (GBC; HBC). The GBCs consist of three types of neuronal progenitors: *Sox2*-expressing neuronal stem cells, *Mash1*-expressing transit amplifying progenitors, and *Ngn1*-expressing INPs. (**C**) Schematic of the neuronal differentiation pathway of OE neuronal progenitor cells. *Sox2*-expressing neuronal stem cells give rise to transit amplifying progenitors expressing *Mash1*, which produce *Ngn1*-expressing immediate neuronal precursors (INPs). INP division produces daughter cells that differentiate into immature ORNs, identified by NCAM immunoreactivity. Immature ORNs eventually mature and express NCAM and olfactory marker protein (OMP) (*See Color Plates*)

early olfactory pit stage, stem and progenitor cell types of the OE are arranged in a concentric, outside-in pattern that reflects the developmental stage of each cell type in the OE lineage (Fig. 3.2). At this stage of development, the outer margin of the invaginating nasal pit (NP) is also marked by expression of an important regulatory signaling molecule of the fibroblast growth factor (FGF) superfamily, FGF8 (Fig. 3.2A, B) [25]. Closest to the *Fgf8*-expressing cells at the inner rim of the invaginating olfactory pit are cells expressing *Mash1*, the earliest committed neuronal progenitors of the OE. Further in toward the center of the pit are the *Ngn1*-expressing INPs; and at the center are *Ncam1*-expressing ORNs (Fig. 3.2A). *Sox2* is expressed throughout the entire neuroepithelium of the invaginating NP, and defines the OE at this early stage. Dual in situ hybridization experiments demonstrate that many of the *Fgf8*-expressing cells at the rim of the invaginating NP also express *Sox2* (Fig. 3.2B), as well as the definitive early OE markers *Pax6* and *Dlx5* [25]. This observation, combined with the fact that apoptosis of this cell population subsequent to loss of *Fgf8* leads to termination of OE neurogenesis and nasal cavity morphogenesis, has led to the view that these early *Sox2/Fgf8*-expressing cells are the primordial neural stem cells of the OE (Fig. 3.2C) [25].

3.3 Molecular Regulation of OE Neurogenesis In Vitro

3.3.1 *FGFs Promote OE Progenitor Cell Divisions*

An ongoing question for neuronal regeneration therapies has been whether most neurogenic niches fail to persist due to neurogenesis-repressive factors, or due to loss of neurogenesis-stimulating factors. Experimental manipulations that selectively ablate ORNs in adult rodents have provided evidence of increased mitotic activity by neuronal progenitors after ORN degeneration; these progenitors re-populate the OE with new ORNs. Interestingly, progenitor cell mitotic activity is re-regulated to low rates once the epithelium recovers, suggesting that progenitors are under tight negative regulation coming from the ORNs themselves [13, 15, 26–28]. Initial attempts using tissue culture methods to identify the molecular signals that regulate these events led to the discovery that the persistent neurogenesis observed in intact OE in vivo is extinguished when the tissue is moved to the culture dish. Specifically, OE progenitor cells were found to undergo terminal division in culture, producing almost exclusively ORNs, and no new progenitor cells [8]. This switch from persistent neurogenesis in vivo to terminal neurogenesis in vitro suggested the loss of a supporting signal or factor present in the surrounding environment of the epithelium. Furthermore, the similarity of this phenomenon to the observation that most other neurogenic niches switch from persistent to terminal neurogenesis around the time of birth, suggested that understanding the signals that maintain the OE's capacity for neurogenesis might shed light on why neurogenesis

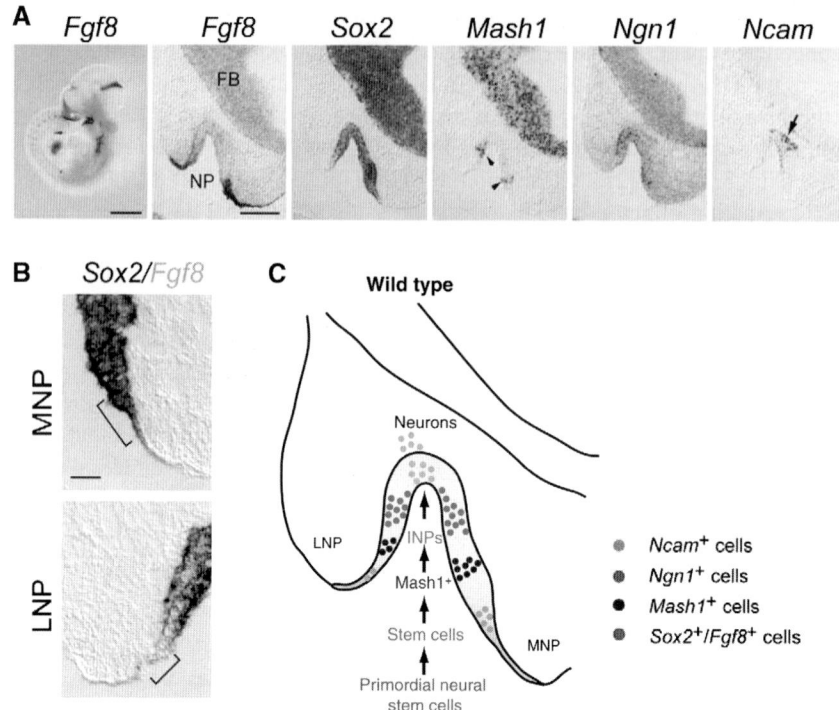

Fig. 3.2 Expression of *Fgf8* and neuronal cell markers in developing OE. (**A**) Six successive images show in situ hybridizations for *Fgf8* (full-length ORF probe) and OE neuronal lineage markers in invaginating nasal pit (NP) at E10.5. In whole-mount in situ hybridization (left-most image), *Fgf8* is detected in commissural plate and olfactory placode, branchial arches, mid-hindbrain junction, and limb and tail buds (Scale bar, 1 mm). In serial sections, locations of neuronal lineage markers within the OE are shown: arrowheads indicate *Mash1*-expressing cells, arrow indicates *Ncam1*-expressing neurons (Scale bar, 200 μm). (**B**) Double label in situ hybridization for *Fgf8* (full-length ORF probe, orange) and *Sox2* (blue) demonstrates overlap of the two markers in a small rim of surface ectoderm and adjacent invaginating neuroepithelium (brackets) (Scale bar, 50 μm). (**C**) Model of peripheral-to-central process of neuronal differentiation in developing OE and origin of *Sox2*-expressing neural stem cells from *Fgf8*-expressing ectoderm. LNP, lateral nasal pit; MNP, medial nasal pit (Adapted from [25]; reprinted courtesy of Development) (*See Color Plates*)

in most of the mammalian nervous system does not persist throughout life. Several molecular signals responsible for promoting neurogenesis in OE have now been identified through tissue culture studies.

FGFs were the first neurogenesis-promoting factors to be identified in OE cultures. When explants of OE purified from late-gestation mouse fetuses were cultured in the presence or absence of different candidate growth factors that were known or suspected to influence proliferation of glial and/or neuronal precursors, all members of the FGF family that were tested (FGF1, -2, -4, -7, and -8) resulted in increased S-phase (^{3}H-thymidine incorporation) labeling indices compared to untreated controls.

Detailed analysis demonstrated that FGFs act to increase the number of divisions through which INPs can progress, prior to terminal differentiation. All INPs – regardless of the number of divisions they have completed – ultimately undergo terminal differentiation to become NCAM-expressing ORNs. This indicates that INPs act as transit amplifying progenitors in the ORN lineage [1, 29, 30].

3.3.2 Stromal Cells Are Required for Proliferation and Neuronal Differentiation of OE Stem Cells In Vitro

The support of OE neurogenesis in vitro through addition of exogenous FGFs suggests that FGFs, or factors with similar action, may be produced by cells or tissues surrounding the OE to support OE neurogenesis in vivo. Identification of such factors could be vital for clinical efforts aimed at stimulating neuronal regeneration from endogenous populations of stem/progenitor cells. The experiments detailed below have shown that olfactory stromal cells secrete factor(s) capable of supporting OE neurogenesis in vitro.

An interesting finding from the series of experiments that tested actions of FGFs on OE neurogenesis in vitro was the observation that there is a rare population of progenitors within the OE that undergoes continual cell division in vitro, but only in the presence of FGFs [13, 29]. Importantly, these cells are capable of producing ORNs, confirming that they are neuronal progenitors. However, both the rarity of these cells, and their capacity for prolonged division in the presence of FGFs, suggested that they represent an early stem or progenitor cell of the OE, possibly the cell population that underlies the persistent neurogenesis observed within the OE in vivo.

To facilitate examination of potential OE neural stem cells, a more direct approach was developed to isolate and culture them [31]. This procedure, called the neuronal colony-forming assay, is illustrated in Fig. 3.3. Immunological panning of a dissociated neuronal cell fraction of OE explants was performed using anti-NCAM-treated Petri dishes (in order to remove postmitotic ORNs), generating a relatively pure (>96%) population of NCAM$^-$ ORN progenitors [27, 31, 32]. Survival of purified neuronal progenitors was dependent on them being cultured over monolayers of feeder cells harvested from the stroma that normally underlies the OE in vivo. Over approximately 1 week in culture, a small fraction of these purified progenitor cells (approximately 1 in 1,000) continued to produce small colonies of cells that contain both proliferating progenitors and differentiated, NCAM-expressing ORNs [31]. Thus, neural stem cells of the OE can be cultured for relatively long periods in vitro, and can produce differentiated ORNs, but their survival and production of downstream progenitors is dependent upon factors present in the OE microenvironment in vivo (i.e. stromal cells) [33–35]. Moreover, using this colony-forming assay, it has been possible to quantify effects of many different signaling molecules on OE neurogenesis in vitro, and then to move on to test the roles for these molecules in vivo.

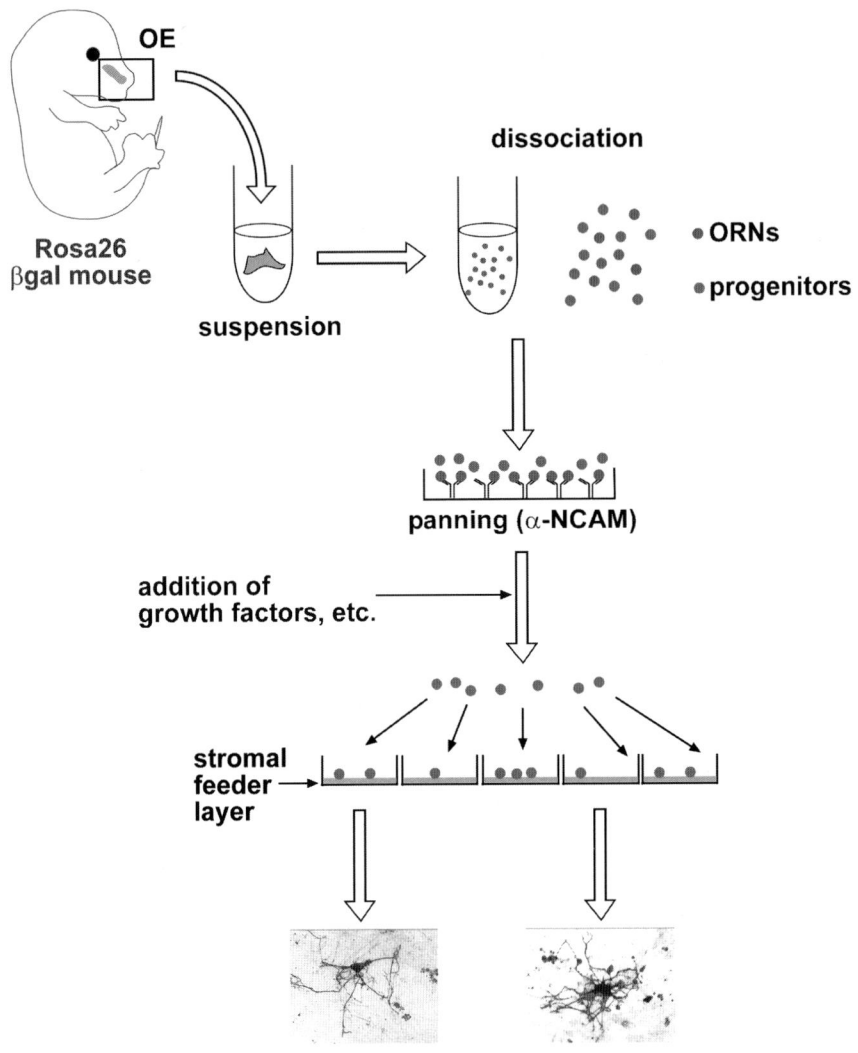

Fig. 3.3 Anti-NCAM immunological panning results in pure population of OE neuronal progenitor cells. OE neuronal cell fractions were resuspended in culture medium and incubated on panning plates for 30 minutes at room temperature in the dark, with intermittent agitation. Panning plates were prepared by coating 100-mm Petri dishes with purified culture supernatant from H28 rat anti-NCAM hybridoma cells. After 30 minutes of immunological panning, cells remaining in suspension were collected, centrifuged, resuspended in culture medium, and plated at various densities on stromal cell feeder layers. The resulting population consists of >96% pure neuronal progenitor cells (*See Color Plates*)

3.3.3 Excess ORNs Inhibit Neurogenesis by Purified OE Stem/Progenitor Cells

In healthy OE, the epithelium undergoes low rates of proliferation and differentiation to replace loss of ORNs due to normal environmental insult (virus, noxious fumes, etc.). However, when the OE sustains massive levels of ORN death by chemical, pharmacological, or surgical (olfactory bulbectomy) manipulation, or naturally through exposure to toxins, progenitor cells respond with a large burst of proliferation [11, 13, 15]. The proliferating progenitor cells generate new ORNs until the OE returns to approximately 70% of its original thickness, after which proliferation rates return to nearly pre-lesioning levels [13, 15, 27]. Over time, the recovering OE regains its correct odorant receptor expression patterns [28]. These experiments demonstrate multiple distinct features of OE neurogenesis in vivo. First, neurogenesis is maintained at a low level, or even repressed, during normal "healthy" conditions. Second, OE neurogenesis is stimulated, or de-repressed, immediately following ORN cell death. Third, as the OE is repopulated with new ORNs, stimulation of neurogenesis ceases, or repression is re-instated. These features of experimentally-induced neurogenesis suggest that when ORN death occurs, (1) a neurogenesis-stimulating factor is expressed or released, or (2) a neurogenesis-repressing factor is lost or decreased. Similarly, when ORNs are regenerated, (1) the neurogenesis-stimulating factor is lost, or (2) the neurogenesis-repressing factor is reinstated.

To determine whether ORNs secrete a factor that has downstream effects on neurogenesis, purified OE stem/progenitor cells were cultured in the presence of excess ORNs. This resulted in a significant *decrease* in the level of neurogenesis [31], clearly indicating that ORNs provide negative feedback to OE progenitor cells through some neurogenesis-repressing factor(s). Interestingly, neurogenesis in these assays is not inhibited by a similar excess of OE stromal cells, suggesting that the repressive factor is specifically produced by differentiated ORNs [31].

3.3.4 Negative Regulation of OE Neurogenesis In Vitro by BMPs

The inhibitory effect of differentiated ORNs on neurogenesis suggests the secretion, by ORNs, of a neurogenesis-inhibiting factor that acts upon the neural stem/progenitor cells that underlie ORNs in the OE in vivo (Fig. 3.1B). Identification of such inhibitory factors could contribute to development of regenerative therapeutic efforts, since removing or antagonizing such factors could significantly increase the efficacy of regenerative therapies.

Bone morphogenetic proteins (BMPs), the largest group of ligands in the TGF-β superfamily, were initially investigated as candidates for molecules that act as negative regulators of OE neurogenesis, for several reasons: BMPs and their receptors are expressed in appropriate regions of the embryonic OE and/or olfactory placode to play a role in regulating OE neurogenesis [36–39]. Furthermore, studies indicate that in other neurogenic niches, BMPs seem to function as neurogenesis-inhibiting signals from the earliest stages of neural development [40–44].

In initial investigations of BMPs, neuronal colony-forming assays were performed in which purified OE neuronal stem/progenitor cells were cultured on stromal feeder layers in the presence or absence of BMPs. BMP4 addition at the time of progenitor cell plating resulted in inhibition of neuronal colony formation [45]. Interestingly, both BMP2, a close relative of BMP4 [46]; and BMP7, a more distantly-related BMP; had equally inhibitory effects [45]. These findings suggest an important role for all three BMP family members in neurogenesis.

To determine whether BMPs act specifically on proliferation of certain progenitor cell types, OE explant cultures were used: progenitor cells proliferate and can be identified easily in such cultures [8, 13, 29]. These studies demonstrated that addition of BMP4 to cultures caused a dramatic reduction in ^{3}H-TdR incorporation by neuronal progenitors, compared to control (untreated) cultures (Fig. 3.4A) [45]. Further experiments showed that this reduction in cell proliferation was due to a failure in development of MASH1$^+$ neuronal progenitors (Fig. 3.4B). This reduction in MASH1$^+$ cells in the explant cultures was not due to cell death (as no increase in apoptosis could be found), but by the stimulation of rapid, proteasome-mediated degradation of existing MASH1 protein [45]. This in turn resulted in a cessation of division by MASH1-expressing progenitors, and subsequent failure of the entire neuronal lineage downstream of the MASH1-expressing cell stage [45].

Interestingly, recent work by others has substantiated and extended these findings. The multiple zinc finger transcription factor *Zfp423/OAZ* (*O/E* associated zinc finger

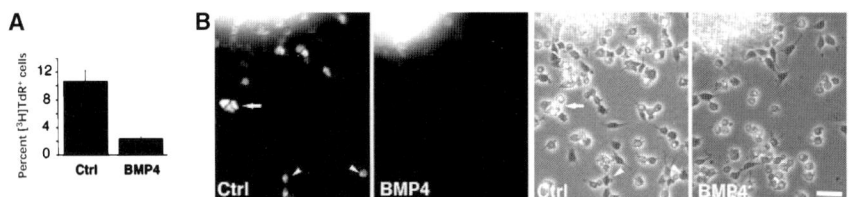

Fig. 3.4 Effects of BMP4 on OE neuronal progenitor cells and ORNs. (**A**) OE explants were cultured for a total of 20 hours in the presence or absence of BMP4 (10 ng/ml), with 1.5 μCi/ml ^{3}H-TdR added for the final 6 hours. The percentage of cells that were ^{3}H-TdR-positive ([^{3}H]TdR$^+$) was determined as the fraction of total migratory cells surrounding each explant that had > five silver grains over the nucleus. Approximately 5,000 migratory cells were counted in each condition. Data are plotted as mean ± s.e. (**B**) Fluorescence and phase-contrast photomicrographs of explant cultures grown for a total of 8 hours in vitro, with or without BMP4 (20 ng/ml) added for the final 2 hours. In control conditions (Ctrl), arrow indicates a cluster of migratory neuronal progenitor cells expressing MASH1; arrowheads indicate examples of individual MASH1-positive cells. In BMP4 (BMP4), no cells have detectable MASH1 immunofluorescence (Scale, 20 μm) (Adapted from [35, 45]; reprinted courtesy of Nature Neuroscience and Development)

protein) has been shown to be a key regulator of ORN maturation that functions downstream of *Mash1* [47]. Examination of $OAZ^{-/-}$ mice showed that OAZ disruption does not affect OE progenitor proliferation, but leads to decreased mature ORNs, impaired axonal targeting and increased apoptosis. Importantly, reintroduction of *OAZ* expression within the mature neuronal layer was sufficient to induce an immature ORN phenotype [47]. OAZ has also been identified as a cofactor of Smad proteins in BMP-signaling [48–50], suggesting that OAZ may play a critical role in integrating extracellular BMP signaling and intracellular transcription factor expression at various stages of ORN differentiation.

3.3.5 Low Concentrations of BMPs Can Promote the Generation of ORNs In Vitro

As discussed above, both administration of BMPs, and addition of excess ORNs, lead to decreased OE neurogenesis in culture. The detection of *Bmp4* and *Bmp7* mRNAs within the OE supports the possibility that BMPs might contribute to the neurogenesis-repressing effect of excess ORNs in culture [35]. Such an effect could have important implications for regenerative therapeutic efforts. If ORNs repress neurogenesis in culture by secreting BMPs, then antagonizing BMP activity by adding secreted protein antagonists, such as noggin [51], to the culture medium should remove the repression of neurogenesis and restore the number of neuronal colonies formed. Surprisingly, addition of noggin alone had a strong inhibitory effect on neurogenesis in neuronal colony-forming assays, even in the absence of any excess ORNs or added BMPs (Fig. 3.5) [35]. Because noggin does not itself signal, but rather binds to and inhibits BMPs from signaling [51, 52], these results suggested that one or more endogenous BMPs (already produced within the neuronal colony-forming assay cultures) promotes neurogenesis. The detection of *Bmp2*, *Bmp4*, and *Bmp7* mRNAs within OE stromal cells supports the possibility that BMPs secreted by stromal cells may support neurogenesis within the OE [35]. In fact, previous experiments had determined that the survival of purified neuronal progenitors depends on factors released from the stromal feeder layer on which they are cultured, since absence of this feeder layer results in stem and progenitor cell death [31].

To determine whether BMPs are responsible for the support of neuronal colony formation provided by stromal cell co-cultures, colony-forming assay cultures were supplemented with conditioned medium from pure stromal cell cultures that had either been (1) pre-cleared of any BMPs using beads coated with recombinant noggin (if any BMPs are responsible for the stimulatory effect of stromal cell conditioned medium, then pre-clearing BMPs from the medium with conjugated noggin should abolish that effect); or (2) control "mock-depleted" (i.e. the medium would still contain any BMPs present, and should still stimulate neurogenesis) conditioned medium. As expected, mock-depleted conditioned medium produced a significant

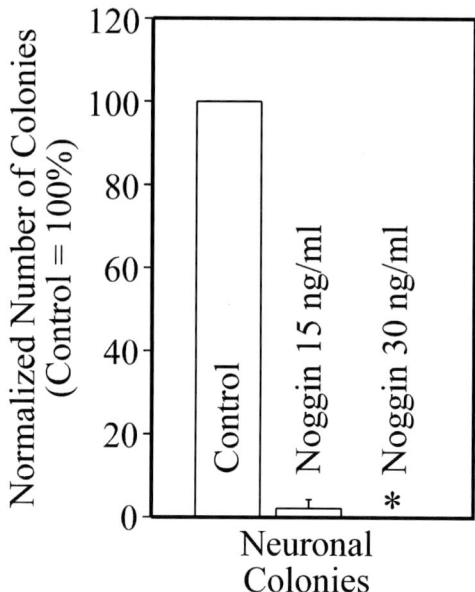

Fig. 3.5 Inhibition of neuronal colony formation by noggin. Numbers of neuronal colonies were normalized to the control (no noggin added) value in a given experiment. These values were expressed as the mean for two independent experiments in a given condition (± range). Asterisk indicates that no neuronal colonies were observed when cultures were treated with 30 ng/ml noggin (Adapted from [35]; reprinted courtesy of Development)

increase in neuronal colony formation when added to colony-forming assays. When noggin-depleted conditioned medium was tested on colony-forming assays, it produced a significantly smaller increase in neuronal colony formation. These findings demonstrated that a portion of the neurogenesis-stimulating signal from stromal cells must derive from BMPs.

3.3.6 Concentration-Dependent Effects of BMPs on Neurogenesis

BMPs have been found previously to produce stimulatory effects on neurogenesis in systems other than OE [40, 43, 53–59]. Interestingly, a detailed study of BMP effects on OE cultures found certain BMPs to be capable of stimulating neurogenesis in OE cultures, when given at very low concentrations. For example, BMP4 produced a significant increase in neuronal colony formation when added to cultures at a concentration of 0.1 ng/ml, indicating that BMP4 can produce opposing, concentration-dependent effects upon OE neurogenesis (promoting at low concentrations; inhibiting at higher concentrations) [35].

How do low levels of BMP4 act to stimulate neurogenesis in neuronal colony-forming assays? The simplest explanation would be that BMP4 stimulates proliferation of OE neuronal progenitors, but this has not been substantiated despite numerous attempts and approaches. Interestingly, it was noted that treatment with 0.1 ng/ml BMP4 improved the appearance of explants, producing more healthy-looking ORNs (Fig. 3.6). Further experiments, using pulse-chase ^{3}H-TdR incorporation paradigms, demonstrated that whereas untreated explant cultures contain very few newly-differentiated NCAM$^+$ ORNs after 4 days in vitro (DIV) [27], cultures treated with low concentrations of BMP4 maintain their ORN population (Fig. 3.6), indicating that BMP4 *promotes the survival* of ORNs at low (Fig. 3.6) but not high (Fig. 3.4) concentrations [35].

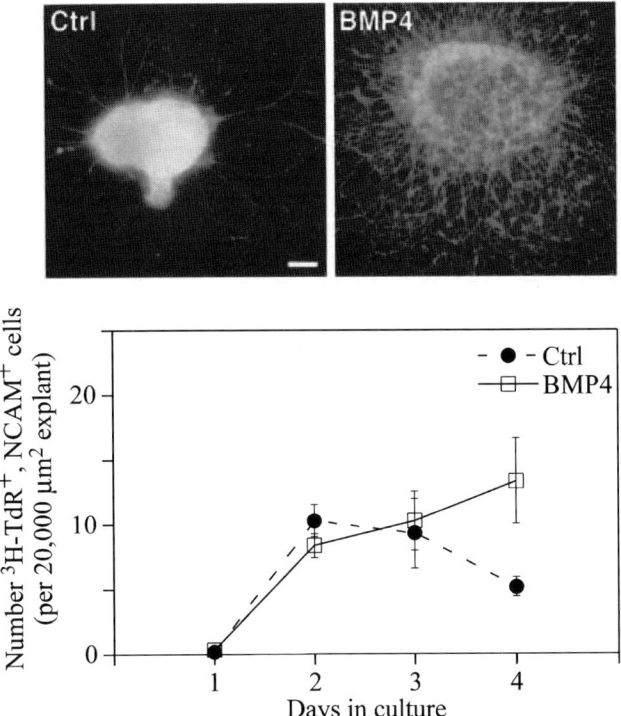

Fig. 3.6 Low-dose BMP4 has a direct effect on olfactory neurogenesis. OE explants were cultured for a total of 96 hours in the presence or absence of 0.1 ng/ml BMP4, and cultures fixed and processed for NCAM immunoreactivity. Fluorescence photomicrographs of OE explants in the two conditions, showing increased numbers of NCAM-positive ORNs surrounding the explant in the presence of BMP4 (Scale bar, 50 μm). Low-dose BMP4 also promotes survival of newly-generated ORNs, quantified from OE explant cultures treated with both BMP4 (0.1 ng/ml) and ^{3}H-TdR. A significant difference in the number of surviving ORNs was observed between control and BMP4-treated cultures after 4 days in vitro (P = 0.02, Student's t-test) (From [45]; reprinted courtesy of Nature Neuroscience) (*See Color Plates*)

3.4   Negative Regulation of Neurogenesis In Vivo and In Vitro

Over 40 years ago, Bullough put forward the hypothesis that tissues produce growth-inhibitory signals, the local concentrations of which directly reflect the mass of the tissue in which they are produced [60]. Such signals were hypothesized to halt cell proliferation when appropriate tissue size had been reached, thereby maintaining cell number appropriate for a tissue's function. Identification of growth and differentiation factor 8 (GDF8)/myostatin, a signaling molecule of the activin/ TGF-β group of the TGF-β superfamily, as an endogenous negative regulator of skeletal muscle development [61, 62]; and growth and differentiation factor 11 (GDF11), a TGF-β closely related in structure to GDF8, as an endogenous negative regulator of neurogenesis in OE [63]; have validated this idea [64]. Indeed, we have found that such feedback inhibition of neurogenesis is important for maintaining neuron number in two different sensory neuroepithelia in mice: the OE and the neural retina [63, 65].

3.4.1   Negative Autoregulation of OE Neurogenesis

Other endogenous factors also contribute to the regulation of OE neurogenesis. Members of both the FGF and TGF-β superfamilies have recently been shown to be expressed in relevant areas of the OE to regulate neurogenesis during development. GDF11, a recently-identified member of the TGF-β superfamily, is expressed in mouse OE beginning at E10.5, and its expression continues through development and into adulthood [18, 63]. Because the closely-related GDF8/myostatin had been shown previously to inhibit the proliferation of muscle progenitor cells [61, 66–68], it was hypothesized that GDF11 might serve a similar role within the OE. Detailed analysis of GDF11 expression showed that *Gdf11* mRNA within the nasal mucosa was confined to the OE proper, with no expression in adjacent respiratory epithelium or underlying stroma. Within the developing OE, *Gdf11* expression is confined to the basal portion of the OE where immature ORNs and their progenitors are localized (Fig. 3.1). Interestingly, the soluble GDF11 signaling antagonist *Follistatin (Fst)* was also found to be expressed throughout the developing OE, as well as the underlying stroma [63]. Examination of *Gdf11* mRNA within the OE of *Mash1*$^{-/-}$ mice (in which INPs and ORNs are absent) found that *Gdf11* expression is essentially lost in the absence of *Mash1* (Fig. 3.7) [63]. Because the OE of *Mash1*$^{-/-}$ mice becomes populated by sustentacular cells and stem cells, but is devoid of ORNs and INPs, *Gdf11* must be expressed by either ORNs themselves or the INPs that are also lost in *Mash1*$^{-/-}$ mice [69].

Does GDF11 affect OE progenitor cell proliferation or survival? Using similar in vitro assays to those described previously, GDF11 was found to inhibit proliferation of OE neuronal progenitor cells, as assayed by ^{3}H-TdR incorporation. Interestingly, GDF11 had no effect on MASH1 expression, nor did it inhibit the

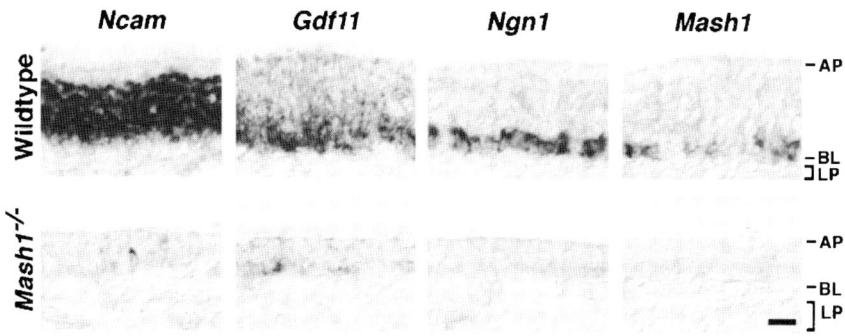

Fig. 3.7 *Gdf11* is expressed by ORNs and their progenitors. OE from E17.5 *Mash1*⁻/⁻ embryos and wild-type littermate was hybridized with probes to *Ncam*, *Gdf11*, *Ngn1*, and *Mash1*. In *Mash1*⁻/⁻ mice the ORN lineage is cut short at an early stage, as *Mash1*-expressing neuronal progenitors initially form, but then undergo apoptosis. Thus, the OE of *Mash1*⁻/⁻ mice is markedly thinner than that of wild-types, and expression of *Ngn1* and *Ncam* is drastically reduced since the epithelium lacks most ORNs and ORN progenitors. *Gdf11* expression is also essentially absent. Since sustentacular cells and horizontal basal cells are still present in *Mash1*⁻/⁻ mice, this indicates that the cells that normally express *Gdf11* must be ORNs and ORN progenitors (Scale, 20 μm; AP, apical surface; BL, basal lamina; LP, lamina propria) (From [63]; reprinted courtesy of Neuron) (*See Color Plates*)

proliferation of *Mash1*-expressing progenitor cells [63], as was found previously for BMP4 [45]. If GDF11 decreases progenitor proliferation in OE explant cultures, but is not acting on MASH1-expressing progenitor cells, then its next most likely site of action is upon the progeny of MASH1-expressing cells – the INPs. Previous studies [29, 35] found that INP proliferation is stimulated by FGF2 treatment. Addition of both FGF2 and GDF11 completely abolished INP proliferation, suggesting that the stimulatory effect of FGF2 on INP proliferation is abrogated by GDF11's effects. GDF11 does not affect INP cell survival, but the increase in expression of the cyclin-dependent kinase inhibitor p27^{Kip1} in these cultures suggests that GDF11 halts INP progression through the cell cycle [63].

Is GDF11 the endogenous factor responsible for feedback inhibition of OE neurogenesis in vivo? To answer this question, we performed genetic experiments in which mice, homozygous for a null allele of *Gdf11*, were analyzed for OE neurogenesis [63]. These genetic experiments confirmed the in vitro results: examination of BrdU incorporation in *Gdf11*-null mice showed significantly higher numbers of BrdU ⁺ cells within the developing OE compared to wild-type animals, reflecting increased OE neurogenesis in the absence of the antineurogenic activity of GDF11. Furthermore, significantly *decreased* numbers of BrdU ⁺ cells were observed within the OE of *Fst*-null mice compared to wild-types, reflecting the increase in GDF11 activity resulting from absence of its endogenous antagonist [63]. Interestingly, *Ngn1* expression within the OE was significantly increased in *Gdf11*-null mice, reflecting increased production of INPs in the absence of GDF11 activity. *Mash1* expression, which marks the progenitor cells that precede INPs within the OE lineage, were unaffected in *Gdf11*-null mice, further supporting the idea that GDF11 acts specifically upon INPs, and not on earlier cell types within the OE lineage [63].

3.4.2 Regulation of Progenitor Cell Competence by GDF11 in Neural Retina

The OE differs from most other mammalian neurogenic tissues in its ability to continually regenerate throughout life. The discovery that GDF11 signaling provides negative autoregulation of OE neurogenesis to allow regeneration, but prevent overgrowth, suggests that a similar signaling mechanism may actively repress neurogenesis within neural tissues considered to be non-regenerative. If this is the case, repressing GDF11 action may unlock a tissue's regenerative potential. Interestingly, both GDF11 and FST are expressed in various areas of the CNS [65, 70–72], such as the dentate gyrus of the hippocampus, the external granule layer of the cerebellum, and the retina. Specifically, recent investigation of the development of the neural retina (considered to be a non-regenerative sensory epithelium) has provided evidence that GDF11/FST signaling plays a unique and important role in the regulation of neural retinal neurogenesis during development [65].

Whereas the ORNs of the OE develop through sequential progression of the OE neural stem cell through various progenitor states, the mammalian retina consists of seven distinct neural cell types, which are all derived from one population of multipotent retinal progenitors [73, 74]. These cells are generated at various stages of retinal development, as the progenitor cells pass through a stereotyped pattern of "competence states" [75–77]. Nearly all retinal cell types are generated prenatally, and retinal neurogenesis in mice ceases completely during the first 2 weeks of life. The production of the various cell types of the retina is controlled by specific expression patterns of various homeobox and basic helix-loop-helix (bHLH) transcription factors [reviewed in 78]. However, the mechanisms governing the expression of these proneural genes are poorly understood.

The identification of GDF11 as a negative regulator of OE neurogenesis [63], and its expression within the developing retina [71], suggested that it might play a role in the regulation of retinal neurogenesis. The *Gdf11* transcript is first expressed in the retina around E12.5 in mice (Fig. 3.8A), when retinal ganglion cells (RGCs) first begin to differentiate [65]. It is expressed throughout the retina, with highest expression in the ganglion cell layer at E15.5, and continues after birth. *Fst* is first detected at E13.5, and similarly exhibits its highest expression within the ganglion cell layer from E15.5 on (Fig. 3.8A). Interestingly, mutant retinas from *Gdf11*-null mice showed obvious morphologic abnormalities, characterized by abnormally high cell density within the ganglion cell layer, and complete lack of the inner plexiform layer (Fig. 3.8B) [65]. Examination of cell marker expression showed expanded expression of the RGC marker *Brn3b*, suggesting that development of this particular cell type is affected in the absence of *Gdf11* (Fig. 3.8B). Furthermore, decreased expression of *Crx1* and *Prox1* transcripts indicated deficient production of early photoreceptors and amacrine cells, respectively [65].

The changes observed within the retinas of *Gdf11*-null animals are reminiscent of those observed within the OE, suggesting that GDF11 is a negative regulator of RGC neurogenesis. However, whereas the *Gdf11*-null OE exhibited significant changes in overall thickness, and in progenitor cell proliferation [63], the retina exhibited no change in overall thickness (Fig. 3.8C) or retinal progenitor proliferation [65]. Because proliferation appears unaffected, the temporal period of RGC genesis was examined via BrdU birthdating, and was found to be significantly expanded (in terms of BrdU-retaining cell number within RGC layer) in the *Gdf11*-null retina (Fig. 3.8C). Experiments using in vitro cultures have shown that GDF11 decreases production of RGCs and increases production of later born cell types: retinal explants cultured in the presence of exogenous GDF11 showed decreased expression of *Brn3b*, and increased expression of *Crx1*. Interestingly, although the RGC population is abnormally expanded in *Gdf11*-null retinas, RGCs appear to differentiate normally, extending axons through the optic chiasm and tracts, which are also abnormally thick (Fig. 3.8D). Neurofilament immunohistochemistry demonstrated an estimated 37% increase in cross-sectional areas of optic nerves in *Gdf11*-null animals compared to wild-types (Fig. 3.8E) [65]. Importantly, the ability of these cells to develop and extend axons along the correct path suggests that they likely can form appropriate connections, often a significant barrier to successful regeneration.

Because retinal progenitor cell proliferation is unchanged in *Gdf11*-null retinas, it appeared that GDF11 influences the competence state of retinal progenitors to produce specific cell types. It was hypothesized that if GDF11 can directly control progenitor cell competence, it might exert such changes through altered expression patterns of the transcription factors that determine competence state. One of the bHLH factors essential to RGC development is *Math5*: in the absence of *Math5* RGC production is severely reduced, and amacrine cell production is increased [79–81]. In *Gdf11*-null retinas, *Math5* expression begins normally, but remains high for an abnormally long period of development, corresponding to the period of prolonged RGC production [65]. The altered expression of *Math5* is accompanied by a delay in the onset of *Mash1* and *NeuroD1*, two transcription factors important for the development of bipolar and amacrine cells [82, 83]. Conversely, *Math5* is prematurely downregulated in *Fst*-null retinas, and *Mash1* expression was detected earlier [65].

3.5   Conclusions and Future Directions

The findings discussed above indicate that, during embryonic development, GDF11 expression within the retina regulates the timing of progenitor cell competence by controlling the expression of genes involved in progenitor cell fate determination (Fig. 3.9). Whereas GDF11 signaling within the OE regulates the production of ORNs through its actions on one specific cell within the OE progenitor cell lineage, its actions within the retina are more complex, affecting a number of cell types,

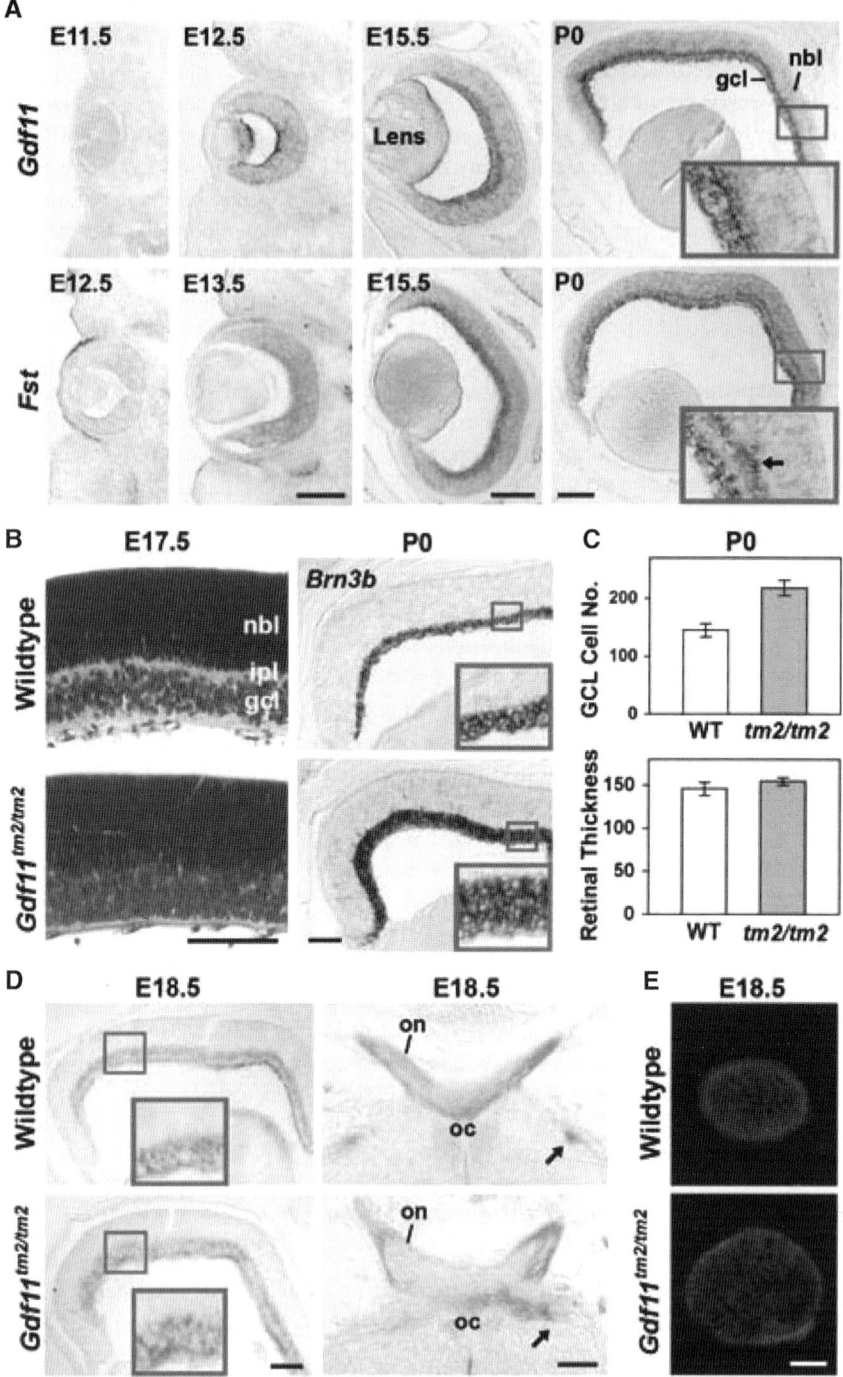

both positively and negatively, by influencing transcription factor expression. In so doing, GDF11 signaling regulates the numbers of specific retinal cell types required to produce a functioning retina. Could GDF11 signaling play a role in the early postnatal switch from continued proliferation of retinal progenitor cells to terminal differentiation? The perinatal lethality of *Gdf11*-null mice has not allowed us to answer this question. However, preliminary attempts at retina-specific disruption of *Fst* indicate that GDF11 signaling continues to play an important role in the regulation of progenitor cells in the postnatal retina [84]. Furthermore, the discovery of a population of retinal stem cells that remains dormant in the ciliary marginal zone well into adulthood [85] suggests the potential to induce endogenous retinal stem cells to divide and regenerate in damaged tissue. Finally, attempts to guide cultured stem or progenitor cells toward particular phenotypes for use in transplantation therapy [86, 87] will be greatly aided by better understanding the molecular signaling that controls the generation and specification of particular cell types. Future experiments aimed at modulation of GDF11 signaling within the retina, both through genetic and pharmacologic means, should provide significant insight into whether retinal stem and progenitor cells can be utilized within the postnatal eye to promote measurable recovery from debilitating injuries and diseases of the eye.

Interestingly, GDF11 has been reported to play a role in early development of a number of tissues, including pancreas [88], kidney [89, 90], muscle [91], bone [91], and spinal cord [92]. Within spinal cord, GDF11 contributes to neuronal subtype specification, similar to its role in retina [92]. GDF11 expression has also been shown to persist into adulthood in discrete regions of the CNS, such as the dentate gyrus of the hippocampus and the external granular layer of the cerebellum [63, 65]. Identifying the role of GDF11 signaling within these regions both during development and in adulthood could have critical implications for the study of neuronal regeneration within the cerebellum and hippocampus.

Current efforts at clinical therapies using stem or progenitor cells to treat neurodegenerative diseases fall under two major themes: (1) directing cultured stem cells to a neural fate and subsequently implanting the derived neural progenitors into areas of need; or (2) focal revival of endogenous stem cells to repopulate damaged areas. Presently, these efforts are significantly hindered by a limited understanding of the

---

Fig. 3.8 *Gdf11* mutants exhibit retinal abnormalities. (**A**) ISH for *Gdf11* and *Fst* in developing mouse retina; nbl, neuroblastic layer; gcl, ganglion cell layer. Arrow in inset indicates *Fst* expression in presumptive amacrine cells (Scale bars, 200 μm) (**B**) Left, hematoxylin-eosin-stained paraffin sections of retina. Right, ISH for *Brn3b*. Insets, higher magnification of *Brn3b*+ gcl (Scale bars, 100 μm) (**C**) Top, increased cell number ($P < 0.01$, student's *t*-test) in *Gdf11*-null retinas. Total cell nuclei in GCL + IPL were counted in 300 μm of central retina in P0 cryosections stained with Hoechst. Bottom, no significant change in central retina thickness. Histograms show mean ± SEM of measurements from four to five animals of each genotype. (**D**) β-galactosidase (X-gal) staining of sections of *Gdf11*-null- and *Gdf11* +/+ -*Tattler-1* embryos (Scale bars, 200 μm; on, optic nerve; oc, optic chiasm) (**E**) Cross sections of dissected optic nerves stained with antibodies to neurofilament (Scale bar, 50 μm) (From [65]; reprinted courtesy of Science) (*See Color Plates*)

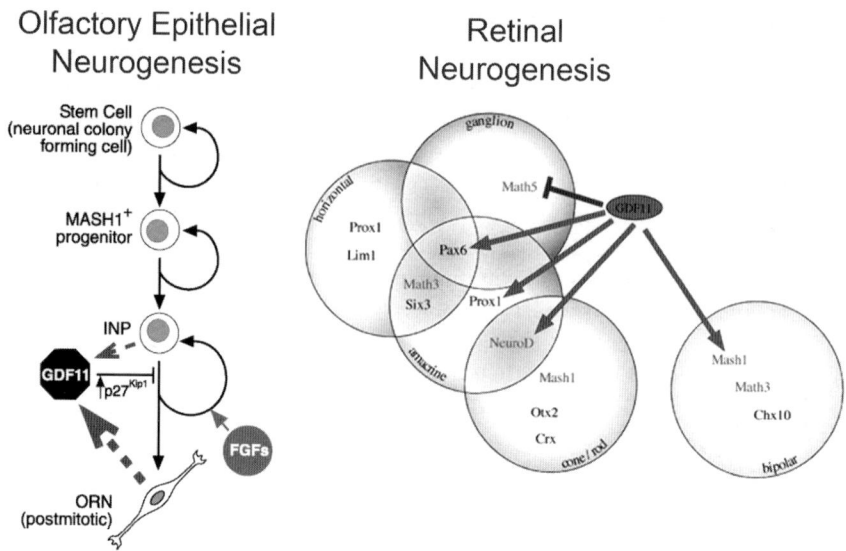

Fig. 3.9 Contrasting roles of GDF11 signaling in OE and retina neurogenesis. In developing OE, GDF11 negatively regulates neuronal production by reversibly blocking the division of *Ngn1*-expressing INPs through increased expression of the cyclin-dependent kinase inhibitor p27^{Kip1}. Loss of ORNs releases INPs from the GDF11-mediated negative regulation, allowing them to increase their proliferation until neuron number is restored. In contrast, GDF11 signaling in retinal neurogenesis specifies retinal cell type specification by regulating retinal progenitor cell competence state. GDF11 suppresses *Math5* expression, and promotes expression of various homeodomain genes such as *Pax6* and bHLH factors such as *NeuroD*, driving progenitors to acquire competence to produce later-born cell types such as amacrine cells and photoreceptors (Adapted from [63, 78] ; reprinted courtesy of Neuron and Genes and Development) (*See Color Plates*)

molecules that regulate stem cell activity, both in terms of endogenous control of stem cells in vivo, and manipulation of cultured stem cells in vitro. Gaining a better understanding of their origin, proliferation, maturation, and phenotypic specification will improve the efficacy of such therapies by increasing the efficiency of generating specific cell types or tissues. Studies of the regulation of olfactory and retinal neurogenesis provide a molecular foundation for future attempts at guiding stem and progenitor cells toward specific cell fates for use in clinical therapies, with the hope that we may eventually harness the full potential of endogenous stem and progenitor cells that might otherwise be incapable of further growth and regeneration.

Acknowledgements This work was supported by March of Dimes; Foundation Fighting Blindness; NIH DC03583; and NIH P50 GM 076516.

References

1. Beites CL, Kawauchi S, Crocker CE, Calof AL (2005) Identification and molecular regulation of neural stem cells in the olfactory epithelium. Exp Cell Res 306:309–316.

2. Taupin P (2006) Adult neural stem cells, neurogenic niches, and cellular therapy. Stem Cell Rev 2:213–219.
3. Farbman AI (1992) Cell Biology of Olfaction. Cambridge, Cambridge University Press.
4. Frisch D (1967) Ultrastructure of mouse olfactory mucosa. Am J Anat 128:87–120.
5. Morrison E, Costanzo R (1992) Morphology of olfactory epithelium in humans and other vertebrates. Microsc Res Technol 23:49–61.
6. Cuschieri A, Bannister LH (1975) The development of the olfactory mucosa in the mouse: electron microscopy. J Anat 119:471–498.
7. Graziadei PPC, Monti Graziadei GA (1979) Neurogenesis and neuron regeneration in the olfactory system of mammals. I. Morphological aspects of differentiation and structural organization of the olfactory sensory neurons. J Neurocytol 8:1–18.
8. Calof AL, Chikaraishi DM (1989) Analysis of neurogenesis in a mammalian neuroepithelium: proliferation and differentiation of an olfactory neuron precursor in vitro. Neuron 3:115–127.
9. Carter LA, MacDonald JL, Roskams AJ (2004) Olfactory horizontal basal cells demonstrate a conserved multipotent progenitor phenotype. J Neurosci 24:5670–5683.
10. Leung CT, Coulombe PA, Reed RR (2007) Contribution of olfactory neural stem cells to tissue maintenance and regeneration. Nat Neurosci 10:720–726.
11. Schwob JE, Youngentob SL, Mezza RC (1995) Reconstitution of the rat olfactoryepithelium after methyl bromide-induced lesion. J Comp Neurol 359:15–37.
12. Caggiano M, Kauer JS, Hunter DD (1994) Globose basal cells are neuronal progenitors in the olfactory epithelium: a lineage analysis using a replication-incompetent retrovirus. Neuron 13:339–352.
13. Gordon MK, Mumm JS, Davis RA, Holcomb JD, Calof AL (1995) Dynamics of MASH1 expression in vitro and in vivo suggest a non-stem cell site of MASH1 action in the olfactory receptor neuron lineage. Mol Cell Neurosci 6:363–379.
14. Mackay-Sim A, Kittel P (1991) Cell dynamics in the adult mouse olfactory epithelium: a quantitative autoradiographic study. J Neurosci 11:979–984.
15. Schwartz Levey M, Chikaraishi DM, Kauer JS (1991) Characterization of potential precursor populations in the mouse olfactory epithelium using immunocytochemistry and autoradiography. J Neurosci 11:3556–3564.
16. Ellis P, Fagan BM, Magness ST, Hutton S, Taranova O, Hayashi S, McMahon A, Rao M, Pevny L (2004) SOX2, a persistent marker for multipotential neural stem cells derived from embryonic stem cells, the embryo or the adult. Dev Neurosci 26:148–165.
17. Graham V, Khudyakov J, Ellis P, Pevny L (2003) SOX2 functions to maintain neural progenitor identity. Neuron 39:749–765.
18. Kawauchi S, Beites C, Crocker CE, Wu HH, Bonnin A, Murray RC, Calof AL (2004) Molecular signals regulating proliferation of stem and progenitor cells in mouse olfactory epithelium. Dev Neurosci 26:166–180.
19. Taranova OV, Magness ST, Fagan BM, Wu Y, Surzenko N, Hutton SR, Pevny LH (2006) SOX2 is a dose-dependent regulator of retinal neural progenitor competence. Genes Dev 20:1187–1202.
20. Wang J, Rao S, Chu J, Shen X, Levasseur DN, Theunissen TW, Orkin SH (2006) A protein interaction network for pluripotency of embryonic stem cells. Nature 444:364–368.
21. Wood HB, Episkopou V (1999) Comparative expression of the mouse Sox1, Sox2 and Sox3 genes from pre-gastrulation to early somite stages. Mech Dev 86:197–201.
22. Cau E, Gradwohl G, Fode C, Guillemot F (1997) Mash1 activates a cascade of bHLH regulators in olfactory neuron progenitors. Development 124:1611–1621.
23. Guillemot F, Lo LC, Johnson JE, Auerbach A, Anderson DJ, Joyner AL (1993) Mammalian achaete-scute homolog 1 is required for the early development of olfactory and autonomic neurons. Cell 75:463–476.
24. Tietjen I, Rihel JM, Cao Y, Koentges G, Zakhary L, Dulac C (2003) Single-cell transcriptional analysis of neuronal progenitors. Neuron 38:161–175.
25. Kawauchi S, Shou J, Santos R, Hebert JM, McConnell SK, Mason I, Calof AL (2005) Fgf8 expression defines a morphogenetic center required for olfactory neurogenesis and nasal cavity development in the mouse. Development 132:5211–5223.

26. Graziadei GA, Graziadei PP (1979) Neurogenesis and neuron regeneration in the olfactory system of mammals. II. Degeneration and reconstitution of the olfactory sensory neurons after axotomy. J Neurocytol 8:197–213.

27. Holcomb JD, Mumm JS, Calof AL (1995) Apoptosis in the neuronal lineage of the mouse olfactory epithelium: regulation *in vivo* and *in vitro*. Dev Biol 172:307–323.

28. Iwema CL, Fang H, Kurtz DB, Youngentob SL, Schwob JE (2004) Odorant receptor expression patterns are restored in lesion-recovered rat olfactory epithelium. J Neurosci 24:356–369.

29. DeHamer MK, Guevara JL, Hannon K, Olwin BB, Calof AL (1994) Genesis of olfactory receptor neurons in vitro: regulation of progenitor cell divisions by fibroblast growth factors. Neuron 13:1083–1097.

30. Goldman SA, Sim F (2005) Neural progenitor cells of the adult brain. Novartis Found Symp 265:66–80.

31. Mumm JS, Shou J, Calof AL (1996) Colony-forming progenitors from mouse olfactory epithelium: evidence for feedback regulation of neuron production. Proc Natl Acad Sci 93:11167–11172.

32. Calof AL, Lander AD (1991) Relationship between neuronal migration and cell- substratum adhesion: laminin and merosin promote olfactory neuronal migration but are anti-adhesive. J Cell Biol 115:779–794.

33. Ahmad S, Stewart R, Yung S, Kolli S, Armstrong L, Stojkovic M, Figueiredo F, Lako M (2007) Differentiation of human embryonic stem cells into corneal epithelial-like cells by in vitro replication of the corneal epithelial stem cell niche. Stem Cells 25:1145–1155.

34. Lensch MW, Daheron L, Schlaeger TM (2006) Pluripotent stem cells and their niches. Stem Cell Rev 2:185–201.

35. Shou J, Murray RC, Rim PC, Calof AL (2000) Opposing effects of bone morphogenetic proteins on neuron production and survival in the olfactory receptor neuron lineage. Development 127:5403–5413.

36. Dewulf N, Verschueren K, Lonnoy O, Moren A, Grimsby S, Vande Spiegle K, Miyazono K, Huylebroeck D, Ten Dijke P (1995) Distinct spatial and temporal expression patterns of two type I receptors for bone mophogenetic proteins during mouse embryogenesis. Endocrinology 136:2652–2663.

37. Helder MN, Ozkaynak E, Sampath KT, Luyten FP, Latin V, Oppermann H, Vukicevic S (1995) Expression pattern of osteogenic protein-1 (bone morphogenetic protein-7) in human and mouse development. J Histochem Cytochem 43:1035–1044.

38. Wu DK, Oh S-H (1996) Sensory organ generation in the chick inner ear. J Neurosci 16:6454–6462.

39. Zhang D, Mehler MF, Song Q, Kessler JA (1998) Development of bone morphogenetic protein receptors in the nervous system and possible roles in regulating trkC expression. J Neurosci 18:3314–3326.

40. Furuta Y, Piston DW, Hogan BL (1997) Bone morphogenetic proteins (BMPs) as regulators of dorsal forebrain development. Development 124:2203–2212.

41. Graham A, Francis-West P, Brickell P, Lumsden A (1994) The signaling molecule BMP4 mediates apoptosis in the rhombencephalic neural crest. Nature 372:684–686.

42. Hawley SH, Wunnenberg-Stapleton K, Hashimoto C, Laurent MN, Watabe T, Blumberg BW, Cho KW (1995) Disruption of BMP signals in embryonic Xenopus ectoderm leads to direct neural induction. Genes Dev 9:2923–2925.

43. Li W, Cogswell CA, LoTurco JJ (1998) Neuronal differentiation of precursors in the neocortical ventricular zone is triggered by BMP. J Neurosci 18:8853–8862.

44. Wilson PA, Hemmati-Brivanlou A (1995) Induction of epidermis and inhibition of neural fate by Bmp-4. Nature 376:331–336.

45. Shou J, Rim PC, Calof AL (1999) BMPs inhibit neurogenesis by a mechanism involving degradation of a transcription factor. Nat Neurosci 2:339–345.

46. Kingsley DM (1994) The TGF-β superfamily: new members, new receptors, and new genetic tests of function in different organisms. Genes Dev 8:133–146.

47. Cheng LE, Reed RR (2007) *Zfp423/OAZ* participates in a developmental switch during olfactory neurogenesis. Neuron 54:547–557.

48. Hata A, Seoane J, Lagna G, Montalvo E, Hemmati-Brivanlou A, Massague J (2000) OAZ uses distinct DNA- and protein-binding zinc fingers in separate BMP-Smad and Olf signaling pathways. Cell 100:229–240.
49. Ku M, Howard S, Ni W, Lagna G, Hata A (2006) OAZ regulates bone morphogenetic protein signaling through Smad6 activation. J Biol Chem 281:5277–5287.
50. Shim S, Bae N, Han JK (2002) Bone morphogenetic protein-4-induced activation of Xretpos is mediated by Smads and Olf-1/EBF associated zinc finger (OAZ). Nucleic Acids Res 30:3107–3117.
51. Zimmerman LB, De Jesus-Escobar JM, Harland RM (1996) The Spemann organizer signal noggin binds and inactivates bone morphogenetic protein 4. Cell 86:599–606.
52. Chang C, Hemmati-Brivanlou A (1999) *Xenopus* GDF6, a new antagonist of noggin and a partner of BMPs. Development 126:3347–3357.
53. Jordan J, Bottner M, Schluesener HJ, Unsicker K, Krieglstein K (1997) Bone morphogenetic proteins: neurotrophic roles for midbrain dopaminergic neurons and implications of astroglial cells. Eur J Neurosci 9:1699–1709.
54. Reissmann E, Ernsberger U, Francis-West PH, Rueger D, Brickell PM, Rohrer H (1996) Involvement of bone morphogenetic protein-4 and bone morphogenetic protein-7 in the differentiation of the adrenergic phenotype in developing sympathetic neurons. Development 122:2079–2088.
55. Schneider C, Wicht H, Enderich J, Wegner M, Rohrer H (1999) Bone morphogenetic proteins are required in vivo for the generation of sympathetic neurons. Neuron 24:861–870.
56. Shah NM, Groves AK, Anderson DJ (1996) Alternative neural crest cell fates are instructively promoted by TGFβ superfamily members. Cell 85:331–343.
57. Varley JE, Maxwell GD (1996) BMP-2 and BMP-4, but not BMP-6, increase the number of adrenergic cells which develop in quail trunk neural crest cultures. Exp Neurol 140:84–94.
58. Varley JE, Wehby RG, Rueger DC, Maxwell GD (1995) Number of adrenergic and Islet- 1 immunoreactive cells is increased in avian trunk neural crest cultures in the presence of human recombinant Osteogenic Protein-1. Dev Dyn 203:434–447.
59. Arkell R, Beddington RSP (1997) BMP-7 influences pattern and growth of the developing hindbrain of mouse embryos. Development 124:1–12.
60. Bullough WS (1965) Mitotic and functional homeostasis: a speculative review. Cancer Res 25:1683–1727.
61. Lee SJ, McPherron AC (1999) Myostatin and the control of skeletal muscle mass. Curr Opin Genet Dev 9:604–607.
62. Zimmers TA, Davies MV, Koniaris LG, Haynes P, Esquela AF, Tomkinson KN, McPherron AC, Wolfman NM, Lee SJ (2002) Induction of cachexia in mice by systemically administered myostatin. Science 296:1486–1488.
63. Wu HH, Ivkovic S, Murray RC, Jaramillo S, Lyons KM, Johnson JE, Calof AL (2003) Autoregulation of neurogenesis by GDF11. Neuron 37:197–207.
64. Gamer LW, Nove J, Rosen V (2003) Return of the chalones. Dev Cell 4:143–144.
65. Kim J, Wu HH, Lander AD, Lyons KM, Matzuk MM, Calof AL (2005) GDF11 controls the timing of progenitor cell competence in developing retina. Science 308:1927–1930.
66. McPherron AC, Lawler AM, Lee SJ (1997) Regulation of skeletal muscle mass in mice by a new TGF-beta superfamily member. Nature 387:83–90.
67. Taylor WE, Bhasin S, Artaza J, Byhower F, Azam M, Willard DH, Jr, Kull FC, Jr, Gonzalez-Cadavid N (2001) Myostatin inhibits cell proliferation and protein synthesis in C2C12 muscle cells. Am J Physiol Endocrinol Metab 280:E221–E228.
68. Thomas M, Langley B, Berry C, Sharma M, Kirk S, Bass J, Kambadur R (2000) Myostatin, a negative regulator of muscle growth, functions by inhibiting myoblast proliferation. J Biol Chem 275:40235–40243.
69. Murray RC, Navi D, Fesenko J, Lander AD, Calof AL (2003) Widespread defects in the primary olfactory pathway caused by loss of Mash1 function. J Neurosci 23:1769–1780.
70. Feijen A, Goumans MJ, van den Eijnden-van Raaij AJ (1994) Expression of activin subunits, activin receptors and follistatin in postimplantation mouse embryos suggests specific developmental functions for different activins. Development 120:3621–3637.

71. Nakashima M, Toyono T, Akamine A, Joyner A (1999) Expression of growth/differentiation factor *11*, a new member of the BMP/TGFb superfamily during mouse embryogenesis. Mech Dev 80:185–189.

72. Roberts VJ, Barth SL (1994) Expression of messenger ribonucleic acids encoding the inhibin/activin system during mid- and late-gestation rat embryogenesis. Endocrinology 134:914–923.

73. Turner DL, Snyder EY, Cepko CL (1990) Lineage-independent determination of cell type in the embryonic mouse retina. Neuron 4:833–845.

74. Wetts R, Fraser SE (1988) Multipotent precursors can give rise to all major cell types of the frog retina. Science 239:1142–1145.

75. Belliveau MJ, Cepko CL (1999) Extrinsic and intrinsic factors control the genesis of amacrine and cone cells in the rat retina. Development 126:555–566.

76. Rapaport DH, Patheal SL, Harris WA (2001) Cellular competence plays a role in photoreceptor differentiation in the developing Xenopus retina. J Neurobiol 49:129–141.

77. Watanabe T, Raff MC (1990) Rod photoreceptor development in vitro: intrinsic properties of proliferating neuroepithelial cells change as development proceeds in the rat retina. Neuron 4:461–467.

78. Harada T, Harada C, Parada LF (2007) Molecular regulation of visual system development: more than meets the eye. Genes Dev 21:367–378.

79. Brown NL, Patel S, Brzezinski J, Glaser T (2001) Math5 is required for retinal ganglion cell and optic nerve formation. Development 128:2497–2508.

80. Kay JN, Finger-Baier KC, Roeser T, Staub W, Baier H (2001) Retinal ganglion cell genesis requires lakritz, a zebrafish atonal homolog. Neuron 30:725–736.

81. Wang SW, Kim BS, Ding K, Wang H, Sun D, Johnson RL, Klein WH, Gan L (2001) Requirement for math5 in the development of retinal ganglion cells. Genes Dev 15:24–29.

82. Hatakeyama J, Tomita K, Inoue T, Kageyama R (2001) Roles of homeobox and bHLH genes in specification of a retinal cell type. Development 128:1313–1322.

83. Morrow EM, Furukawa T, Lee JE, Cepko CL (1999) NeuroD regulates multiple functions in the developing neural retina in rodent. Development 126:23–36.

84. Hamilton JA, Kim J, Calof AL (Sept. 2007) GDF11-FST Regulation of Retinal Neurogenesis in Normal and Ocular Mutant Mice. *Pacific Ocular Regenerative Biology Conference XII.*

85. Tropepe V, Coles BL, Chiasson BJ, Horsford DJ, Elia AJ, McInnes RR, van der Kooy D (2000) Retinal stem cells in the adult mammalian eye. Science 287:2032–2036.

86. Lamba DA, Karl MO, Ware CB, Reh TA (2006) Efficient generation of retinal progenitor cells from human embryonic stem cells. Proc Natl Acad Sci USA 103:12769–12774.

87. MacLaren RE, Pearson RA, MacNeil A, Douglas RH, Salt TE, Akimoto M, Swaroop A, Sowden JC, Ali RR (2006) Retinal repair by transplantation of photoreceptor precursors. Nature 444:203–207.

88. Dichmann DS, Yassin H, Serup P (2006) Analysis of pancreatic endocrine development in GDF11-deficient mice. Dev Dyn 235:3016–3025.

89. Esquela AF, Lee SJ (2003) Regulation of metanephric kidney development by growth/differentiation factor 11. Dev Biol 257:356–370.

90. Oxburgh L, Chu GC, Michael SK, Robertson EJ (2004) TGFbeta superfamily signals are required for morphogenesis of the kidney mesenchyme progenitor population. Development 131:4593–4605.

91. Gamer LW, Cox KA, Small C, Rosen V (2001) Gdf11 is a negative regulator of chondrogenesis and myogenesis in the developing chick limb. Dev Biol 229:407–420.

92. Liu JP, Laufer E, Jessell TM (2001) Assigning the positional identity of spinal motor neurons: rostrocaudal patterning of Hox-c expression by FGFs, Gdf11, and retinoids. Neuron 32:997–1012.

Chapter 4
Epigenetic Control of Neural Stem Cell Self-Renewal and Specification

GuoQiang Sun, Chunnian Zhao, and Yanhong Shi*

Abstract Neural stem cells have the ability to self-renew and to differentiate. Epigenetic control has been shown to play an important role in regulating both. Recent progress in epigenetics provides novel perspective on regulation of neural stem cell maintenance and fate-specification, which, in turn, offers new strategies to combat neurodegenerative diseases using stem cell-based therapies. In this chapter, we attempt to cover recent advances in this exciting area with three aspects of epigenetic control: histone modification, DNA methylation and microRNAs. Understanding regulatory mechanisms of neural stem cell self-renewal and specification will offer new tools for clinical application of neural stem cells in the treatment of neurodegenerative diseases and brain injury.

Keywords Neural stem cells, epigenetics, histone modification, DNA methylation, microRNAs, nuclear receptor, TLX (NR2E1)

4.1 Introduction

Neural stem cells of the mammalian central nervous system (CNS) persist in the subventricular zone (SVZ) as well as in the hippocampal dentate gyrus [1]. These cells have the ability to self-renew and differentiate into all three major neural subtypes: astrocytes, oligodendrocytes and neurons. Substantial progress in neural stem cell research in the past decade has yielded a wealth of information regarding the mechanism of self-renewal and fate-specification. Recent evidence suggested epigenetic control as a key mechanism to maintain the cells in the "stemness" state as well as to convert the cells into lineage restricted progenitor cells or terminally differentiated mature cells [2–4].

Division of Neurosciences, and Center for Gene Expression and Drug Discovery, Beckman Research Institute of City of Hope, 1500 E. Duarte Rd, Duarte, CA 91010, USA

*Corresponding Author:
e-mail: yshi@coh.org

Y. Shi, D.O. Clegg (eds.) *Stem Cell Research and Therapeutics*,
© Springer Science+Business Media B.V. 2008

Epigenetics, coined by Conrad Waddington, is the study of reproducible, stable and ideally, heritable changes in gene expression that occur without a change in DNA sequence. Thus neural stem cell differentiation may be thought to be the change of "epigenetic landscape", the sum of epigenetic changes at the cellular level, as described by Waddington.

Molecular mechanisms that control epigenetic changes can be loosely categorized as chromatin/histone modification, DNA methylation, and small RNAs, such as small interfering RNAs (siRNAs) and microRNAs (miRNAs). Chromatin is the packaging structure of genetic material, DNA, through association with histone proteins. The nucleosome, the basic repeating unit of chromatin, consists of 146 bp of DNA wrapped around an octameric histone core containing four basic histones: H2A, H2B, H3, and H4. Nucleosomal DNA can be further compacted by association with the linker histone H1 and additional nonhistone proteins, as well as by higher order looping and folding of the chromatin fiber. This organization of chromatin restricts free physical access of nuclear factors to the DNA. It is now clear that post-translational modifications of histone proteins can alter chromatin conformation and play direct regulatory roles in gene expression. Tremendous diversity in the histone/nucleosome structures can be generated by more than 100 post-translational modifications, such as acetylation, phosphorylation, methylation and ubiquitination. These modifications occur primarily at specific positions within the amino-terminal histone tails [2]. Considering so many possible combinations of modifications that can occur on a variety of sites on histones, it has been proposed that different combinations of histone modifications may result in distinct outcomes in terms of chromatin-regulated functions. This idea was formally proposed as the Histone Code Hypothesis [5] (Fig. 4.1).

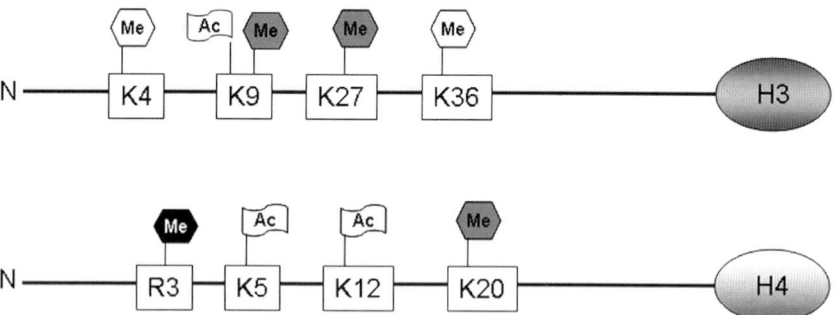

Fig. 4.1 Histone modification and histone code. The N-terminal domains of histone H2A, H2B, H3 and H4 are depicted as horizontal lines. Relevant lysines and arginines are shown as boxes. Acetylations (Ac) and methylations (Me) are indicated in the symbol. Acetylation of histones H3, H4, and methylation of histone H3 lysine 4 (H3K4) and H3 lysine 36 (H3K36) are marks for transcriptional activation (in white), while methylation of H3 lysine 9 (H3K9), H3 lysine 27 (H3K27), and H4 lysine 20 (H4K20) are associated with transcriptional repression (in gray). Methylation of H4 arginine 3 (H4R3) can be either active or repressive (in black). Many additional modifications occur but are omitted for simplicity

Lysine acetylation and methylation in the histone tail is the primary site for histone modification. While lysine acetylation almost always correlates with chromatin accessibility and transcriptional activity, lysine methylation can have different effects depending on which residue is modified. Lysine residues can be mono-, di-, or tri-methylated. Methylation of histone H3 lysine 4 (H3K4) and H3 lysine 36 (H3K36) is associated with transcribed chromatin. In contrast, methylation of H3 lysine 9 (H3K9), H3 lysine 27 (H3K27), and H4 lysine 20 (H4K20) generally correlates with repression [2]. Distinct histone modifications can influence each other and may also interact with DNA methylation, in part through the activities of protein complexes that bind modified histones or methylated cytosines.

Histone modifications, including acetylation, methylation and phosphorylation, are reversible and dynamic and are often associated with inducible expression of individual genes. In this chapter, we focus on the recent studies investigating the mechanisms of epigenetics in neural stem cell self-renewal and specification in the mammalian nervous system.

4.2   Histone Modification in Neural Stem Cells

In general, acetylation of the histone tail disrupts the electrostatic interaction between positively charged amino acids from the histone tail and negative charges from phosphate groups in DNA, leading to decompression of the chromatin structure, allowing access to transcription factors, and ultimately, gene activation. Conversely, histone deacetylation leads to gene repression. Histone acetylation is mediated by an enzyme, histone acetylase (HAT) while histone deacetylation is catalyzed by another enzyme, histone deacetylase (HDAC). Mammalian HDACs can be classified based on their structure and homology to yeast HDACs. Each class has a distinct expression pattern. Class I HDACs (HDAC1, 2, 3, 8, and 11) are ubiquitously expressed, while Class II HDACs (HDAC4, 5, 7, and 9) display more tissue-specific expression patterns. Class II HDACs contain an amino-terminal extension that can interact with other transcriptional cofactors and convey response to extracellular stimuli [6].

Several studies have clearly demonstrated that histone acetylation plays a key role in fate decision of neural stem cells [4, 7, 8]. In a recent study, we demonstrated the role of HDACs in adult neural stem cell maintenance and self-renewal through interaction with a nuclear receptor, TLX [7]. TLX is expressed in neural stem cells in both embryonic and adult brains and is required for the maintenance of self-renewal of neural stem cells [9, 10]. TLX null mice have smaller brains with reduced olfactory bulbs and hippocampi [9]. In our recent study [7], TLX was shown to recruit histone deacetylases (HDACs) to its downstream target genes in neural stem cells, leading to repression of TLX target gene expression. TLX interacts with HDAC3 and HDAC5 in neural stem cells through a conserved cofactor binding motif. Two TLX target genes, the cyclin-dependent kinase inhibitor, p21(CIP1/WAF1)(p21), and the tumor suppressor gene, pten, are regulated by TLX and HDAC interaction in neural stem cells. Both genes are involved in neural stem/ progenitor cell proliferation [11–13]. Either inhibition of HDAC activity or knockdown of HDAC expression induced p21 and pten gene expression and decreased neural stem cell proliferation [7]. This study suggests that the complex, containing both TLX and HDAC, is required for neural stem cell proliferation, because expression of a TLX peptide containing the minimal HDAC interaction domain is sufficient to induce TLX target gene expression and reduced neural stem cell proliferation. Collectively, these findings demonstrate a novel mechanism for neural stem cell proliferation through transcriptional repression of p21 and pten gene expression by TLX-HDAC interactions (Fig. 4.2). It remains to be determined whether the TLX-HDAC complex contains other mediators or co-regulators. TLX is an orphan nuclear receptor, of which the ligand has not been identified. The discovery of TLX ligands remains a tremendous interest both for elucidation of the mechanism of TLX function in neural stem cells as well as for developing therapeutic tools to treat neurodegenerative diseases.

It has also been shown that inhibitors of histone deacetylases promote neuronal fate of adult hippocampal neural progenitors, and suppress the fate for astrocytes and oligodendrocytes through induction of neurogenic transcription factors, including NeuroD [8, 14]. In another example, HADC activity is important in the process of myelination in the developing corpus callosum [15]. The first two weeks of postnatal development is a critical stage for propagation of progenitor cells of

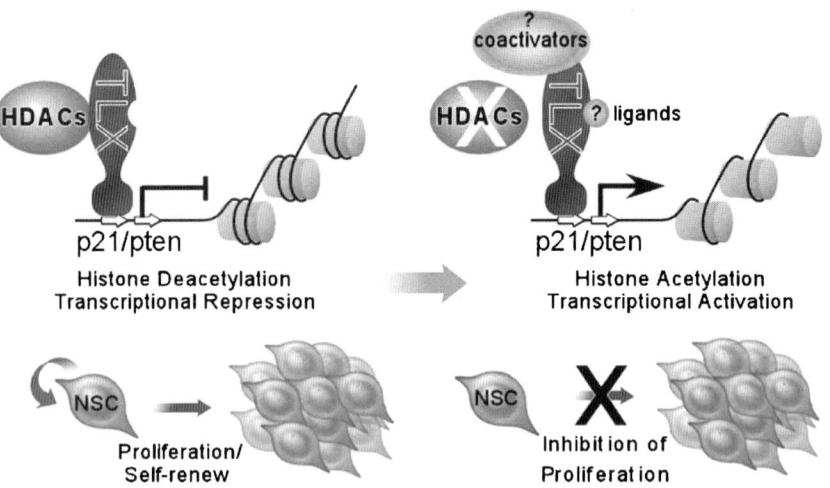

Fig. 4.2 Orphan nuclear receptor TLX partners with HDACs to regulate neural stem cell proliferation and self-renewal. Nuclear receptor TLX binds to its target genes, such as the cyclin-dependent kinase inhibitor, p21, and the tumor suppressor gene, pten. In the absence of ligand, TLX recruits the histone deacetylase complex (HDACs) to the target gene promoters and represses target gene expression. Release or inhibition of HDACs and /or recruitment of coactivator complex activates p21 and pten gene expression, which leads to inhibition of proliferation and induction of neural differentiation (*See Color Plates*)

myelin-forming oligodendrocytes. During the third week, after myelination has ensued, the progenitor cells differentiate. Administration of a HDAC inhibitor during the first two weeks inhibits oligodendrocyte progenitors from differentiating and results in significant hypomyelination. However, after the onset of myelination, the inhibitor has no effect on the myelination process [15], presumably because the reversible deacetylation of lysine residue in H3 is replaced by the more stable methylation of H3K9 and expression of HP1α protein, a signature of compacted chromatin [15].

The relevance of HDACs in neural stem cells is complicated by a recent report, in which a HDAC inhibitor was shown to convert lineage-committed oligodendrocyte progenitor cells into multipotent neural stem cells. Four compounds possessing such capability, all HDAC inhibitors, were identified by unbiased high-throughput screening from a drug library of about 40,000 [16]. This study presents an interesting possibility that the treatment of cells with an HDAC inhibitor may function to open the chromosome as a priming event, and that the fate decision of the cell depends on the availability of certain factors within the cell. In this study, some cells differentiated from neural stem cells to neurons or glia cells, while in other cases, glia progenitor cells de-differentiated into neural stem cells.

The connection of neural stem cells to the polycomb group (PcG), a histone modification complex, has been established by several recent studies. PcG proteins maintain transcriptional silence in a process that is thought to involve trimethylation of histone H3 at Lys27 (H3K27). The PcG gene family includes two distinct complexes: polycomb repression complex1 and 2 (PRC1 and PRC2). PRC2 is involved in the initiation of transcriptional silencing through two enzymatic activities: histone deacetylase and histone methyltransferase. Histone methyltransferases in PRC2 can methylate histone H3K9 and H3K27, and histone H1K26. One of the key subunits of the PRC1 complex is Bmi-1. Bmi-1 is essential for the self-renewal of neural stem cells [17–19]. Deficiency in the polycomb family transcriptional repressor Bmi-1 leads to progressive postnatal growth retardation and neurological defects. In the absence of Bmi-1, the cyclin-dependent kinase inhibitor gene p16^{Ink4a} is elevated in neural stem cells, reducing the rate of proliferation. p16^{Ink4a} deficiency partially reverses the self-renewal defect in Bmi-1 null neural stem cells. This conserved requirement for Bmi-1 to promote self-renewal and to repress p16^{Ink4a} expression suggests that a common mechanism regulates the self-renewal and postnatal persistence of diverse types of stem cells. However, the mechanism of how other PcG complex components interact with Bmi-1 and regulate neural stem cell proliferation and differentiation remains to be determined [20].

Recently, two nuclear receptor corepressors SMRT (silencing mediate of retinoid and thyroid hormone receptors) and NCoR (nuclear receptor repressor corepressor) have been shown to play important roles in the maintenance of neural stem cell fate [21, 22]. SMRT and NCoR are paralogs of one another and function in similar fashions. Initially, both NCoR and SMRT make direct contact with repression motifs in the ligand binding domain of nuclear receptors in the absence of ligand, which leads to the assembly of a larger array of additional corepressors such as mSin3 and HDACs. When the ligands are available, the corepressor complex is replaced by coactivator complexes, which possess HAT activity, as well as other chromatin remodeling complexes [23]. The expression pattern of SMRT is primarily in the ventricular zone of embryonic brains, where the multipotent neural stem cell resides. NCoR has a broader distribution, with expression throughout the dorsal cortex [21]. Genetic knockout of the NCoR gene in cortical progenitor cells results in impaired self-renewal and spontaneous differentiation into astrocyte-like cells [22], whereas SMRT deletion in cortical progenitor cells gives rise to all three neural cell types: neurons, astrocytes and oligodendrocytes. Chromatin immunoprecipitation assay indicates that SMRT was preferentially recruited to the promoter of neuronal gene *Dcx* [21]. One of the nuclear receptors, retinoic acid receptor α (RARα), interacts with SMRT in the absence of ligand and represses target gene expression. In the presence of RARα ligand, SMRT is released from the promoter of target genes [24]. Retinoic acid signaling has been implicated in patterning and differentiation in telecephelon development [25, 26]. In cortical progenitor cells, SMRT maintains neural stem cells partially by repressing RARα target gene, *jmjd3*, a jumonjiC family of specific histone H3 trimethyl K27 (H3K27me3) demethylase. Expression of *jmjd3* is involved in activating components of neuronal differentiation. These studies suggest an elegant mechanism for retinoic acid signaling in neural stem cell differentiation through epigenetic regulation [21].

4.3   DNA Methylation in Neural Stem Cells

DNA methylation is now considered vital for brain development and neuronal maturation [27, 28]. The most common DNA methylation in mammals is the methylation of cytosine in the $5'$ position of CpG dinucleotides (named CpG island). DNA methylation is involved in several biological processes: maintenance of chromatin structure in repressive status such as genomic imprinting, X chromosome inactivation, and chromatin remodeling. Clusters of CpG dimers, a characteristic structure located in the regulatory regions of many genes, can serve as a target for gene expression [29]. DNA methylation level is mainly controlled by DNA methyltransferases (DNMTs), while DNA demethylase is still elusive. DNA methylation-dependent gene silencing is mediated by DNMTs. There are two major categories of DNMT: DNMT1 and DNMT3 (DNMT3a, and DNMT3b). DNMT1 is a maintenance methyltransferase, which methylates CpGs on semimethylated DNA, whereas DNMT3a and DNMT3b function as de novo DNA methyltransferases, targeting unmethylated CpGs to establish new methylation patterns [27, 30, 31].

DNMT1 expression is high in postmitotic neurons [27]. Treatment of undifferentiated progenitor cells with a demethylating agent such as 5-azadeoxycytidine or retinoic acid can initiate differentiation into mature neurons. DNMT1 null mice are embryonic lethal. Conditional knockout of DNMT1 using a Cre/LoxP system showed that DNMT1 deficiency in postmitotic neurons had no effect on levels of global methylation during postnatal life [32]. However DNMT1 is required for survival of neural precursors [33].

Both DNMT3a and DNMT3b are expressed in the developing nervous system [28, 34, 35]. DNMT3b exhibits expression in early embryonic and neural progenitor cells during neurogenesis [31], whereas DNMT3a is expressed in perinatal and adult stages in all neural lineages. In addition, mutations in DNMT3b result in human ICF syndrome (immunodeficiency, centromeric instability, facial anomalies) [31].

DNMT3b has been shown to regulate neural differentiation by recruiting HDAC2 in PC12 cells, a cell line derived from neuroendocrine tumors and capable of differentiating into neuronal cells [36]. PC12 can be induced into neuronal lineage by neurotrophic factors, such as nerve growth factor (NGF). Knock-down DNMT3b expression in PC12 cells resulted in interference in neuronal differentiation and maintenance of the cells in the proliferative state.

DNA methylation has also been shown to regulate STAT3 target gene expression. Activation of STAT3 is critical for neural development. Demethylation of CpG in STAT3 binding sites has been identified on the promoter of glial fibrillary acidic protein (GFAP) gene, a marker for astrocytes, when cells are committed to neural lineage, while hypermethylation of CpG has been shown on the GFAP promoter in non-neural cells generated from embryonic stem cells. Demethylation on the promoter of astrocyte-specific genes has been shown to be an important mechanism for the transition of pluripotent stem cells to cells of neural lineage [20, 37].

DNA methylation regulates gene expression through two mechanisms: (1) methylation at CpG sites blocks the binding of transcription factors and leads to transcriptional inactivation; and (2) methyl-CpGs are bound by a family of methyl-CpG binding proteins (MBDs), including MBD1, MBD2, MBD3, MBD4, and MeCP2 (methyl CpG binding protein 2). Binding of MBDs and further recruitment of histone deacetylase (HDAC) repressor complexes results in histone deacetylation and inactive chromatin structures that are repressive for transcription. The most extensively studied member of this family is MeCP2, mutation of which causes neurological deficits in both humans (Rett Syndrome) and rodents. Adult neurogenesis can be controlled and stimulated by a group of chemicals called neurotrophins. One well-studied neurotrophin is brain-derived neurotrophic factor (BDNF). Its transcription increases dramatically upon membrane depolarization. It has been shown that MeCP2 binds to BDNF promoter to repress BDNF expression in quiescent neurons. Upon membrane depolarization, MeCP2 becomes phosphorylated, which triggers dissociation of MeCP2 from binding to 5mCpG site in BNDF promoter, thereby activating the transcription [38, 39]. The importance of MBDs in central nervous system is reflected from the phenotype of MBD mutant mice. Mice lacking MBD1 have deficits in adult neurogenesis and hippocampal function [40], while mice lacking MBD2 show only mild maternal behavior deficits. MBD3 null mice die at an early embryonic stage. Mice deficient in MBD4, a mismatch repair enzyme, show deficits in DNA repair and increased tumor formation [32].

4.4   Chromatin Remodeling Complexes in Neural Stem Cells

The transition from neural stem cells to neurons requires a spectrum of changes at the epigenetic level, resulting in activation of neuron-specific genes. Many genes are associated with neuronal functions, including neurotransmitters and their receptors, molecules for vesicle trafficking and release, guide cues involved in axonal growth, and synaptogenesis and neuronal trophic factors. These genes are repressed in dividing progenitors during the developing stages of the nervous system by a transcription factor REST [repressor element 1 (RE1) silencing transcription factor]. REST binds to 21 bp RE1 site that is present in the regulatory regions of many neuronal-specific genes. REST is also known as neuron restrictive silence factor (NRSF), which was originally identified as a key regulator in neurogenesis [41]. Originally, REST was believed to be a silencer of neuronal genes in neural stem cells and other non-neuronal cells. During development of the neural tube, REST is expressed in the ventricular zone of the neuroepithilium, whereas in the adult central nervous system, expression of REST is abundant in hippocampus, midbrain and hindbrain. REST can act as an anchor for the recruitment of multiple chromatin-modifying enzymes, facilitating interactions among individual enzymes that regulate gene expression. REST-mediated gene repression is achieved by the recruitment of two separate corepressor complexes, mSin3 and CoREST [42–44]. The mSin3 complex contains HDAC1, HDAC2, HDCA4 and HDAC5. The CoREST complex contains HDAC1 and HDAC2, a histone H3K4 demethylase LSD1, the chromatin-remodeling enzyme BRG1, Histone H3K9 methylase-G9a and MeCP2 (Fig. 4.3). A recent study revealed that REST acts not only as a silencer but also as a repressor [45]. REST can recruit distinct corepressor complexes on different promoters in embryonic hippocampal neural stem cells. Interestingly, when REST occupies the promoters, it can create a subtle and balanced local epigenetic environment, which contains both repressive local epigenetic signatures, such as a low degree of H4 and H3K9 acetylation at the majority of RE1, and active signatures, such as increased level of dimethylation of H3K9 [45]. These data suggest that REST maintains neural stem cells in the repressive state; meanwhile, the repression is in the open state which is ready to be reversed once the differentiation signal is available.

REST complex has been demonstrated to regulate neural stem cells through small RNA [46]. A 20-nucleotide dsRNA has been identified that contains an RE1 sequence in adult rat hippocampal neural stem cells. The dsRNA is present at low levels in rat neuronal progenitor cells and at higher levels in mature neurons, but is absent from astrocytes [46]. Interestingly, this dsRNA specifically blocks the function of REST, since overexpression of dsRNA in neural stem cells results in induction of REST target genes. The mechanism of dsRNA action is not clear, probably through recruitment of other factors, which can convert REST complex into REST activator. One such factor can be the histone acetyltransferase CBP, since CBP was shown to be present in REST target gene promoter [46]. Recently a novel REST binding motif has been identified. A much larger gene network related to neuronal functions utilizing serial analysis of chromatin occupancy (SACO) has been uncovered [47].

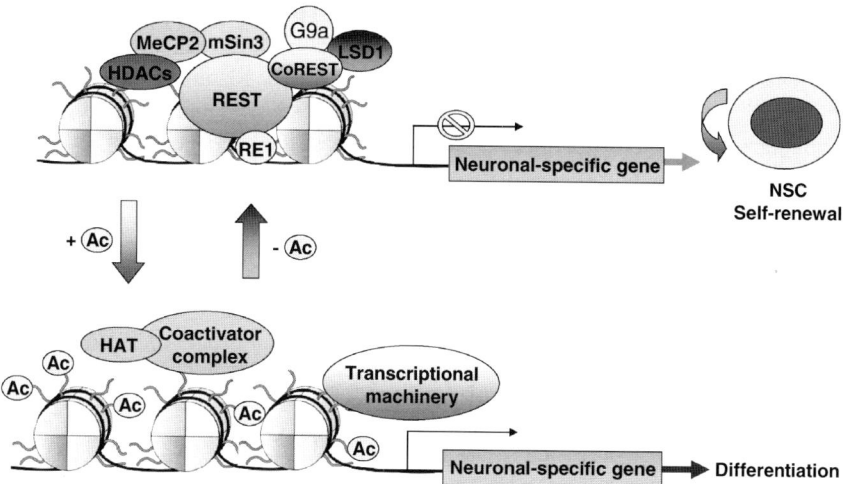

Fig. 4.3 Chromatin remodeling factors in neural stem cells. In neural stem/progenitor cells, REST (repressor element 1 silencing transcription factor) binds to a recognition site RE1 on the neuronal-specific gene promoter. REST can recruit two major complexes: mSin3 complex and CoREST complex. The mSin3 complex includes MeCP2 (methyl CpG binding protein 2) and HDACs (histone deacetylases). The CoREST complex contains HDACs, LSD1 (histone lysine specific demethylase 1) and histone H3K9 methylase G9a. Under the repressive state the neuronal gene expression is suppressed. When the complex was replaced by coactivators in neuronal-lineage cells, the neuron-specific genes are activated. Acetylations (Ac), neural stem cell (NSC) (*See Color Plates*)

Another chromatin remodeling complex, nBAF (neural Brg/Brm associated factor) complex has been shown to regulate genes critical for dendrite growth during development through Ca2 +-responsive dendrite regulator CREST [48]. Deletion of BAF53b, an nBAF complex component in mouse, leads to perinatal lethal and dramatic defects in dendritic arborization, suggesting that BAF53b and nBAF complexes control a transcriptional program of dendritic development. Indeed, the nBAF complex occupies the promoter of Ephexin1 gene, which plays important roles in axon growth [49, 50]. Two BAF subunits, Brg/Brm, possess ATPase activity, which uses energy derived from ATP-hydrolysis to regulate nucleosome mobility and chromatin accessibility.

Chromatin remodeling complex is a regulatory platform involved in self-renewal and specification of neural stem cells, the importance of which has been recently recognized and appreciated. The coordination of these multiple effects presents a challenge as well as opportunities in the study of neural stem cells.

4.5   MicroRNA in Neural Stem Cells

MicroRNAs (miRNAs) are newly discovered regulators in the gene expression networks. miRNAs are approximately 22 nucleotide (nt) non-coding RNAs that are transcribed in the nucleus by RNA polymerase II. The primary transcripts of miRNAs are processed in the nucleus by RNase III endonuclease, Drosha, into 60–75 neocleotides, and are subsequently exported to the cytoplasm and are further cleaved into mature miRNAs by Dicer, a cytoplasmic RNase III-type protein. Mature miRNAs are then transferred to Argonaute proteins in the RNA-induced silencing complex (RISC), where they direct and form imperfect base pairing with the target gene mRNA 3′ UTR (untranslated regions), leading to translational interruption, and in some case inducing mRNA degradation [51].

Recent studies indicate that miRNAs have a pivotal function in cell differentiation and the maintenance of stem cell populations. Knockout of Dicer1 leads to embryonic lethality and abolishment of stem cell populations; while Argonaute family members are required for maintaining germline stem cells in various species, suggesting miRNAs as a new class of regulators in stem cell self-renewal.

Currently, more than 5,000 miRNAs have been annotated in the database, about 500 of which are of human origin. Around 70% of identified miRNAs are found expressed in the brain [51–53]. The expression pattern of miRNAs in the brain is not only spatiotemporal but also cell type-specific, implying their essential roles in the development of the nervous system. Distinct sets of miRNAs are specifically expressed in pluripotent cells but not in adult tissues [54, 55]. miRNAs have been shown to specify cell fates in the nervous system in worms [56, 57] and determine brain morphogenesis in zebrafish [58]. Distinct expression patterns of miRNAs have been detected during mammalian brain development, suggesting a role of miRNA in mammalian neural development. Several miRNAs, including miR-124a, miR-128 and miR-9, which are expressed exclusively in the brain, and let-7 which expresses ubiquitously, play important roles in mammalian neurogenesis [59].

miRNAs act as repressors in gene regulation. Each miRNA can repress more than one target, while multiple binding sites of miRNA exist in individual mRNA [51]. During differentiation, progenitor cells express families of miRNAs in a sequential manner, resulting in lineage-specific changes in the translation of subsets of transcripts. Among these miRNAs, mir-124 and mir-128 were preferentially expressed in neurons. In contrast, mir-23 was restricted to astrocytes; mir-26 and mir-29 were more strongly expressed in astrocytes than neurons [60]. By targeting lineage-specific genes, miRNAs participate in the determination of cell fate. Let-7 and lin-4 co-regulate *hunchback*, a gene involved in differentiation of neuroblasts. *Senseless,* which controls sensory organ precursor selection in flies, is targeted by miR-9a. Knockdown of miR-9a in flies led to extra sense organs, whereas overexpression of miR-9a contributed to massive loss of sensory organ precursors.

Recent studies suggest the interaction of miRNAs with another type of regulator, transcription factors, and provide evidence on how miRNAs fit into the gene regulatory network. Transcription factors are crucial in neuronal and glial differentiation. For example, transcription repressor REST has binding motifs for two brain-specific miRNAs, miR-124 and miR-9, while REST was found to repress a family of mouse miRNA genes, including miR-124 and miR-9 [61, 62], suggesting a double negative regulatory loop between REST and these miRNAs. miR-124 is upregulated during neuronal differentiation when REST leaves its binding sites on miR-124 promoter, and the induced miR-124 could further suppress REST expression and maintain the identity of differentiated neuronal cells.

4.6 Perspectives

We are just beginning to unveil the complex regulatory network of gene expression by epigenetics. Recent advancement of epigenetic research provides insight into neural stem cell maintenance and differentiation as well as nervous system development, and also holds tremendous potential for the development of stem cell-based therapies for neurodegenerative diseases. Since the epigenetic status of each individual may vary, one future goal might be the manipulation of the epigenetic landscape to yield customized neurons or glia for individualized therapies.

Acknowledgements We thank Ms. Jill Brantley and Emily Sun for proof reading this manuscript. This work was supported by Whitehall Foundation, the Margret E. Early Medical Trust, James S. McDonnell Foundation, NIH NINDS R01NS059546 and R21NS053350. GS is a Herbert Horvitz Postdoctoral Fellow. Y.S. is a Kimmel Scholar.

References

1. Gage FH. (2000) Mammalian neural stem cells. Science; 287:1433–1438.
2. Bernstein BE, Meissner A, Lander ES. (2007) The mammalian epigenome. Cell; 128:669–681.
3. Hsieh J, Gage FH. (2004) Epigenetic control of neural stem cell fate. Current opinion in genetics & development; 14:461–469.
4. Shi Y, Sun G, Zhao C, Stewart R. (2008) Neural stem cell self-renewal. Critical reviews in oncology/hematology; 65:43–53.
5. Jenuwein T, Allis CD. (2001) Translating the histone code. Science; 293:1074–1080.
6. Thiagalingam S, Cheng KH, Lee HJ, et al. (2003) Histone deacetylases: unique players in shaping the epigenetic histone code. Annals of the New York Academy of Sciences; 983:84–100.
7. Sun G, Yu RT, Evans RM, Shi Y. (2007) Orphan nuclear receptor TLX recruits histone deacetylases to repress transcription and regulate neural stem cell proliferation. Proceedings of the National Academy of Sciences of the United States of America; 104:15282–15287.
8. Hsieh J, Nakashima K, Kuwabara T, Mejia E, Gage FH. (2004) Histone deacetylase inhibition-mediated neuronal differentiation of multipotent adult neural progenitor cells. Proceedings of the National Academy of Sciences of the United States of America; 101:16659–16664.
9. Shi Y, Chichung Lie D, Taupin P, et al. (2004) Expression and function of orphan nuclear receptor TLX in adult neural stem cells. Nature; 427:78–83.
10. Li W, Sun G, Yang S, et al. (2008) Nuclear receptor TLX regulates cell cycle progression in neural stem cells of the developing brain. Molecular endocrinology; 22:56–64.
11. Groszer M, Erickson R, Scripture-Adams DD, et al. (2001) Negative regulation of neural stem/progenitor cell proliferation by the Pten tumor suppressor gene in vivo. Science; 294:2186–2189.
12. Qiu J, Takagi Y, Harada J, et al. (2004) Regenerative response in ischemic brain restricted by p21cip1/waf1. The Journal of experimental medicine; 199:937–945.
13. Kippin TE, Martens DJ, van der Kooy D. (2005) p21 loss compromises the relative quiescence of forebrain stem cell proliferation leading to exhaustion of their proliferation capacity. Genes & development; 19:756–767.

14. Siebzehnrubl FA, Buslei R, Eyupoglu IY, et al. (2007) Histone deacetylase inhibitors increase neuronal differentiation in adult forebrain precursor cells. Experimental brain research. Experimentelle Hirnforschung. Experimentation cerebrale; 176:672–678.

15. Shen S, Li J, Casaccia-Bonnefil P. (2005) Histone modifications affect timing of oligodendrocyte progenitor differentiation in the developing rat brain. The Journal of cell biology; 169:577–589.

16. Lyssiotis CA, Walker J, Wu C, et al. (2007) Inhibition of histone deacetylase activity induces developmental plasticity in oligodendrocyte precursor cells. Proceedings of the National Academy of Sciences of the United States of America; 104:14982–14987.

17. Zencak D, Lingbeek M, Kostic C, et al. (2005) Bmi1 loss produces an increase in astroglial cells and a decrease in neural stem cell population and proliferation. The Journal of neuroscience; 25:5774–5783.

18. Molofsky AV, Pardal R, Iwashita T, et al. (2003) Bmi-1 dependence distinguishes neural stem cell self-renewal from progenitor proliferation. Nature; 425:962–967.

19. Molofsky AV, He S, Bydon M, Morrison SJ, Pardal R. (2005) Bmi-1 promotes neural stem cell self-renewal and neural development but not mouse growth and survival by repressing the p16Ink4a and p19Arf senescence pathways. Genes & development; 19:1432–1437.

20. Takizawa T, Nakashima K, Namihira M, et al. (2001) DNA methylation is a critical cell-intrinsic determinant of astrocyte differentiation in the fetal brain. Developmental cell; 1:749–758.

21. Jepsen K, Solum D, Zhou T, et al. (2007) SMRT-mediated repression of an H3K27 demethylase in progression from neural stem cell to neuron. Nature; 450:415–419.

22. Hermanson O, Jepsen K, Rosenfeld MG. (2002) N-CoR controls differentiation of neural stem cells into astrocytes. Nature; 419:934–939.

23. Privalsky ML. (2004) The role of corepressors in transcriptional regulation by nuclear hormone receptors. Annual review of physiology; 66:315–360.

24. Hong SH, Privalsky ML. (1999) Retinoid isomers differ in the ability to induce release of SMRT corepressor from retinoic acid receptor-alpha. The Journal of biological chemistry; 274:2885–2892.

25. Mark M, Ghyselinck NB, Chambon P. (2006) Function of retinoid nuclear receptors: lessons from genetic and pharmacological dissections of the retinoic acid signaling pathway during mouse embryogenesis. Annual review of pharmacology and toxicology; 46:451–480.

26. Maden M. (2002) Retinoid signalling in the development of the central nervous system. Nature reviews; 3:843–853.

27. Feng J, Fouse S, Fan G. (2007) Epigenetic regulation of neural gene expression and neuronal function. Pediatric research; 61:58R–63R.

28. Sharma RP, Grayson DR, Guidotti A, Costa E. (2005) Chromatin, DNA methylation and neuron gene regulation – the purpose of the package. Journal of psychiatry & neuroscience; 30:257–263.

29. Li E. (2002) Chromatin modification and epigenetic reprogramming in mammalian development. Nature reviews. Genetics; 3:662–673.

30. Wu H, Sun YE. (2006) Epigenetic regulation of stem cell differentiation. Pediatric research; 59:21R–25R.

31. Okano M, Bell DW, Haber DA, Li E. (1999) DNA methyltransferases Dnmt3a and Dnmt3b are essential for de novo methylation and mammalian development. Cell; 99:247–257.

32. Fan G, Martinowich K, Chin MH, et al. (2005) DNA methylation controls the timing of astrogliogenesis through regulation of JAK-STAT signaling. Development; 132:3345–3356.

33. Fan G, Beard C, Chen RZ, et al. (2001) DNA hypomethylation perturbs the function and survival of CNS neurons in postnatal animals. Journal of neuroscience research; 21:788–797.

34. Feng J, Chang H, Li E, Fan G. (2005) Dynamic expression of de novo DNA methyltransferases Dnmt3a and Dnmt3b in the central nervous system. Journal of neuroscience research; 79:734–746.

35. Watanabe D, Suetake I, Tajima S, Hanaoka K. (2004) Expression of Dnmt3b in mouse hematopoietic progenitor cells and spermatogonia at specific stages. Gene expression patterns; 5:43–49.

36. Bai S, Ghoshal K, Datta J, et al. (2005) DNA methyltransferase 3b regulates nerve growth factor-induced differentiation of PC12 cells by recruiting histone deacetylase 2. Molecular and cellular biology; 25:751–766.
37. Shimozaki K, Namihira M, Nakashima K, Taga T. (2005) Stage- and site-specific DNA demethylation during neural cell development from embryonic stem cells. Journal of neurochemistry; 93:432–439.
38. Chen WG, Chang Q, Lin Y, et al. (2003) Derepression of BDNF transcription involves calcium-dependent phosphorylation of MeCP2. Science; 302:885–889.
39. Martinowich K, Hattori D, Wu H, et al. (2003) DNA methylation-related chromatin remodeling in activity-dependent BDNF gene regulation. Science; 302:890–893.
40. Zhao X, Ueba T, Christie BR, et al. (2003) Mice lacking methyl-CpG binding protein 1 have deficits in adult neurogenesis and hippocampal function. Proceedings of the National Academy of Sciences of the United States of America; 100:6777–6782.
41. Ballas N, Mandel G. (2005) The many faces of REST oversee epigenetic programming of neuronal genes. Current opinion in neurobiology; 15:500–506.
42. Jepsen K, Hermanson O, Onami TM, et al. (2000) Combinatorial roles of the nuclear receptor corepressor in transcription and development. Cell; 102:753–763.
43. Naruse Y, Aoki T, Kojima T, Mori N. (1999) Neural restrictive silencer factor recruits mSin3 and histone deacetylase complex to repress neuron-specific target genes. Proceedings of the National Academy of Sciences of the United States of America; 96:13691–13696.
44. Ooi L, Wood IC. (2007) Chromatin crosstalk in development and disease: lessons from REST. Nature review. Genetics; 8:544–554.
45. Greenway DJ, Street M, Jeffries A, Buckley NJ. (2007) RE1 Silencing transcription factor maintains a repressive chromatin environment in embryonic hippocampal neural stem cells. Stem cells; 25:354–363.
46. Kuwabara T, Hsieh J, Nakashima K, Taira K, Gage FH. (2004) A small modulatory dsRNA specifies the fate of adult neural stem cells. Cell; 116:779–793.
47. Otto SJ, McCorkle SR, Hover J, et al. (2007) A new binding motif for the transcriptional repressor REST uncovers large gene networks devoted to neuronal functions. Journal of neuroscience research; 27:6729–6739.
48. Wu JI, Lessard J, Olave IA, et al. (2007) Regulation of dendritic development by neuron-specific chromatin remodeling complexes. Neuron; 56:94–108.
49. Sahin M, Greer PL, Lin MZ, et al. (2005) Eph-dependent tyrosine phosphorylation of ephexin1 modulates growth cone collapse. Neuron; 46:191–204.
50. Shamah SM, Lin MZ, Goldberg JL, et al. (2001) EphA receptors regulate growth cone dynamics through the novel guanine nucleotide exchange factor ephexin. Cell; 105:233–244.
51. Bartel DP. (2004) MicroRNAs: genomics, biogenesis, mechanism, and function. Cell; 116:281–297.
52. Du T, Zamore PD. (2005) microPrimer: the biogenesis and function of microRNA. Development; 132:4645–4652.
53. Wienholds E, Plasterk RH. (2005) MicroRNA function in animal development. FEBS letters; 579:5911–5922.
54. Houbaviy HB, Murray MF, Sharp PA. (2003) Embryonic stem cell-specific MicroRNAs. Developmental Cell; 5:351–358.
55. Suh MR, Lee Y, Kim JY, et al. (2004) Human embryonic stem cells express a unique set of microRNAs. Developmental biology; 270:488–498.
56. Johnston RJ, Hobert O. (2003) A microRNA controlling left/right neuronal asymmetry in Caenorhabditis elegans. Nature; 426:845–849.
57. Chang S, Johnston RJ, Jr., Frokjaer-Jensen C, Lockery S, Hobert O. (2004) MicroRNAs act sequentially and asymmetrically to control chemosensory laterality in the nematode. Nature; 430:785–789.
58. Giraldez AJ, Cinalli RM, Glasner ME, et al. (2005) MicroRNAs regulate brain morphogenesis in zebrafish. Science; 308:833–838.

59. Krichevsky AM, Sonntag KC, Isacson O, Kosik KS. (2006) Specific microRNAs modulate embryonic stem cell-derived neurogenesis. Stem cells; 24:857–864.
60. Smirnova L, Grafe A, Seiler A, et al. (2005) Regulation of miRNA expression during neural cell specification. The European journal of neuroscience; 21:1469–1477.
61. Wu J, Xie X. (2006) Comparative sequence analysis reveals an intricate network among REST, CREB and miRNA in mediating neuronal gene expression. Genome biology; 7:R85.
62. Conaco C, Otto S, Han JJ, Mandel G. (2006) Reciprocal actions of REST and a microRNA promote neuronal identity. Proceedings of the National Academy of Sciences of the United States of America; 103:2422–2427.

Chapter 5
Neural Stem Cells and Neurogenic Niche in the Adult Brain

Xuekun Li, Basam Z. Barkho, and Xinyu Zhao*

Abstract The discovery of adult neurogenesis has greatly advanced our knowledge of the human brain. During the past 50 years, the regulatory mechanisms and potential functions of this intriguing process have been extensively investigated. Our current knowledge supports the model that adult neurogenesis is regulated by both intrinsic genetic and epigenetic programs and extrinsic microenvironment and stimuli. This intricate molecular network has profound roles in controlling the self-renewal and multipotency of neural stem cells, the cellular basis of adult neurogenesis. In this review, we will summarize the current knowledge and our recent work in understanding adult neurogenesis with emphasis on answering two questions: how intrinsic epigenetic mechanisms, mediated through histone modifications, non-coding RNAs, and DNA methylation, define the signature of adult neural stem cells, and how extrinsic effects of growth factors, cytokines, and chemokines contribute to the adult neurogenic niche.

Keywords Adult neurogenesis, neural stem cells, epigenetics, DNA methylation, cytokine, migration

5.1 Introduction

Neural stem cells (NSCs) are multipotent cells that are characterized by their abilities to self-renew and to generate differentiated cells in the nervous system. Neurogenesis is defined as the process of generating new neurons from NSCs, which consists of the proliferation and fate determination of NSCs, migration and survival of young neurons, and maturation and integration of newly matured

---

Department of Neurosciences, University of New Mexico School of Medicine, Albuquerque, NM 87131, USA

*Corresponding Author:
MSC 08 4740, 915 Camino de Salud NE, Albuquerque, NM 87131-0001
e-mail: xzhao@salud.unm.edu

neurons [1]. Since the discovery of adult neurogenesis, neuroscientists and developmental biologists have been exploring the regulatory mechanisms and functions
of this fascinating process. Our current knowledge supports the model that adult
neurogenesis is regulated by both intrinsic programs and extrinsic modulators.
Intrinsic programs include genes, genetic background, and epigenetic modifications that are essential for controlling NSC self-renewal and multipotency. Extrinsic
factors include both the microenvironment where NSCs physically reside and the
stimuli that NSCs receive due to endocrinal, physiological and pathological changes
(see a recent review by [2]). Although many significant advances have been made,
more challenges are ahead of us in understanding how these regulatory mechanisms
coordinately modulate neurogenesis and define neurogenic niche in adult mammalian brains. In this review, we will summarize our current knowledge of neurogenesis in the adult mammalian brain, with focus on the emerging function of epigenetic
mechanisms in regulating NSC intrinsic properties and the potential roles of injury-
induced cytokines and chemokines in modulating neurogenic niche.

5.2   Neurogenesis in the Adult Brain

The discovery of adult neurogenesis has completely changed our opinion about the
potential of adult brains. It was Joseph Altman who initiated this breakthrough [3,
4] and his 1965 publication in the Journal of Comparative Neurology is widely
considered as the inaugural study in the field of adult neurogenesis [5]. Michael
Kaplan further confirmed the presence of neurogenesis in the adult hippocampus
and olfactory bulb using electron microscopy [6]. The finding of ongoing neurogenesis in adult songbirds by Fernando Nottebohm has provided the first evidence
for the potential functions of adult neurogenesis [7]. In 1992, Reynolds and Weiss
isolated neural stem/progenitor cells (NSPCs) from adult mouse brains, therefore
providing the cellular basis for adult neurogenesis [8]. However, the identity of
NSCs in vivo is still a controversial issue due to lack of a well-characterized marker
that is specific for NSCs. To date, it is well accepted that adult mammalian brains
have two regions with persistent neurogenic capabilities: one is the subventricular
zone (SVZ) in the lateral ventricle and another one is the subgranular zone (SGZ)
in the dentate gyrus of the hippocampus. The presence of neurogenesis in these two
regions has been demonstrated in many species including primates [9, 10] and
humans [11, 12]. Why only these two regions have the ability to generate new neurons in the adult brain is a fundamental question remaining to be answered.

5.2.1   Neurogenesis in the SVZ

In 1993, Marla Luskin found that some cells from the anterior SVZ of neonatal rat
pups exclusively generate neuronal progenitor cells, and these cells migrate along a

restricted pathway referred to as rostral migratory stream (RMS) to the olfactory bulb [13]. Later, it was found that this chain migration also exists in the adult mouse [14] and primate brain [9, 10]. Although an earlier study failed to demonstrate a RMS structure and chain migration in human brains [15], a recent study, using more refined techniques, has clearly shown that human brains also have a RMS where migratory cells express PSA-NCAM, a marker for neuroblast [11]. The identity of NSCs in the adult SVZ is not fully clear. SVZ has at least four types of cells that are involved in neurogenesis [16]. A small number of slow dividing glial fibrillary acidic protein (GFAP)-positive cells (GFAP-positive, Type B cells) could be NSCs because these cells give rise to rapidly dividing transient amplifying cells (Type C cells), which in turn produce neuronal progenitor cells (Type A cells or neuroblasts) [17–19]. Neuroblasts derived from SVZ stem cells express immature neuronal markers DCX, PSA-NCAM, and Type III β-tubulin (TuJI) and tangentially migrate along the RMS to the olfactory bulb [13, 14]. During the migration, these cells continue to divide, but the cell cycle is lengthened [20]. When they arrive at the end of the RMS, residing in the core of olfactory bulb, they exit from the RMS, switch to a radial migration pattern, and differentiate into mature interneurons in the granule layer and periglomerular layer of the olfactory bulb [13, 14].

5.2.2 Neurogenesis in the SGZ

In the SGZ of the hippocampus, some GFAP-positive cells have also been shown to be slow dividing NSCs [21]. These GFAP-positive NSCs proliferate in the SGZ and produce new neurons, which migrate into the granule cell layer and become mature granule neurons in the dentate gyrus [1]. It was proposed that the neurogenic process in the SGZ could be separated into six developmental stages [22]: The NSCs, similar to the Type B cells in SVZ (stage 1), generate transient amplifying progenitor cells (type IIa, IIb, and III cells) that then differentiate into immature neurons and establish initial connections with other cells (stage 5). At stage 6, immature neurons become mature granule neurons and form functional synapses. From the initial differentiation of NSCs to the synaptic integration of new neurons takes about 2–4 weeks (see a recent review [1]). During this process, cells at different stages can be distinguished by stage-specific markers (Table 5.1).

5.2.3 Neurogenesis in Other Adult Brain Regions

In healthy adult brains, the presence of neurogenesis in regions other than the SGZ and SVZ is still controversial. Several studies demonstrated the presence of neurogenesis in the neocortex of healthy adult primates [23, 24], whereas other studies contradict these findings [25, 26]. Neurogenesis in adult substantia nigra [27] is also contradicted by other studies [28–31]. One study found neurogenesis in adult

Table 5.1 Histological markers that are commonly used for cell lineage analysis (This table was created based on published literature [1, 22, 106, 140–142])

Cell types	Histological marker
Neural stem cells	GFAP, Nestin, Prominin, SOX-2
Proliferating cells	Ki-67, BrdU, PCNA
Immature neurons	β-Tubulin, DCX, PSA-NCAM
Radial glia	GLAST, RC2
Mature neurons	NeuN, MAP-2, NF, BLBP
Astrocytes	GFAP, S-100β, GLAST, Vimentin
Oligodendrocyte precursors	NG2
Oligodendrocytes	O4, MBP, RIP

GFAP, Glial fibrillary acidic protein; BrdU, 5-bromo-2-deoxyuridine; PCNA, proliferating cell nuclear antigen; DCX, doublecortin; PSA-NACM, polysialiclyliated neural cell adhesion molecule; GLAST, glutamine transporter; NeuN, neuronal neuclei; MAP2, microtuble-associated protein 2; NF, neurofilament; BLBP, brain lipid binding protein; O4, oligodendrocyte 4; MBP, myelin basic protein.

hypothalamus [32], which has yet to be further confirmed. The inconsistency of some of these data could be due to technical issues in staging neurons that are double labeled with the proliferation marker BrdU.

5.2.4 Functions of Adult Neurogenesis

The most exciting aspect of adult neurogenesis is its potential function. The meaning of 'function' can be understood at two levels. First, the new neurons could integrate into the existing neural networks and contribute to synaptic plasticity in normal adult brains. Second, under pathological conditions, such as disease or injury, new neurons could replace the injured neurons and participate in functional recovery.

The hippocampus is one of the most plastic regions in the adult brain, likely due to its role as a short-term information processing and storage site during adult learning and memory [33]. Intriguingly, there seems to be a positive correlation between the levels of adult hippocampal neurogenesis and the ability of hippocampus-dependent learning and memory. Extensive studies have shown that both hippocampal neurogenesis and adult learning are modulated by many physiological or pathological conditions [2]. For example, mice living in an enriched environment have more new neurons in the adult hippocampus as well as improved hippocampal-dependent learning abilities. This effect was also found in aged mice [34]. Furthermore, voluntary physical exercise (wheel running) promotes both adult hippocampal neurogenesis and learning [35]. Hormonal (e.g., estrogen) and antidepressant treatments lead to increased hippocampal neurogenesis and learning, whereas depression, chronic drug abuse, neural inflammation, and cell proliferation inhibitor result in decreased neurogenesis and learning [2, 36–39]. On the other hand, more new neurons are not always good, as in the case of epilepsy [40–42]. Therefore, direct evidence supporting the functional outcome of adult hippocampal neurogenesis is still lacking.

Neural injuries can lead to increased neurogenesis [2]. Stroke results in localized cell death. Recent experimental findings raise the possibility that functional improvement after stroke may be achieved through neuronal replacement by endogenous NSCs residing in the adult brain. The primary evidence is that, at 1 week following brain injury, there is increased cell proliferation in the SVZ of adult rodents. At 2 weeks post-injury, newly-generated cells have traveled from the SVZ and RMS into the damaged area (distances up to 2 mm in length), where some have been found to express mature neuronal markers at later time points [43–46] and to form synapses [47]. Since progenitor cells localized in striatal parenchyma could also be activated by growth factors, some of these new cells might originate locally at the striatal parenchyma [48, 49]. These studies suggest a compensatory role of neurogenesis which may contribute to functional recovery after brain injury [43, 44]. However, the number of neurons generated from endogenous NSCs is extremely small (approximately 0.2% of the lost striatal neurons) and the survival of these new neurons in the lesion area is minimal, posing a great challenge for therapeutic applications.

To prove that adult neurogenesis is functional, it is essential to demonstrate that new neurons form functional synapses and integrate into neural networks. Using retroviral marking, immunohistology, electrophysiological recording, and electron microscopy, several research groups have found that, at 4 weeks post-labeling, some of the new granule neurons have integrated into the neural network and exhibit electrophysiological properties similar to other mature granule neurons [50–53]. Interestingly, the development of these new neurons in the adult brains recapitulates that in the embryonic brains, with immature neurons displaying excitatory GABA current and mature neurons exhibiting inhibitory GABA current [52, 54]. Whether these new neurons contribute to the functional outcome of adult brains remains to be investigated.

5.3 Intrinsic Genetic and Epigenetic Regulation of Neurogenesis

The intrinsic mechanisms controlling the self-renewal and fate specification of adult NSCs are complex and not well understood. It was found that mice of different genetic backgrounds exhibit distinct levels of adult neurogenesis both in standard housing conditions and during voluntary physical exercise [55, 56], suggesting that heritable genetic and epigenetic programs are modulating adult neurogenesis. At single gene levels, many growth and cell cycle related genes are directly involved in the regulation of adult NSCs [1]. For example, cell growth and tumor suppressor phosphatase, PTEN, is critical in regulating the proliferation of NSCs, and its mutation leads to increased NSC self-renewal [57], neuronal positioning, and cell migration [58], and subsequently an enlarged brain size [59]. The basic helix-loop-helix proteins,

Hairy/Enhancer of split family protein Hes1 and Hes5, inhibit neuronal differentiation and promote astrocyte differentiation of NSCs [60, 61], whereas Hes6 enhances neuronal fate determination and represses astrocyte differentiation [62]. Cell cycle inhibitors p21 and p27 inhibit the proliferation of NSCs and are essential for normal CNS development [63, 64]. Mutation of Ataxia Telangiectasia Mutated, a DNA repair protein, leads to genomic instability and reduced neuronal differentiation of adult NSCs [65]. Orphan steroid receptor TLX maintains adult NSCs in a proliferative and undifferentiated state, and TLX-null NSCs fail to proliferate [66].

Recently, epigenetic mechanisms have come to the center stage of neurogenic regulations. Epigenetic mechanisms refer to meiotically and mitotically heritable changes in gene expression that are not coded in the DNA sequence itself [67]. In mammals, epigenetic mechanisms include DNA methylation [68], histone modification [69], and noncoding RNAs-mediated gene regulations [70].

5.3.1   Histone Modification

In eukaryotic cells, the basic unit of chromatin is formed by 146 base pairs of DNA wrapping around the histone octamer. The core histones H2A, H2B, H3, and H4 are subject to dozens of different modifications, including acetylation, methylation, and phosphorylation. Among these modifications, lysine (K) acetylation and methylation are the best-understood [71]. Initial histone modification studies focused largely on histone acetylation that is catalyzed by two opposing enzymes, histone acetyltransferease (HAT) and histone deacetylase (HDAC). At least eight HATs and nine HDACs have been identified in mammals [72]. The activities of HATs and HDACs can directly affect adult NSCs and adult neurogenesis. For example, neuron-specific genes share the conserved 21–23-base pair DNA response element, RE-1 (repressor element 1). Neuronal restricted silencing factor (NRSF or REST) binds to RE-1 and forms a complex that represses non-neuronal gene expression by recruiting HDAC1/2 and Sin3A [73–76]. Treatment of adult NSPCs by volporic acid (VPA), a HDAC inhibitor and antiepileptic medicine, leads to reduced proliferation, increased neuronal differentiation, and decreased astrocyte and oligodendrocyte differentiation through activating a pan-neuronal transcription factor NeuroD1 [77]. More recently, Jessberger et al. further confirmed that VPA treatment attenuates seizure-induced aberrant neurogenesis through regulating NRSF and HDACs [78]. In the developing brain, VPA administration also induces the significant hypomyelination and delays the differentiation of oligodendrocytes through inhibiting the activity of HDACs [79]. Histone methylation plays an important role in embryonic stem cell (ESC) development, cell fate determination, and X-chromosome inactivation [80, 81]. The patterns of histone H3K4 methylation (an active chromatin mark), H3K27 methylation (a temporary inactive chromatin mark), and H3K9 methylation (a long term repressive chromatin mark) define the chromatin state of NSCs [82]. Mutation of Bmi-I, a component of polycomb group proteins with H3K27 methylase activity, results in reduced self-renewal of adult

NSCs [83]. The chromatin state of NSCs is distinct from those of ESCs or differentiated cell types [82]. It is likely that during NSC differentiation, the chromatin state that defines the NSC signature shifts towards the chromatin states corresponding to those of more differentiated cell types, therefore, the epigenetic landscapes could be a much more precise marker for stem cell signature than the expression patterns of single genes.

5.3.2 Non-coding Small RNAs

In 1960s, messenger RNAs (mRNAs) were demonstrated to carry the genetic information, while ribosomal RNAs (rRNAs) and transfer RNAs (tRNAs) that did not code protein but facilitated protein synthesis were termed non-coding RNAs. Today, the non-coding RNA world has changed dramatically as new members, such as small nuclear RNAs (snRNAs), microRNAs (miRNAs), small nucleolar RNAs (snoRNAs), short interfering RNAs (siRNAs), repeat-associated small interfering RNAs (rasiRNAs) and others have been discovered [84]. The biological functions of most of these newly discovered noncoding RNAs are still unclear. The biogenesis and functions of microRNAs (miRNAs) are among the best studied noncoding RNAs. The gene coding miRNA is transcribed into primary miRNA by RNA polymerase II, and primary miRNA is then processed by RNase III Drosha into 70–100 nucleotide precursor miRNA. Precursor miRNA is transported into cytoplasm by exportin-5, and further processed by RNase III Dicer to form mature miRNA [85]. Mature miRNAs are single-stranded and composed of 20–25 nucleotides. Nearly 500 known human miRNA sequences have been identified. miRNA incorporates into a multi-protein complex known as RNA-induced silencing complex (RISC). miRNA directs RISC to the target mRNAs based on sequence homology, which leads to either degradation of mRNA or the translational suppression of target genes [85, 86, 87]. miRNAs are especially abundant in the brain, play crucial roles in nervous system development, and are involved in multiple cellular activities, including developmental timing, cell death, cell specification, cell proliferation, homeostasis, apoptosis, and neural patterning [86, 87]. It has been shown that the expression patterns of small RNAs undergo dynamic changes during the differentiation of human ESCs into neuronal progenitors and mature neurons [88, 89]. Exogenous expression of neuronal-enriched miR124a and miR9 in ESCs inhibit their differentiation into astrocytes by modulating the STAT3 pathway that is critical for astrocyte differentiation [90]. In addition, miR124a can also down-regulate the expression of small C-terminal domain phosphatase 1 (an anti-neuronal phosphatase) and promote pro-neuronal RNA splicing and thus neurogenesis [91, 92]. Studies have also revealed critical modulatory roles of miRNAs in neuronal synapse development by regulating protein synthesis at synaptic terminals [93, 94]. Since each miRNA can target multiple mRNAs and each mRNA can be regulated by several miRNAs, miRNA, as well as other noncoding small RNAs, may create another dimension of complexity in the regulatory mechanisms of adult neurogenesis.

5.3.3 DNA Methylation

DNA methylation is a covalent modification of cytosine at the position C5 in CpG dinucleotides. In mammals, over 70% of CpG dinucleotides are methylated and nearly all DNA methylation occurs on CpG dinucleotides. Unmethylated CpG patches are usually found in the promoters and the first exons, termed CpG islands [95]. DNA methylation is catalyzed by three DNA methyltransferases (DNMTs). The *de novo* establishment of DNA methylation relies on DNMT3a and 3b, whereas, the maintenance of DNA methylation depends on DNMT1 that specifically recognizes semi-methylated DNA and methylates the remaining strand [96]. Mammalian DNA methylation has been implicated in a diverse range of cellular functions, including tissue-specific gene expression, cell differentiation, genomic imprinting, and X chromosome inactivation [97]. DNA methylation represses gene expression by either directly blocking the binding of transcription factors [98] or by recruiting a family of methylated-CpG binding proteins (MBDs) many of which share homology only in their methyl-CpG binding (MBD) domains [97].

The MBD protein family includes MBD1, MBD2, MBD3, MBD4, MeCP2, Keiso, and several newly discovered members [99]. MBD1/Mbd1 is a multifunctional protein that is localized in both euchromatin and heterochromatin. MBD1 has two DNA-binding domains; the MBD domain specifically recognizes methylated CpGs, and a zinc finger (CXXC3) domain specifically binds unmethylated CpG. The presence of two DNA binding domains in MBD1 may contribute to higher affinity and specificity in binding DNA sequences [100]. The transcriptional repression by MBD1 can be facilitated by several putative cofactors [101], and it is likely that MBD1 represses transcription through various mechanisms, depending on the genes and cell types. However, despite great effort, few MBD1 target genes have been identified. Moreover, although recent literature suggests that each MBD protein may have its own preferred binding sites in the genome [102], current available structure-function data have not provided sequence specificity other than CpGs. Although extensive *in vitro* analyses have suggested a role for MBD1 in transcriptional repression [103], chromatin assembly [103, 104], and heterochromatin structure maintenance, the biological function of MBD1 is not well understood [105].

In adult mouse brain, Mbd1 is localized in both neurons and a subset of nestin-positive immature cells in the germinal zone of the hippocampus (SGZ) [106], suggesting that Mbd1 may regulate the functions of adult NSPCs. Mbd1 mutant (*Mbd1*$^{-/-}$) mice develop normally into adulthood, with no detectable developmental defect, except for mild reduction in forebrain weight, indicating that early development of the brain may be suboptimal in the absence of Mbd1. In the *Mbd1*$^{-/-}$ hippocampus, cell proliferation level is normal, but the survival of newborn cells is significantly reduced and the neuronal differentiation capacity of newborn cells is also decreased. As a possible consequence, *Mbd1*$^{-/-}$ dentate gyrus has reduced cell density. In addition, adult *Mbd1*$^{-/-}$ mice have spatial learning deficits and markedly reduced dentate gyrus-specific long term potentiation, a proposed cellular mechanism for learning and memory [106]. Recently, we have found that these mice also exhibit increased anxiety, depression, and reduced social interaction (Allan and Zhao, unpublished results), suggesting that Mbd1 is involved in multiple brain pathways and functions. At a cellular level, NSPCs isolated from adult $Mbd1^{-/-}$ mice have a reduced neuronal differentiation capacity in vitro, consistent with our in vivo findings [106]. In addition, $Mbd1^{-/-}$ NSPCs have increased genomic instability and increased expression of endogenous stem cell mitogen fibroblast growth factor (Fgf-2). Fgf-2 is a potent growth factor for a large number of cell types and its over-expression has been found in many transformed tumor cells including glioma cells with possible NSC origin [107]. We hypothesized that Mbd1 regulates the expression of endogenous Fgf-2 in adult NSPCs, and therefore affects the neuronal differentiation of adult NSPCs. To test his hypothesis, we acutely knocked down Mbd1 in NSPCs using lentivirus expressing Mbd1-RNAi and found that this manipulation led to increased Fgf-2 levels. On the other hand, when we over-expressed exogenous Mbd1 in adult NSPCs using lentivirus, we found that Fgf-2 levels were decreased. Furthermore, we determined that Fgf-2 expression in adult NSPCs is modulated by DNA methylation (data not shown), and DNA methylation of the Fgf-2 promoter was decreased in $Mbd1^{-/-}$ NSPCs, which could be responsible for increased Fgf-2 levels in these cells. To study the functional significance of abnormally high levels of Fgf-2 in $Mbd1^{-/-}$ NSPCs, we infected NSPCs with lentivirus over-expressing recombinant Fgf-2. We found that the Fgf-2-expressing lentivirus-infected NSPCs exhibited higher levels of proliferation (data not shown) and lower levels of neuronal differentiation compared to control GFP-expressing lentivirus-infected NSPCs. These data suggest that the levels of mitogen Fgf-2 expressed intrinsically by adult NSPCs are modulated by Mbd1 and DNA methylated-mediated epigenetic regulation. Such regulation could have a significant role in regulating NSPC differentiation and proliferation.

5.4 Extrinsic Factors Contribute to the Neurogenic Niche

A fundamental question in understanding adult neurogenesis is why only the SVZ and SGZ have neurogenic capabilities in healthy adult mammalian brains. One possible reason is that these two regions comprise a special niche that is permissive for neurogenesis [19, 108]. This proposal is supported by the following: First, a subpopulation of GFAP-positive "astrocytes" in the SVZ and SGZ are found to be NSCs, but astrocytes outside the SVZ and SGZ do not exhibit neurogenic potential under normal conditions [17, 109]. Second, multipotent neuroprogenitors (NSPCs) can be isolated from many different adult brain regions, including postmortem human white matter [110, 111]. These multipotent progenitors can differentiate into both neurons and glia when transplanted into neurogenic regions but into only glia when grafted into other non-neurogenic brain regions [108, 112]. Third, certain classical signaling pathways that play critical roles during the embryonic brain development, including Wnt [113], Notch [114], and Shh [115], are still active in the adult SGZ and SVZ [15, 19, 116]. Fourth, using gene expression profiling, we have identified groups of genes that are differentially expressed in neurogenic (adult dentate gyrus) versus non-neurogenic regions (adult CA1 and adult spinal cord) [117]. Finally, astrocytes derived from neurogenic tissues can support neuronal differentiation of cultured NSPCs while those derived from non-neurogenic tissues inhibit neuronal differentiation of NSPCs [118]. In the following text, we dissect some components of the neurogenic niche.

5.4.1 Growth Factor and Neurovascular Components of Stem Cell Niche

In the SGZ and SVZ, fast proliferating neural progenitors are frequently localized near blood vessels, and were found in clusters associated with the vasculature, suggesting a possible interaction between NSCs and blood vessels [119]. Administration of exogenous vascular endothelial growth factor (VEGF) not only promotes the proliferation of vascular endothelial cells, but also increases the number of immature neuronal cells [120–122]. Endothelial cells could release soluble factors that stimulate self-renewal, inhibit differentiation, and enhance neuronal production of NSPCs [123]. It has been demonstrated that DCX-positive neuroblasts are in close proximity to the endothelial cells of vasculature, suggesting a possible mechanism by which the neuroblasts migrate along the endothelial cell trails to reach the olfactory bulb [43]. Furthermore, a conditioned medium from endothelial cells has been shown to induce NSPC differentiation into endothelial cells, suggesting a possible role of adult NSCs in angiogenesis [124].

5.4.2 Extrinsic Cytokines and Chemokines Contribute to the Neurogenic Niche

During embryonic neurogenesis, neurons are formed before glia. However, NSCs and new neurons in adult brains are in intimate contact with surrounding glia [108]. In a landmark study, Song et al demonstrated that astrocytes isolated from neurogenesis-supporting tissues (newborn and adult hippocampus or newborn spinal cord) promote in vitro neuronal differentiation of adult NSPCs, while astrocytes isolated from neurogenesis-inhibiting tissues (adult spinal cord or adult skin fibroblasts) inhibit neurogenesis [118]. To identify the genes that are responsible for the differential effects of these astrocytes, we performed gene expression arrays and found that 36.6% detectable genes are differentially expressed among these primary astrocytes [125]. To determine whether the genes differentially expressed in neurogenesis supporting tissues [117, 126] and astrocytes [125] are critical in defining the neurogenic niche, we studied the effects of a subset of these genes that express either secreted or cell surface proteins on NSC differentiation and proliferation. Interestingly, many of them encode cytokines, chemokines, and inflammation-related proteins. Among the cytokines, interleukin (IL) 1β (20 ng/ ml) and IL-6 (20 ng/ml) are highly expressed by neurogenesis-promoting astrocytes, and both of them could enhance neuronal differentiation without affecting NSPC proliferation and survival [125]. Because the majority of candidate neurogenesis-promoting cytokines did not show significant effect on NSPC neuronal differentiation when applied alone, we also tested several different combinations of these cytokines.

We used NSPCs infected by lentivirus-expressing luciferase driven by an early pan neuronal transcription factor, NeuroD1 to screen for the best combinations of these factors that could promote neurogenesis. We then further confirmed these results using immunostaining and stereological quantification. We found that a combination of IL-1β, IL-6, vascular cell adhesion molecule-1 (VCAM-1), interferon-induced protein 10 (IP-10, also known as CXCL10), cathepsin S, and TGF-β2 had the strongest effect on NSPC neuronal differentiation (Fig. 5.1). The effect of this combination was significantly higher than IL-1β or IL-6 alone. Our data suggest that inflammatory cytokines could promote neurogenesis and be a necessary component for adult neurogenic niche. In a separate study, Palmer's group has shown that, when treated with high levels of IL-6 (60 ng/ml) for longer periods of time (similar to chronic neural inflammation), NSPCs had reduced neurogenesis

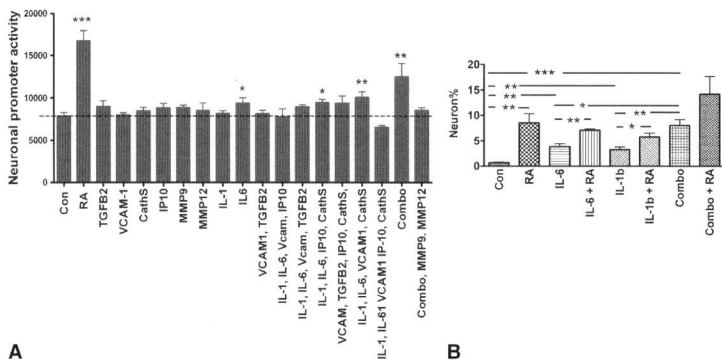

Fig. 5.1 A combination of factors expressed at higher levels by neurogenesis-promoting astrocytes and tissues promote neuronal differentiation of NSPCs. (**A**) The combination of IL-1β, IL-6,VCAM1, IP-10, cathepsin S, and TGF-β2 (Combo), enhanced NeuroD1 promoter activity in NSPCs, analyzed by luciferase activity assays (*, p < 0.05; **, p < 0.01; ***, p < 0.001, n = 14. unpaired, two-tailed, student's t-test). (**B**) IL-1 β, IL-6, and Combo could promote neuronal differentiation of NSPCs indicated by the percentage of TuJ1-positive neurons, as analyzed by immunofluorescent staining and quantification. "Combo" was significantly more potent than IL-1β and IL-6 alone (*, p < 0.05; **, p < 0.01; ***, p < 0.001. unpaired, two-tailed, student's t-test)

[127]. In addition, ciliary neurotrophic factor (CNTF) and cardiotrophin-1 (CT-1), two members of the IL-6 family, led to reduced neurogenesis, but increased glial genesis in adult NSPCs [128, 129]. Therefore, cytokines at the neurogenic niche could have differential effects on adult NSCs, depending on the concentration and context. On the other hand, the adult neurogenic niche could also be defined by the absence of neurogenic inhibitory factors. IGFBP6, a negative regulator of IGF signaling pathway with high specificity for binding IGF-II [130], and decorin, an extracellular proteoglycan that can inhibit several cytokines including TGFβ2 [131], have higher expression levels in neurogenesis-inhibitory tissues/astrocytes and these two factors inhibited the neuronal differentiation of adult NSPCs in our in vitro assays [125]. Other neurogenesis-inhibitory factors, such as NOGO, ephrin-A5 and MAG, have been found in regions that do not support neurogenesis [132]. In addition, BMP signaling inhibits neurogenesis and promotes glial genesis, which is antagonized by Noggin, secreted by adult ependymal cells at the SVZ [133]. Pigment epithelium–derived factor (PEDF) is expressed by ependymal and endothelial cells in adult SVZ, and has been shown to promote NSC self-renewal both in vitro and in vivo [134]. Intraventricular administration of PEDF could activate the slowly dividing NSCs without changing their proliferation rate [134]. Therefore, specific positive and negative factors are essential for specifying neurogenic niche in adult brains.

As described above, ischemic injuries lead to increased neurogenesis in the adult brain. Neuroblasts generated in the SVZ migrate to the ischemic area of striatum [46]. Extensive efforts have been devoted to understanding this injury-induced neurogenic response with the hope that we can develop therapeutic methods to repair neurological injuries [2]. It is currently known that during brain injuries, there is an increase in the number and amount of cytokines and chemokines in and around the injured area. In the CNS, chemokines are typically known for a role in cell migration during brain development. For example, stromal cell-derived factor 1 (SDF-1) has been shown to have an obligatory role in neuronal migration during the formation of the granule-cell layer of the cerebellum [135]. However, upon neuroinflammatory injury, such as multiple sclerosis or stroke, chemokines have been reported to attract inflammatory cells to cause cell death in the diseased or

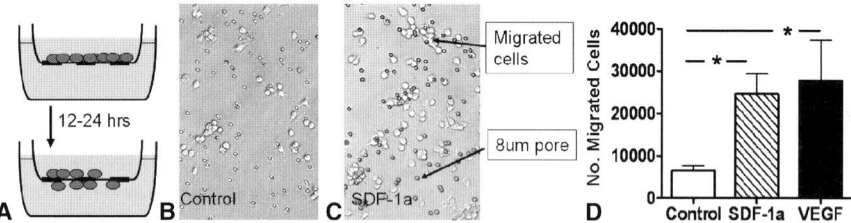

Fig. 5.2 Cytokines promote the migration of NSPC-derived cells. (**A**) A schematic drawing illustrates the in vitro cell migration assay. (**B–D**) SDF-α and VEGF promote the migration of NSPCs-derived cells. **B** and **C** are phase contrast photos showing migrated cells in the bottom chambers of control (**B**) and SDF-α treated (**C**) cells; **D** is quantification of migrated cells in control (no chemokines added), SDF-α, and VEGF treated samples (*, p < 0.05, n = 4)

injured regions. These injury-induced factors have been shown to be produced by reactive cells, such as astrocytes and immune cells within the lesion area. But several of these factors have displayed chemo-attractive roles for other cells after brain injury. For instance, both SDF-1α and VEGF have been well-characterized to attract NSC-derived cells [136–138]. Both embryonic and adult NSCs express the receptors for SDF-1α (CXCR4) and VEGF (VEGF-R2) [139], further supporting the notion that these chemokines have an important role in regulating the migration of NSC-derived cells. Using a modified Boyden chamber assay, we have demonstrated that adult NSCs migrate towards higher concentrations of SDF1 and VEGF (Fig. 5.2). Using this in vitro system, we are defining the molecular signature of migratory cells with the goal of optimizing the neurogenic potential in response to injury cues.

5.5 Concluding Remarks

Previous studies have confirmed the presence of neurogenesis in adult mammalian brains, demonstrated the integration of newborn neurons into the neural network, and established the concept of intrinsic programs and extrinsic niche for NSC regulation. However, critical questions remain regarding the identity of NSCs in vivo, the biological function of adult neurogenesis, and the factors or combination of factors that define the identify of NSCs and direct their fate choices. The regulation of adult neurogenesis and adult NSCs are complex (Fig. 5.3). We anticipate that, during the next few years, emerging new high

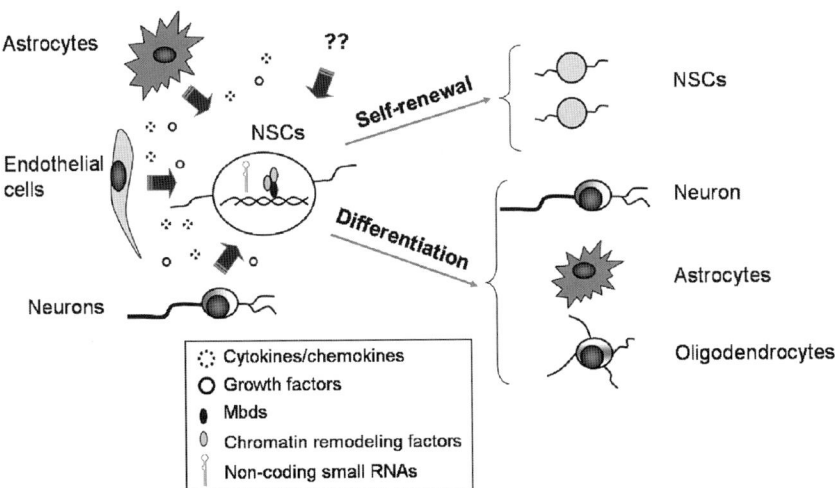

Fig. 5.3 Intrinsic programs and extrinsic niche that may regulate the self-renewal and multipotency of adult NSCs

throughput and high sensitivity technologies will significantly help us to unveil the intricate intrinsic and extrinsic molecular networks that regulate adult neurogenesis.

Acknowledgement This work was funded by NIH/NIMH, NIH/NCRR/COBRE, International Rett Syndrome Foundation, Oxnard Foundation, and UNM School of Medicine.

References

1. Ming, G. L. & Song, H. (2005) Adult neurogenesis in the mammalian central nervous system. Annu Rev Neurosci 28, 223–50.
2. Zhao, X., Schaffer, D. & Gage, F. (2004) *Stem cells in the Nervous System: Functional and Clinical Implications* (Springer, Berlin/Heidelberg, Germany).
3. Altman, J. (1962) Are new neurons formed in the brains of adult mammals? Science 135, 1127–8.
4. Altman, J. (1963) Autoradiographic investigation of cell proliferation in the brains of rats and cats. Anat Rec 145, 573–91.
5. Altman, J. & Das, G. D. (1965) Autoradiographic and histological evidence of postnatal hippocampal neurogenesis in rats. J Comp Neurol 124, 319–35.
6. Kaplan, M. S. & Hinds, J. W. (1977) Neurogenesis in the adult rat: electron microscopic analysis of light radioautographs. Science 197, 1092–4.
7. Alvarez-Buylla, A. & Nottebohm, F. (1988) Migration of young neurons in adult avian brain. Nature 335, 353–4.
8. Reynolds, B. A. & Weiss, S. (1992) Generation of neurons and astrocytes from isolated cells of the adult mammalian central nervous system. Science 255, 1707–10.
9. Pencea, V., Bingaman, K. D., Freedman, L. J. & Luskin, M. B. (2001) Neurogenesis in the subventricular zone and rostral migratory stream of the neonatal and adult primate forebrain. Exp Neurol 172, 1–16.
10. Kornack, D. R. & Rakic, P. (2001) The generation, migration, and differentiation of olfactory neurons in the adult primate brain. Proc Natl Acad Sci U S A 98, 4752–7.
11. Curtis, M. A., Kam, M., Nannmark, U., Anderson, M. F., Axell, M. Z., Wikkelso, C., Holtas, S., van Roon-Mom, W. M., Bjork-Eriksson, T., Nordborg, C., Frisen, J., Dragunow, M., Faull, R. L. & Eriksson, P. S. (2007) Human neuroblasts migrate to the olfactory bulb via a lateral ventricular extension. Science 315, 1243–9.
12. Eriksson, P. S., Perfilieva, E., Bjork-Eriksson, T., Alborn, A. M., Nordborg, C., Peterson, D. A. & Gage, F. H. (1998) Neurogenesis in the adult human hippocampus. Nat Med 4, 1313–7.
13. Luskin, M. B. (1993) Restricted proliferation and migration of postnatally generated neurons derived from the forebrain subventricular zone. Neuron 11, 173–89.
14. Lois, C., Garcia-Verdugo, J. M. & Alvarez-Buylla, A. (1996) Chain migration of neuronal precursors. Science 271, 978–81.
15. Sanai, N., Tramontin, A. D., Quinones-Hinojosa, A., Barbaro, N. M., Gupta, N., Kunwar, S., Lawton, M. T., McDermott, M. W., Parsa, A. T., Manuel-Garcia Verdugo, J., Berger, M. S. & Alvarez-Buylla, A. (2004) Unique astrocyte ribbon in adult human brain contains neural stem cells but lacks chain migration. Nature 427, 740–4.
16. Doetsch, F., Garcia-Verdugo, J. M. & Alvarez-Buylla, A. (1997) Cellular composition and three-dimensional organization of the subventricular germinal zone in the adult mammalian brain. J Neurosci 17, 5046–61.
17. Doetsch, F., Caille, I., Lim, D. A., Garcia-Verdugo, J. M. & Alvarez-Buylla, A. (1999) Subventricular zone astrocytes are neural stem cells in the adult mammalian brain. Cell 97, 703–16.

18. Alvarez-Buylla, A., Herrera, D. G. & Wichterle, H. (2000) The subventricular zone: source of neuronal precursors for brain repair. Prog Brain Res 127, 1–11.
19. Alvarez-Buylla, A. & Lim, D. A. (2004) For the long run: maintaining germinal niches in the adult brain. Neuron 41, 683–6.
20. Smith, C. M. & Luskin, M. B. (1998) Cell cycle length of olfactory bulb neuronal progenitors in the rostral migratory stream. Dev Dyn 213, 220–7.
21. Seri, B., Garcia-Verdugo, J. M., McEwen, B. S. & Alvarez-Buylla, A. (2001) Astrocytes give rise to new neurons in the adult mammalian hippocampus. J Neurosci 21, 7153–60.
22. Kempermann, G., Jessberger, S., Steiner, B. & Kronenberg, G. (2004) Milestones of neuronal development in the adult hippocampus. Trends Neurosci 27, 447–52.
23. Gould, E., Vail, N., Wagers, M. & Gross, C. G. (2001) Adult-generated hippocampal and neocortical neurons in macaques have a transient existence. Proc Natl Acad Sci U S A 98, 10910–7.
24. Gould, E., Reeves, A. J., Graziano, M. S. & Gross, C. G. (1999) Neurogenesis in the neocortex of adult primates. Science 286, 548–52.
25. Kornack, D. R. & Rakic, P. (2001) Cell proliferation without neurogenesis in adult primate neocortex. Science 294, 2127–30.
26. Koketsu, D., Mikami, A., Miyamoto, Y. & Hisatsune, T. (2003) Nonrenewal of neurons in the cerebral neocortex of adult macaque monkeys. J Neurosci 23, 937–42.
27. Zhao, M., Momma, S., Delfani, K., Carlen, M., Cassidy, R. M., Johansson, C. B., Brismar, H., Shupliakov, O., Frisen, J. & Janson, A. M. (2003) Evidence for neurogenesis in the adult mammalian substantia nigra. Proc Natl Acad Sci U S A 100, 7925–30.
28. Lie, D. C., Dziewczapolski, G., Willhoite, A. R., Kaspar, B. K., Shults, C. W. & Gage, F. H. (2002) The adult substantia nigra contains progenitor cells with neurogenic potential. J Neurosci 22, 6639–49.
29. Chen, Y., Ai, Y., Slevin, J. R., Maley, B. E. & Gash, D. M. (2005) Progenitor proliferation in the adult hippocampus and substantia nigra induced by glial cell line-derived neurotrophic factor. Exp Neurol 196, 87–95.
30. Cooper, O. & Isacson, O. (2004) Intrastriatal transforming growth factor alpha delivery to a model of Parkinson's disease induces proliferation and migration of endogenous adult neural progenitor cells without differentiation into dopaminergic neurons. J Neurosci 24, 8924–31.
31. Frielingsdorf, H., Schwarz, K., Brundin, P. & Mohapel, P. (2004) No evidence for new dopaminergic neurons in the adult mammalian substantia nigra. Proc Natl Acad Sci U S A 101, 10177–82.
32. Kokoeva, M. V., Yin, H. & Flier, J. S. (2007) Evidence for constitutive neural cell proliferation in the adult murine hypothalamus. J Comp Neurol 505, 209–20.
33. Squire, L. R. (1993) The hippocampus and spatial memory. Trends Neurosci 16, 56–7.
34. Kempermann, G., Kuhn, H. G. & Gage, F. H. (1998) Experience-induced neurogenesis in the senescent dentate gyrus. J Neurosci 18, 3206–12.
35. van Praag, H., Kempermann, G. & Gage, F. H. (1999) Running increases cell proliferation and neurogenesis in the adult mouse dentate gyrus. Nat Neurosci 2, 266–70.
36. Karten, Y. J., Olariu, A. & Cameron, H. A. (2005) Stress in early life inhibits neurogenesis in adulthood. Trends Neurosci 28, 171–2.
37. Malberg, J. E., Eisch, A. J., Nestler, E. J. & Duman, R. S. (2000) Chronic antidepressant treatment increases neurogenesis in adult rat hippocampus. J Neurosci 20, 9104–10.
38. Perera, T. D., Coplan, J. D., Lisanby, S. H., Lipira, C. M., Arif, M., Carpio, C., Spitzer, G., Santarelli, L., Scharf, B., Hen, R., Rosoklija, G., Sackeim, H. A. & Dwork, A. J. (2007) Antidepressant-induced neurogenesis in the hippocampus of adult nonhuman primates. J Neurosci 27, 4894–901.
39. Shors, T. J., Miesegaes, G., Beylin, A., Zhao, M., Rydel, T. & Gould, E. (2001) Neurogenesis in the adult is involved in the formation of trace memories. Nature 410, 372–6.
40. Overstreet-Wadiche, L. S., Bromberg, D. A., Bensen, A. L. & Westbrook, G. L. (2006) Seizures accelerate functional integration of adult-generated granule cells. J Neurosci 26, 4095–103.

41. Parent, J. M. (2007) Adult neurogenesis in the intact and epileptic dentate gyrus. Prog Brain Res 163, 529–817.
42. Parent, J. M., Valentin, V. V. & Lowenstein, D. H. (2002) Prolonged seizures increase proliferating neuroblasts in the adult rat subventricular zone-olfactory bulb pathway. J Neurosci 22, 3174–88.
43. Ohab, J. J., Fleming, S., Blesch, A. & Carmichael, S. T. (2006) A neurovascular niche for neurogenesis after stroke. J Neurosci 26, 13007–16.
44. Jin, K., Wang, X., Xie, L., Mao, X. O., Zhu, W., Wang, Y., Shen, J., Mao, Y., Banwait, S. & Greenberg, D. A. (2006) Evidence for stroke-induced neurogenesis in the human brain. Proc Natl Acad Sci U S A 103, 13198–202.
45. Parent, J. M., Vexler, Z. S., Gong, C., Derugin, N. & Ferriero, D. M. (2002) Rat forebrain neurogenesis and striatal neuron replacement after focal stroke. Ann Neurol 52, 802–13.
46. Kokaia, Z. & Lindvall, O. (2003) Neurogenesis after ischaemic brain insults. Curr Opin Neurobiol 13, 127–32.
47. Yamashita, T., Ninomiya, M., Hernandez Acosta, P., Garcia-Verdugo, J. M., Sunabori, T., Sakaguchi, M., Adachi, K., Kojima, T., Hirota, Y., Kawase, T., Araki, N., Abe, K., Okano, H. & Sawamoto, K. (2006) Subventricular zone-derived neuroblasts migrate and differentiate into mature neurons in the post-stroke adult striatum. J Neurosci 26, 6627–36.
48. Palmer, T. D., Ray, J. & Gage, F. H. (1995) FGF-2-responsive neuronal progenitors reside in proliferative and quiescent regions of the adult rodent brain. Mol Cell Neurosci 6, 474–86.
49. Pencea, V., Bingaman, K. D., Wiegand, S. J. & Luskin, M. B. (2001) Infusion of brain-derived neurotrophic factor into the lateral ventricle of the adult rat leads to new neurons in the parenchyma of the striatum, septum, thalamus, and hypothalamus. J Neurosci 21, 6706–17.
50. van Praag, H., Schinder, A. F., Christie, B. R., Toni, N., Palmer, T. D. & Gage, F. H. (2002) Functional neurogenesis in the adult hippocampus. Nature 415, 1030–4.
51. Schmidt-Hieber, C., Jonas, P. & Bischofberger, J. (2004) Enhanced synaptic plasticity in newly generated granule cells of the adult hippocampus. Nature 429, 184–7.
52. Ge, S., Goh, E. L., Sailor, K. A., Kitabatake, Y., Ming, G. L. & Song, H. (2006) GABA regulates synaptic integration of newly generated neurons in the adult brain. Nature 439, 589–93.
53. Zhao, C., Teng, E. M., Summers, R. G., Jr., Ming, G. L. & Gage, F. H. (2006) Distinct morphological stages of dentate granule neuron maturation in the adult mouse hippocampus. J Neurosci 26, 3–11.
54. Laplagne, D. A., Esposito, M. S., Piatti, V. C., Morgenstern, N. A., Zhao, C., van Praag, H., Gage, F. H. & Schinder, A. F. (2006) Functional convergence of neurons generated in the developing and adult hippocampus. PLoS Biol 4, e409.
55. Kempermann, G. & Gage, F. H. (2002) Genetic influence on phenotypic differentiation in adult hippocampal neurogenesis. Brain Res Dev Brain Res 134, 1–12.
56. Kempermann, G., Kuhn, H. G. & Gage, F. H. (1997) Genetic influence on neurogenesis in the dentate gyrus of adult mice. Proc Natl Acad Sci U S A 94, 10409–14.
57. Li, L., Liu, F., Salmonsen, R. A., Turner, T. K., Litofsky, N. S., Di Cristofano, A., Pandolfi, P. P., Jones, S. N., Recht, L. D. & Ross, A. H. (2002) PTEN in neural precursor cells: regulation of migration, apoptosis, and proliferation. Mol Cell Neurosci 20, 21–9.
58. Marino, S., Krimpenfort, P., Leung, C., van der Korput, H. A., Trapman, J., Camenisch, I., Berns, A. & Brandner, S. (2002) PTEN is essential for cell migration but not for fate determination and tumourigenesis in the cerebellum. Development 129, 3513–22.
59. Groszer, M., Erickson, R., Scripture-Adams, D. D., Dougherty, J. D., Le Belle, J., Zack, J. A., Geschwind, D. H., Liu, X., Kornblum, H. I. & Wu, H. (2006) PTEN negatively regulates neural stem cell self-renewal by modulating G0-G1 cell cycle entry. Proc Natl Acad Sci U S A 103, 111–6.
60. Wu, Y., Liu, Y., Levine, E. M. & Rao, M. S. (2003) Hes1 but not Hes5 regulates an astrocyte versus oligodendrocyte fate choice in glial restricted precursors. Dev Dyn 226, 675–89.
61. Ishibashi, M., Ang, S. L., Shiota, K., Nakanishi, S., Kageyama, R. & Guillemot, F. (1995) Targeted disruption of mammalian hairy and Enhancer of split homolog-1 (HES-1) leads to

up-regulation of neural helix-loop-helix factors, premature neurogenesis, and severe neural tube defects. Genes Dev 9, 3136–48.

62. Jhas, S., Ciura, S., Belanger-Jasmin, S., Dong, Z., Llamosas, E., Theriault, F. M., Joachim, K., Tang, Y., Liu, L., Liu, J. & Stifani, S. (2006) Hes6 inhibits astrocyte differentiation and promotes neurogenesis through different mechanisms. J Neurosci 26, 11061–71.

63. Siegenthaler, J. A. & Miller, M. W. (2005) Transforming growth factor beta 1 promotes cell cycle exit through the cyclin-dependent kinase inhibitor p21 in the developing cerebral cortex. J Neurosci 25, 8627–36.

64. Doetsch, F., Verdugo, J. M., Caille, I., Alvarez-Buylla, A., Chao, M. V. & Casaccia-Bonnefil, P. (2002) Lack of the cell-cycle inhibitor p27Kip1 results in selective increase of transit-amplifying cells for adult neurogenesis. J Neurosci 22, 2255–64.

65. Allen, D. M., van Praag, H., Ray, J., Weaver, Z., Winrow, C. J., Carter, T. A., Braquet, R., Harrington, E., Ried, T., Brown, K. D., Gage, F. H. & Barlow, C. (2001) Ataxia telangiectasia mutated is essential during adult neurogenesis. Genes Dev 15, 554–66.

66. Shi, Y., Chichung Lie, D., Taupin, P., Nakashima, K., Ray, J., Yu, R. T., Gage, F. H. & Evans, R. M. (2004) Expression and function of orphan nuclear receptor TLX in adult neural stem cells. Nature 427, 78–83.

67. Levenson, J. M. & Sweatt, J. D. (2005) Epigenetic mechanisms in memory formation. Nat Rev Neurosci 6, 108–18.

68. Reik, W., Dean, W. & Walter, J. (2001) Epigenetic reprogramming in mammalian development. Science 293, 1089–93.

69. Jenuwein, T. & Allis, C. D. (2001) Translating the histone code. Science 293, 1074–80.

70. Bernstein, E. & Allis, C. D. (2005) RNA meets chromatin. Genes Dev 19, 1635–55.

71. Bernstein, B. E., Meissner, A. & Lander, E. S. (2007) The mammalian epigenome. Cell 128, 669–81.

72. Miremadi, A., Oestergaard, M. Z., Pharoah, P. D. & Caldas, C. (2007) Cancer genetics of epigenetic genes. Hum Mol Genet 16 Spec No 1, R28–R49.

73. Ballas, N., Grunseich, C., Lu, D. D., Speh, J. C. & Mandel, G. (2005) REST and its corepressors mediate plasticity of neuronal gene chromatin throughout neurogenesis. Cell 121, 645–57.

74. Lunyak, V. V., Burgess, R., Prefontaine, G. G., Nelson, C., Sze, S. H., Chenoweth, J., Schwartz, P., Pevzner, P. A., Glass, C., Mandel, G. & Rosenfeld, M. G. (2002) Corepressor-dependent silencing of chromosomal regions encoding neuronal genes. Science 298, 1747–52.

75. Lunyak, V. V. & Rosenfeld, M. G. (2005) No rest for REST: REST/NRSF regulation of neurogenesis. Cell 121, 499–501.

76. Rice, J. C. & Allis, C. D. (2001) Histone methylation versus histone acetylation: new insights into epigenetic regulation. Curr Opin Cell Biol 13, 263–73.

77. Hsieh, J., Nakashima, K., Kuwabara, T., Mejia, E. & Gage, F. H. (2004) Histone deacetylase inhibition-mediated neuronal differentiation of multipotent adult neural progenitor cells. Proc Natl Acad Sci U S A 101, 16659–64.

78. Jessberger, S., Nakashima, K., Clemenson, G. D., Jr., Mejia, E., Mathews, E., Ure, K., Ogawa, S., Sinton, C. M., Gage, F. H. & Hsieh, J. (2007) Epigenetic modulation of seizure-induced neurogenesis and cognitive decline. J Neurosci 27, 5967–75.

79. Shen, S., Li, J. & Casaccia-Bonnefil, P. (2005) Histone modifications affect timing of oligodendrocyte progenitor differentiation in the developing rat brain. J Cell Biol 169, 577–89.

80. Plath, K., Fang, J., Mlynarczyk-Evans, S. K., Cao, R., Worringer, K. A., Wang, H., de la Cruz, C. C., Otte, A. P., Panning, B. & Zhang, Y. (2003) Role of histone H3 lysine 27 methylation in X inactivation. Science 300, 131–5.

81. Torres-Padilla, M. E., Parfitt, D. E., Kouzarides, T. & Zernicka-Goetz, M. (2007) Histone arginine methylation regulates pluripotency in the early mouse embryo. Nature 445, 214–8.

82. Mikkelsen, T. S., Ku, M., Jaffe, D. B., Issac, B., Lieberman, E., Giannoukos, G., Alvarez, P., Brockman, W., Kim, T. K., Koche, R. P., Lee, W., Mendenhall, E., O'Donovan, A., Presser, A., Russ, C., Xie, X., Meissner, A., Wernig, M., Jaenisch, R., Nusbaum, C., Lander, E. S. & Bernstein, B. E. (2007) Genome-wide maps of chromatin state in pluripotent and lineage-committed cells. Nature 448, 553–60.

83. Molofsky, A. V., He, S., Bydon, M., Morrison, S. J. & Pardal, R. (2005) Bmi-1 promotes neural stem cell self-renewal and neural development but not mouse growth and survival by repressing the p16Ink4a and p19Arf senescence pathways. Genes Dev 19, 1432–7.

84. Mattick, J. S. & Makunin, I. V. (2005) Small regulatory RNAs in mammals. Hum Mol Genet 14 Spec No 1, R121–32.

85. Bartel, D. P. (2004) MicroRNAs: genomics, biogenesis, mechanism, and function. Cell 116, 281–97.

86. Ambros, V. (2004) The functions of animal microRNAs. Nature 431, 350–5.

87. Kosik, K. S. (2006) The neuronal microRNA system. Nat Rev Neurosci 7, 911–20.

88. Wu, H., Xu, J., Pang, Z. P., Ge, W., Kim, K. J., Blanchi, B., Chen, C., Sudhof, T. C. & Sun, Y. E. (2007) Integrative genomic and functional analyses reveal neuronal subtype differentiation bias in human embryonic stem cell lines. Proc Natl Acad Sci U S A 104, 13821–6.

89. Landgraf, P., Rusu, M., Sheridan, R., Sewer, A., Iovino, N., Aravin, A., Pfeffer, S., Rice, A., Kamphorst, A. O., Landthaler, M., Lin, C., Socci, N. D., Hermida, L., Fulci, V., Chiaretti, S., Foa, R., Schliwka, J., Fuchs, U., Novosel, A., Muller, R. U., Schermer, B., Bissels, U., Inman, J., Phan, Q., Chien, M., Weir, D. B., Choksi, R., De Vita, G., Frezzetti, D., Trompeter, H. I., Hornung, V., Teng, G., Hartmann, G., Palkovits, M., Di Lauro, R., Wernet, P., Macino, G., Rogler, C. E., Nagle, J. W., Ju, J., Papavasiliou, F. N., Benzing, T., Lichter, P., Tam, W., Brownstein, M. J., Bosio, A., Borkhardt, A., Russo, J. J., Sander, C., Zavolan, M. & Tuschl, T. (2007) A mammalian microRNA expression atlas based on small RNA library sequencing. Cell 129, 1401–14.

90. Krichevsky, A. M., Sonntag, K. C., Isacson, O. & Kosik, K. S. (2006) Specific microRNAs modulate embryonic stem cell-derived neurogenesis. Stem Cells 24, 857–64.

91. Visvanathan, J., Lee, S., Lee, B., Lee, J. W. & Lee, S. K. (2007) The microRNA miR-124 antagonizes the anti-neural REST/SCP1 pathway during embryonic CNS development. Genes Dev 21, 744–9.

92. Makeyev, E. V., Zhang, J., Carrasco, M. A. & Maniatis, T. (2007) The MicroRNA miR-124 promotes neuronal differentiation by triggering brain-specific alternative pre-mRNA splicing. Mol Cell 27, 435–48.

93. Ashraf, S. I. & Kunes, S. (2006) A trace of silence: memory and microRNA at the synapse. Curr Opin Neurobiol 16, 535–9.

94. Schratt, G. M., Tuebing, F., Nigh, E. A., Kane, C. G., Sabatini, M. E., Kiebler, M. & Greenberg, M. E. (2006) A brain-specific microRNA regulates dendritic spine development. Nature 439, 283–9.

95. Jones, P. A. & Takai, D. (2001) The role of DNA methylation in mammalian epigenetics. Science 293, 1068–70.

96. Jaenisch, R. & Bird, A. (2003) Epigenetic regulation of gene expression: how the genome integrates intrinsic and environmental signals. Nat Genet 33 Suppl, 245–54.

97. Bird, A. (2002) DNA methylation patterns and epigenetic memory. Genes Dev 16, 6–21.

98. Takizawa, T., Nakashima, K., Namihira, M., Ochiai, W., Uemura, A., Yanagisawa, M., Fujita, N., Nakao, M. & Taga, T. (2001) DNA methylation is a critical cell-intrinsic determinant of astrocyte differentiation in the fetal brain. Dev Cell 1, 749–58.

99. Klose, R. J. & Bird, A. (2006) Genomic DNA methylation: the mark and its mediators. Trends Biochem Sci 31, 89–97.

100. Jorgensen, H. F., Ben-Porath, I. & Bird, A. P. (2004) Mbd1 is recruited to both methylated and nonmethylated CpGs via distinct DNA binding domains. Mol Cell Biol 24, 3387–95.

101. Fujita, N., Watanabe, S., Ichimura, T., Ohkuma, Y., Chiba, T., Saya, H. & Nakao, M. (2003) MCAF mediates MBD1-dependent transcriptional repression. Mol Cell Biol 23, 2834–43.

102. Klose, R. J., Sarraf, S. A., Schmiedeberg, L., McDermott, S. M., Stancheva, I. & Bird, A. P. (2005) DNA binding selectivity of MeCP2 due to a requirement for A/T sequences adjacent to methyl-CpG. Mol Cell 19, 667–78.

103. Fujita, N., Watanabe, S., Ichimura, T., Tsuruzoe, S., Shinkai, Y., Tachibana, M., Chiba, T. & Nakao, M. (2003) Methyl-CpG binding domain 1 (MBD1) interacts with the Suv39h1-HP1 heterochromatic complex for DNA methylation-based transcriptional repression. J Biol Chem 278, 24132–8.

104. Sarraf, S. A. & Stancheva, I. (2004) Methyl-CpG binding protein MBD1 couples histone H3 methylation at lysine 9 by SETDB1 to DNA replication and chromatin assembly. Mol Ceil 15, 595–605.

105. Setoguchi, H., Namihira, M., Kohyama, J., Asano, H., Sanosaka, T. & Nakashima, K. (2006) Methyl-CpG binding proteins are involved in restricting differentiation plasticity in neurons. J Neurosci Res 84, 969–79.

106. Zhao, X., Ueba, T., Christie, B. R., Barkho, B., McConnell, M. J., Nakashima, K., Lein, E. S., Eadie, B. D., Willhoite, A. R., Muotri, A. R., Summers, R. G., Chun, J., Lee, K. F. & Gage, F. H. (2003) Mice lacking methyl-CpG binding protein 1 have deficits in adult neurogenesis and hippocampal function. Proc Natl Acad Sci U S A 100, 6777–82.

107. Ueba, T., Kaspar, B., Zhao, X. & Gage, F. H. (1999) Repression of human fibroblast growth factor 2 by a novel transcription factor. J Biol Chem 274, 10382–7.

108. Gage, F. H. (2002) Neurogenesis in the adult brain. J Neurosci 22, 612–3.

109. Garcia, A. D., Doan, N. B., Imura, T., Bush, T. G. & Sofroniew, M. V. (2004) GFAP-expressing progenitors are the principal source of constitutive neurogenesis in adult mouse forebrain. Nat Neurosci 7, 1233–41.

110. Palmer, T. D., Markakis, E. A., Willhoite, A. R., Safar, F. & Gage, F. H. (1999) Fibroblast growth factor-2 activates a latent neurogenic program in neural stem cells from diverse regions of the adult CNS. J Neurosci 19, 8487–97.

111. Goldman, S. A. & Sim, F. (2005) Neural progenitor cells of the adult brain. Novartis Found Symp 265, 66–80; discussion 82–97.

112. Shihabuddin, L. S., Horner, P. J., Ray, J. & Gage, F. H. (2000) Adult spinal cord stem cells generate neurons after transplantation in the adult dentate gyrus. J Neurosci 20, 8727–35.

113. Lie, D. C., Colamarino, S. A., Song, H. J., Desire, L., Mira, H., Consiglio, A., Lein, E. S., Jessberger, S., Lansford, H., Dearie, A. R. & Gage, F. H. (2005) Wnt signalling regulates adult hippocampal neurogenesis. Nature 437, 1370–5.

114. Tanigaki, K., Nogaki, F., Takahashi, J., Tashiro, K., Kurooka, H. & Honjo, T. (2001) Notch1 and Notch3 instructively restrict bFGF-responsive multipotent neural progenitor cells to an astroglial fate. Neuron 29, 45–55.

115. Ahn, S. & Joyner, A. L. (2005) In vivo analysis of quiescent adult neural stem cells responding to Sonic hedgehog. Nature 437, 894–7.

116. Kuo, C. T., Mirzadeh, Z., Soriano-Navarro, M., Rasin, M., Wang, D., Shen, J., Sestan, N., Garcia-Verdugo, J., Alvarez-Buylla, A., Jan, L. Y. & Jan, Y. N. (2006) Postnatal deletion of Numb/Numblike reveals repair and remodeling capacity in the subventricular neurogenic niche. Cell 127, 1253–64.

117. Zhao, X., Lein, E. S., He, A., Smith, S. C., Aston, C. & Gage, F. H. (2001) Transcriptional profiling reveals strict boundaries between hippocampal subregions. J Comp Neurol 441, 187–96.

118. Song, H., Stevens, C. F. & Gage, F. H. (2002) Astroglia induce neurogenesis from adult neural stem cells. Nature 417, 39–44.

119. Palmer, T. D., Willhoite, A. R. & Gage, F. H. (2000) Vascular niche for adult hippocampal neurogenesis. J Comp Neurol 425, 479–94.

120. Cao, L., Jiao, X., Zuzga, D. S., Liu, Y., Fong, D. M., Young, D. & During, M. J. (2004) VEGF links hippocampal activity with neurogenesis, learning and memory. Nat Genet 36, 827–35.

121. Fabel, K., Fabel, K., Tam, B., Kaufer, D., Baiker, A., Simmons, N., Kuo, C. J. & Palmer, T. D. (2003) VEGF is necessary for exercise-induced adult hippocampal neurogenesis. Eur J Neurosci 18, 2803–12.

122. Jin, K., Zhu, Y., Sun, Y., Mao, X. O., Xie, L. & Greenberg, D. A. (2002) Vascular endothelial growth factor (VEGF) stimulates neurogenesis in vitro and in vivo. Proc Natl Acad Sci U S A 99, 11946–50.

123. Shen, Q., Goderie, S. K., Jin, L., Karanth, N., Sun, Y., Abramova, N., Vincent, P., Pumiglia, K. & Temple, S. (2004) Endothelial cells stimulate self-renewal and expand neurogenesis of neural stem cells. Science 304, 1338–40.

124. Wurmser, A. E. & Gage, F. H. (2002) Stem cells: cell fusion causes confusion. Nature 416, 485–7.

125. Barkho, B. Z., Song, H., Aimone, J. B., Smrt, R. D., Kuwabara, T., Nakashima, K., Gage, F. H. & Zhao, X. (2006) Identification of astrocyte-expressed factors that modulate neural stem/progenitor cell differentiation. Stem Cells Dev 15, 407–21.

126. Lein, E. S., Zhao, X. & Gage, F. H. (2004) Defining a molecular atlas of the hippocampus using DNA microarrays and high-throughput in situ hybridization. J Neurosci 24, 3879–89.

127. Monje, M. L., Toda, H. & Palmer, T. D. (2003) Inflammatory blockade restores adult hippocampal neurogenesis. Science 302, 1760–5.

128. Chojnacki, A., Shimazaki, T., Gregg, C., Weinmaster, G. & Weiss, S. (2003) Glycoprotein 130 signaling regulates Notch1 expression and activation in the self-renewal of mammalian forebrain neural stem cells. J Neurosci 23, 1730–41.

129. Song, M. R. & Ghosh, A. (2004) FGF2-induced chromatin remodeling regulates CNTF-mediated gene expression and astrocyte differentiation. Nat Neurosci 7, 229–35.

130. Bienvenu, G., Seurin, D., Grellier, P., Froment, P., Baudrimont, M., Monget, P., Le Bouc, Y. & Babajko, S. (2004) Insulin-like growth factor binding protein-6 transgenic mice: postnatal growth, brain development, and reproduction abnormalities. Endocrinology 145, 2412–20.

131. Hausser, H., Groning, A., Hasilik, A., Schonherr, E. & Kresse, H. (1994) Selective inactivity of TGF-beta/decorin complexes. FEBS Lett 353, 243–5.

132. Popa-Wagner, A., Carmichael, S. T., Kokaia, Z., Kessler, C. & Walker, L. C. (2007) The response of the aged brain to stroke: too much, too soon? Curr Neurovasc Res 4, 216–27.

133. Lim, D. A., Tramontin, A. D., Trevejo, J. M., Herrera, D. G., Garcia-Verdugo, J. M. & Alvarez-Buylla, A. (2000) Noggin antagonizes BMP signaling to create a niche for adult neurogenesis. Neuron 28, 713–26.

134. Ramirez-Castillejo, C., Sanchez-Sanchez, F., Andreu-Agullo, C., Ferron, S. R., Aroca-Aguilar, J. D., Sanchez, P., Mira, H., Escribano, J. & Farinas, I. (2006) Pigment epithelium-derived factor is a niche signal for neural stem cell renewal. Nat Neurosci 9, 331–9.

135. Asensio, V. C. & Campbell, I. L. (1999) Chemokines in the CNS: plurifunctional mediators in diverse states. Trends Neurosci 22, 504–12.

136. Imitola, J., Park, K. I., Teng, Y. D., Nisim, S., Lachyankar, M., Ourednik, J., Mueller, F. J., Yiou, R., Atala, A., Sidman, R. L., Tuszynski, M., Khoury, S. J. & Snyder, E. Y. (2004) Stem cells: cross-talk and developmental programs. Philos Trans R Soc Lond B Biol Sci 359, 823–37.

137. Zhang, H., Vutskits, L., Pepper, M. S. & Kiss, J. Z. (2003) VEGF is a chemoattractant for FGF-2-stimulated neural progenitors. J Cell Biol 163, 1375–84.

138. Tettamanti, G., Malagoli, D., Benelli, R., Albini, A., Grimaldi, A., Perletti, G., Noonan, D. M., de Eguileor, M. & Ottaviani, E. (2006) Growth factors and chemokines: a comparative functional approach between invertebrates and vertebrates. Curr Med Chem 13, 2737–50.

139. Tran, P. B., Ren, D., Veldhouse, T. J. & Miller, R. J. (2004) Chemokine receptors are expressed widely by embryonic and adult neural progenitor cells. J Neurosci Res 76, 20–34.

140. Shibata, T., Yamada, K., Watanabe, M., Ikenaka, K., Wada, K., Tanaka, K. & Inoue, Y. (1997) Glutamate transporter GLAST is expressed in the radial glia-astrocyte lineage of developing mouse spinal cord. J Neurosci 17, 9212–9.

141. Toresson, H., Mata de Urquiza, A., Fagerstrom, C., Perlmann, T. & Campbell, K. (1999) Retinoids are produced by glia in the lateral ganglionic eminence and regulate striatal neuron differentiation. Development 126, 1317–26.
142. Ellis, P., Fagan, B. M., Magness, S. T., Hutton, S., Taranova, O., Hayashi, S., McMahon, A., Rao, M. & Pevny, L. (2004) SOX2, a persistent marker for multipotential neural stem cells derived from embryonic stem cells, the embryo or the adult. Dev Neurosci 26, 148–65.

Chapter 6
Progressing Neural Stem Cell Lines to the Clinic

Kenneth Pollock and John D. Sinden

Abstract In recent years, prospects for treating serious neurological disorders have improved with the development of cell therapy as a viable therapeutic strategy. Initial clinical studies on cell implantation therapy in the brain used primary fetal tissue but progress has been made in developing expanded cell lines from somatic neural stem cells and embryonic stem cells. In addition, neural stem cell lines have been established by means of genetic modification to generate immortalized clonal lines including the use of conditional immortalization. These cells and cell lines provide the raw materials for the manufacture of investigational medicinal products for use in early clinical trials. The use of conditional immortalization technologies is particularly attractive for cell therapy products by enabling long term expansion. Cell lines for therapeutic application in neurological disease have been developed by ReNeuron using the c-mycER technology including one line, CTX0E03, that is in late pre-clinical development for the treatment of stroke.

Keywords Stem cells, neurodegenerative disease, implantation, immortalizing technology, regulatory issues

6.1 Introduction: Clinical Indications for Transplant Therapy

Many severe neurological disorders including stroke, Alzheimer's, Parkinson's and Huntington's diseases are characterized by the loss of neuronal tissue, giving rise to deficits in cognitive and motor function. In the case of stroke, non-specific hypoxic brain damage occurs in the territory supplied by a transiently blocked cerebral artery. In contrast, Parkinson's disease (PD) results from the selective degeneration of the dopaminergic neurons in the substantia nigra that project into the

ReNeuron Ltd, 10 Nugent Road, Surrey Research Park, Guildford, GU2 7AF, UK
e-mail: Kenny-pollock@reneuron.com, John-sinden@reneuron.com

Y. Shi, D.O. Clegg (eds.) *Stem Cell Research and Therapeutics*,
© Springer Science+Business Media B.V. 2008

striatum, which have a role in fine motor control of skeletal muscle. Huntington's disease (HD) is similar to PD in that it results in degeneration of a selective neuronal pathway, namely, the loss of medium spiny striatal output neurons in the caudate and putamen regions, together with some less specific cortical atrophy. HD is an autosomal dominant disease associated with extended polyglutamine repeats on the Huntington protein, but how this gives rise to pathology is unknown [1]. Although diverse in origin and extent, these neurological conditions share a common prognosis. There are no cures available to reverse established pathology, and current treatments are by and large targeted at relief of peripheral symptoms through physiotherapy and drug therapy.

In recent years, prospects for the treatment of neurological diseases have improved with the development of cell implantation therapy as a real option to replace, repair and regenerate damaged brain tissue. How such implanted cells might work in different neurological disorders is an ongoing area of investigation for researchers in the field, but it is becoming increasingly clear that trophic support of host neurons at risk from dying from the disease process may be as important as direct replacement of dead or dying cells. In contrast to most other adult tissues in the body, the brain has limited capacity for self repair and the incidence of stem cells that might support recovery in the brain is extremely low and localized to particular regions such as the hippocampal dentate gyrus and forebrain subventricular zone [2, 3]. With this limited capacity for endogenous repair in mind, progress has been made in recent years towards the establishment of neural stem cell lines that could be used in the manufacture of new medicinal products for the treatment of severe neurodegenerative diseases. The development of cell based therapeutics presents a challenge that includes harnessing appropriate biological characteristics and developing a manufacturing process that retains the required quality attributes of a medicinal product all the way from initial isolation and expansion of primary cells through to drug product formulation immediately prior to implantation in the patient. These considerations are underpinned by the requirement to meet regulatory safety and efficacy standards for the manufacture of cell therapies prior to clinical trials approval. For a review on meeting FDA expectations for cell therapy products see [4]. In particular, recent legislation has been introduced in both the US and Europe covering the quality standards of human cells and tissues for use in medicinal products. These include the introduction of Good Tissue Practice (GTP) in the US [5] and the human tissues and cells directive (EUTCD) [6] in Europe.

Here we discuss the underlying biological profiles of appropriate cells and cell lines, the manufacturing strategies for establishing banks and production lots of cells, and the regulatory hurdles to overcome when progressing neural stem cell lines from a research base into the clinic. In particular, we will focus on development of allogeneic products that would be available to a large number of patients. A key example for discussion is progression of a neural stem cell therapy (ReN001) currently in late pre-clinical development at ReNeuron for the treatment of ischemic stroke.

The development of neural stem cells for neurological disorders will rely predominantly on direct implantation of cell therapy product into the brain. This in itself has required the development of neurosurgical techniques including stereotaxic implantation in combination with MRI scanning to target precisely the delivery of cells into the appropriate anatomical region of the brain [7]. An alternative approach for clinical delivery of cells to the brain is by intravenous infusion. Pre-clinical studies in rodents have demonstrated functional recovery in animal models of neurological disease following systemic delivery of stem cells [8, 9] suggesting that this approach could be developed for the treatment of patients with stroke, if cells were non-residents in tissues outside the brain. However solutions to these problems will come in time, the immediate requirement is to develop cell lines that are efficacious.

6.2 Early Success and Proof of Concept

6.2.1 Primary Fetal Tissue

Transplantation of neural cells for neurological disease has been validated with both animal and human derived sources of tissue in both animal models of disease and early clinical trials. These early experimental studies have shown that grafted primary fetal cells survive and exert positive effects in animal models of PD [10, 11], Alzheimer's disease [12], HD [13, 14] and ischemic brain damage [15, 16].

In humans, implantation of cells into the CNS as therapy was also pioneered using primary fetal tissue as the source of neural cells. Some early successes have been reported in anecdotal, open or single study clinical reports, in both PD [17, 18] and HD patients [19, 20] but placebo-controlled double blinded transplant studies in both of these diseases have not demonstrated consistent benefits to patients in terms of the primary endpoints measured in these studies [21, 22]. However, the use of primary fetal tissue has provided anecdotal proof of concept data for neural transplant therapy in humans and tested the surgical feasibility of safe CNS implantation. However, the ethical issues and practical problems surrounding supply and use of fetal material on a regular basis consigns such approaches to the periphery of mainstream medicine. Problems include requirements for several donor fetuses, graft heterogeneity in transplant surgery, limited time frames for safety assessments of donors and cells for adventitious agents, and the physical tendency of grafted cells to remain clumped around the site of implantation rather than integrating into host brain structures [23]. Overall, these studies have also highlighted the severe limitations in conducting clinical trials with heterogeneous material of variable quality that makes the interpretation of clinical outcomes difficult. One alternative to the use of human fetal tissue is the use of xenografts in the form of fetal porcine tissue which circumvents ethical concerns associated with human fetal tissue, and allows a consistent supply of material with associated quality assurance. This approach was initially developed by Diacrin Inc. (now GenVec Inc.) who progressed this material as a potential therapeutic product (LGE cells). Pre-clinical studies in animal models of stroke, HD and PD [24–26] culminated in a clinical trial in a limited number of stroke patients [27]. Prior to implant, cells were treated with an anti-MHC class I F (ab')2 fragment designed to render the cells less open to host immune responses by masking porcine MHC Class 1 expression, and obviating the need for immunosuppressive agent administration to the patients. Although some positive clinical outcomes were reported, the FDA terminated the study after two patients suffered adverse events, most likely secondary to the implant procedure. Further progress with porcine xenografts has also been hindered by the existence of endogenous porcine retrovirus that could potentially infect humans [28]. Nonetheless, the use of human or porcine fetal transplants has further demonstrated the feasibility of direct implantation of primary cell based therapeutics directly into a patient's brain.

6.2.2 Embryonic Stem Cells

Enthusiasm for treating neurological disease with exogenous cell therapy has recently been fuelled by increasing knowledge of the potentiality and flexibility of embryonic stem (ES) cells, and the possibilities for guiding them towards specific mature neuronal phenotypes. Hence, ES cells might be used to generate tailor-made replacement cells for specific neurological disorders, e.g., nigro-striatal dopaminergic neurons for PD or medium spiny neurons for HD. ES cells can be directed towards differentiation into tissue-specific phenotypes including neurons, since many of the necessary fate-determining factors such as sonic hedgehog and FGF8 have been identified [29, 30].

Recent studies with murine [31] and primate [32] embryonic stem (ES) cells have successfully demonstrated functional recovery in animal models of PD, where recovery depends on release of dopamine by grafted cells. It is important to consider whether to graft these expanding cell populations as stem cells, or to induce cell differentiation prior to implantation. Differentiation of stem cells before grafting, or biasing cells towards a specific mature phenotype, avoids the risk of continued division in vivo and provides the exciting possibility of grafts enriched for particular cell types, notably dopaminergic (DA) cells for treatment of PD. Grafting of primary mesencephalic fetal tissue for PD has suffered from low survival of DA cells in vivo (typically 5–10%). Grafting of unmodified ES cells, while providing sufficient numbers of tyrosine hydroxylase-positive (TH+) cells to promote recovery from motor asymmetry (as shown by amphetamine-induced rotation bias), resulted in tumor formation in 20% of animals, so would not be clinically appropriate [11]. Enrichment of TH + cells within grafts has been the goal of many laboratories and has been pursued using a variety of culture conditions, treatment with anti-apoptotic and anti-inflammatory agents, or co-grafting of trophic factors [33], with some promising evidence for enhanced survival and efficacy. However, the strategy of transfecting ES cells with the Nurr1 gene to promote dopaminergic differentiation [31] appears to be highly promising for specific PD treatment.

The greatest strength of ES cells as source material for cell therapy product development, namely self replication with the capability to differentiate along a tissue /lineage specific pathway, is also the greatest weakness in that, at best, ES cells can be an infinite source of raw material that can become any cell type in the body and, at worst, ES cells can be considered as a risk through inappropriate cell division and or inappropriate cell differentiation. While ES cells may offer the potential to generate neural cell types to order, this technology is still in its infancy with respect to broad clinical applications.

The critical points to be addressed therefore are expansion capability in vitro [34, 35], long term control of phenotype, and control of differentiation prior to implantation and also following implantation in a patient. Moreover, much of the ethical and legal wrangling surrounding the use and exploitation of ES cells for research, for clinical applications and as commercial drug products remains to be resolved both in the US and Europe. From a biological perspective, safety concerns over the use of ES cells derived on mouse feeder cells and the tendency of ES cells to develop unstable karyotype in long term culture [31] are being addressed by the ES cell community. Leading the commercial charge with respect to specific product development is the biotechnology company Geron which has developed the process of expansion and differentiation of human ES cell lines for therapeutic applications and is progressing an ES derived cell line towards an IND submission for the treatment of spinal cord injury [36].

6.2.3 Somatic Neural Stem Cells

Neural stem cells isolated from fetal brain tissue or adult sources provide transplant material with more immediate relevance for neurological disorders than ES cells. These "somatic" neural stem cells have already progressed further down lineage-specific pathways of development than ES cells, but provide more suitable starting material for the isolation and establishment of multipotent neural stem cell lines. This is because they are easier to obtain, easier to grow in cultivation and less constrained by differing international legal frameworks than ES cells. The possibility of deriving expanded cell lines from human tissue is of major clinical importance. Nevertheless, this brings its own ethical and regulatory constraints and considerations for progressing these lines to clinical trials. In particular, the introduction of GTP and EUTCD regulations, mentioned earlier, has raised the regulatory standards required for procuring and processing human tissue.

The challenges for using expanded neurosphere cultures as the basis of a therapeutic product, or expansion of any somatic stem cells, are in establishing a manufacturing process that generates sufficient numbers of cells consistently and reproducibly to allow treatment of a large number of patients. Both rodent and human somatic stem cells respond to epidermal growth factor (EGF) and fibroblast growth factor (FGF-2) and can be cultured as monolayers or free-floating neurospheres [34, 35, 37, 38,]. As one example, a population of cholinergic neurons was generated from expanded fetal neural stem cells following engraftment into adult rats [39], demonstrating the innate capability of transplanted neurosphere cells to differentiate into an appropriate cell type. A further refinement of the neurosphere approach has been exploited by the biotechnology company Stem Cells Inc. (SCI). Using a proprietary technology, neural stem cell populations have been obtained using positive selection for the stem cell marker CD133 [40] followed by growth factor expansion in vitro. Cell lines expanded this way have shown good engraftment in animal models of stroke [41] and in spinal cord injury [42]. This approach has been used successfully to generate banks of cells providing sufficient material for preclinical safety and efficacy testing. This has culminated in a successful IND submission for the treatment of Batten disease, an inherited, fatal disorder that begins in early childhood. Under the IND, SCI have so far implanted these cells into six Batten patients [43] and continue to develop this approach for other therapeutic applications. However, it remains to be seen if a single stage expansion to generate a bank of drug substance/product can provide consistent and reproducible supplies of material for clinical trials in larger patient populations. In addition, for therapies that require multiple batches of cells processed from different donors to cover a large number of patients, each batch of cells may require repeat regulatory submission and/or extensive product release testing prior to clinical use.

Additional sources of adult stem cells for grafting into the CNS have been suggested including bone marrow [44], umbilical cord blood [45, 46] and cadaveric CNS [47]. Following the considerable scientific interest in understanding and manipulating adult stem cells, their application to the development of stem cell therapies is progressing with applications in other disease indications, including stroke [48].

6.3   Stem Cells as a Standardised Therapeutic Product

Whatever the source of cells for transplantation – primary fetal, embryonic or expanded somatic neural stem cells, it is clear that real clinical and industrial progress in human neural stem cell transplantation therapy is dependent upon the availability of cell lines with established provenance, that are able to expand quickly and serve as a sustainable resource, available on demand to a broad population of patients. The standard model for achieving this objective is to progress cell expansion/manufacturing through a cell banking process in line with procedures used for the manufacture of biologicals. An example of such cell banking is shown in Fig. 6.1. This approach will ensure a sustainable supply of standardized material from pre-clinical safety studies all the way to BLA (Biologics License Applications) submission and marketing authorization. In order to achieve this goal, cell lines must be generated with appropriate biological characteristics (tissue or cell-specific phenotype) and must be sufficiently robust to survive a scaleable manufacturing process (in culture flasks, cell factories or bioreactors) to make 'master' and 'working' cell banks of frozen vials of cells from which reproducible clinical lots of drug

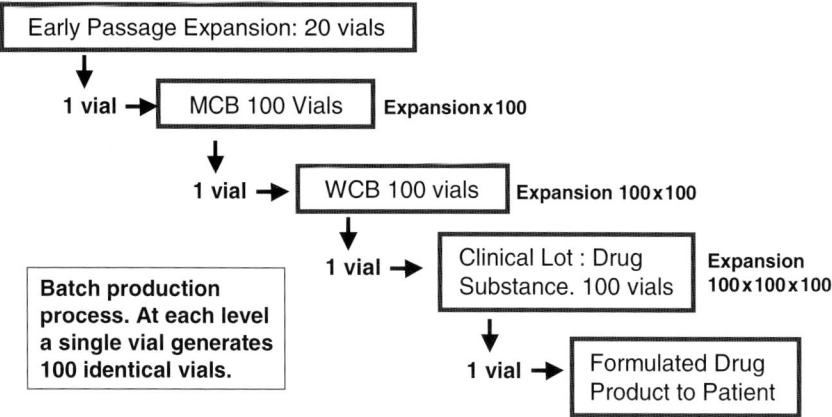

Fig. 6.1 Generic cell banking process. Stem cell lines are isolated by cloning and expanded in culture to generate an early passage stock. Cells are subsequently expanded through several passages and replicate vials of cells cryopreserved in liquid nitrogen as a master cell bank (MCB). One vial of cells is recovered, expanded in culture and cryopreserved to generate a working cell bank (WCB). A third expansion generates cells that are cryopreserved as a clinical lot. Finally cells are recovered and formulated as product for delivery to the patients. Using the approach shown, a million-fold expansion of one original vial can be achieved. Sufficient material is available such that cell banks are then tested to meet safety and performance specifications (*See Color Plates*)

substance and commercially viable drug product batches can be derived. An early example of this approach for the treatment of neurological disease is the development of LBS (Layton Biosciences) Neurons for the treatment of stroke. These cells, derived from the N- era-2 carcinoma cell line, have shown benefit in animal models of stroke [49], have been manufactured to cGMP (Current Good Manufacturing Practice) standards, and have shown some functional improvement in stroke patients [50] following implantation. However, LBS neurons are a tumor-derived cell line and concerns have been raised raise over longterm safety following implantation. No further clinical studies have been carried out on this product.

6.3.1 Immortalized Cell Lines

An established approach to enable long term expansion of neural stem cell lines in culture is the derivation cell lines that are "immortalized" through genetic modification [51]. Several technologies have been applied to the generation of cell lines within the neural stem cell field, including telomerase reverse transcriptase (hTERT), SV40 large T antigen, and the *myc* proto-oncogenes. These transgenes are generally introduced into primary cells using retroviral transduction followed by clonal selection.

In normal cells, the loss of hTERT and the progressive loss in telomere length eventually results in cell senescence [52]. Over-expression of hTERT enables continuous cell division without the concomitant reduction in telomere length that can give rise to cell senescence or genetic instability, which is the curse of many expanded cell populations in vitro. hTERT over-expression has been used successfully to generate neuronally restricted immortalized progenitor cells derived from human fetal spinal cord [53]. In this study, lineage restricted neural progenitor cells were obtained that survived over 150 population doublings while retaining a normal karyotype. Following implantation into the CNS in rodents, these cells survived in vivo for several months without associated tumor formation. However, over-expression of hTERT is associated with tumor cells and the use of this technology in an unregulated fashion remains a safety concern.

A solution to this problem is the use of *conditional* immortalizing genes which have a mechanism for turning on and off the gene product as required. Conditional immortalization involves transduction of cells with immortalizing oncogenes [54], which can be switched on to permit cell division in vitro, but can then be switched off in vivo. A pioneering example of this approach was the use of the temperature sensitive mutant allele (tsA58) of the simian virus 40 large T antigen (SV40 TAg), which maintains stem cells in continued division in "cold" (33°C) culture conditions, but switches off division at normal body temperature (37–39°C), allowing cells to undergo growth arrest and differentiate into mature phenotypes after grafting into the brain. Clonal cell lines developed from the fetal neuroepithelial (E14) tissue from the H-2Kb-tsA58 transgenic mouse [55] have shown successful conditional immortalization, with cells dividing in culture, and differentiating into all CNS cell types at higher temperatures in vitro and in vivo [56, 57]. One of these transgenic mouse-derived neural stem cell lines, MHP-36, has been extensively tested in vivo and has shown efficacy in a range of animal models, including stroke, PD and Alzheimer's disease. Subsequently, tsT conditionally immortalized cell lines have been generated by retroviral transduction of both human and mouse fetal brain tissue. Unfortunately, many of these cell lines failed to engraft and survive in the CNS in animal models and displayed abnormal karyotypes making them unsuitable candidates for clinical applications.

Perhaps the best-known technology for generating immortalized cell lines for neural applications is c-myc. Over-expression of the *myc* oncogenes has long been established as suitable for immortalizing fetal neural cells [58, 59]. Such lines have enabled long-term expansion in culture, with spontaneous differentiation upon growth factor removal. One key advantage of *myc* is that it up-regulates a number of growth control genes that help the cell maintain genetic stability during extended periods of cell division. These genes include hTERT, itself an immortalizing gene as described earlier, and histone deacetylases, which maintain chromatin integrity [60]. However, when implanted into animals, there is some evidence that neural stem cell lines immortalized with the v-myc gene can continue to proliferate inappropriately in vivo as seen by Ki67 staining [61]. The use of *myc* immortalized cell lines for therapeutic application in neurological disorders is therefore constrained by the safety risk associated with a tendency to cause tumors following engraftment.

A number of such lines of human origin have now been established, but all remain within the research domain [62, 63]. We have developed a v-myc immortalized human ventral mesencephalon derived stem cell line, *ReNcell® VM*, that demonstrates both high content dopaminergic differentiation and action potential generation in culture [64]. However, the introduction of regulatable *myc* genes can nullify oncogene-associated tumor risk by providing a chemical switch to turn the function of the *myc* gene on and off. Such regulatable transgenes have been engineered for some time and include the tetracycline transactivator/repressor system developed in the early 1990s [65]. Using this approach, Hoshimaru [58] developed a conditionally immortalized rat hippocampal cell line; addition of tetracycline to the media turned off v-myc expression and allowed the cells to differentiate into mature neurons. More recently, the "tet-on" technology has been applied to human mesencephalon to generate the dopaminergic cell line, MESC2.10, conditionally immortalized with v-myc [66]. A cell line such as this works well at a research level in this case to generate competent dopaminergic neurons, but addition of a drug such as tetracycline to differentiate cells into neurons in vivo and in a clinical scenario is not practical. As an alternative, a human neural stem cell line, HB2-G2, has been developed, that grows in the presence of doxycyclin but undergoes growth arrest and differentiates into neurons when this drug is withdrawn from the medium. The unregulated version of this v-myc immortalized cell line has shown behavioral recovery in animal models of stroke and lysosomal storage disease [67]. However, there are no reports to date of clinical development of such lines.

6.3.2 c-MycER Conditional Immortalization

An alternative conditional immortalizing technology for generating neural stem cell lines for clinical applications is c-mycER[TAM]. Originally developed as a c-myc-estrogen receptor fusion protein, the transgene was modified with the introduction of a point mutation on the estrogen binding domain to retain high affinity binding for a synthetic drug, 4-hydroxy tamoxifen (4-OHT), while losing affinity for native estradiol [68, 69]. In the presence of 4-OHT and growth factors (EGF and bFGF), c-mycER[TAM] protein remains transcriptionally active in the cell nucleus, maintaining cell division. When 4-OHT and growth factors are withdrawn, either in vitro or following formulation for grafting in vivo, the c-mycER[TAM] fusion protein remains in the cytoplasm, and is thereby inactive. Use of an inactive mutant estrogen receptor means that c-mycER[TAM] is not responsive to hormonal estrogen, other sex hormones or steroids or even phenols in the growth media. The protein-based functional regulation of myc protein confers greater control than other forms of pro-drug-based transcriptional regulation. The structure of the transgene is shown in Fig. 6.2. The reality of this technology is to enable longterm expansion of clonally-derived neural stem cell lines in culture at a reasonable rate while retaining genetic and phenotypic stability. Removal of 4-OHT and exogenous growth factors, as would occur during implantation in vivo, allows the

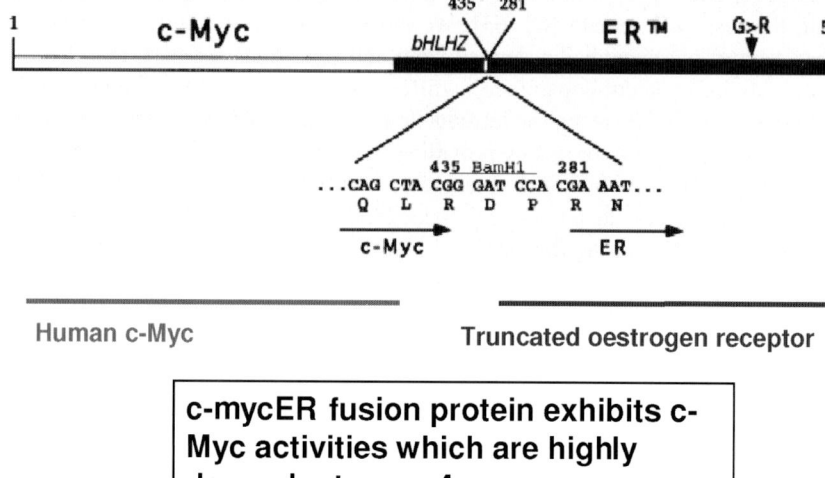

Fig. 6.2 The mycER[TAM] transgene. The transgene comprises the sequence of human c-myc, fused with the ligand binding domain of the estradiol receptor but containing the point mutation to confer ligand binding selective for 4-hydroxy tamoxifen (*See Color Plates*)

cells to differentiate through asymmetric cell division and undergo growth arrest. For neural stem cells this would give rise to post-mitotic neurons, astrocytes and oligodendrocytes. The c-mycER[TAM] is beneficial on two fronts: it supports cell line expansion at a reasonable rate for manufacturing and provides a safety switch in the cells post implantation.

Using this technology, ReNeuron has established a strategy for generating conditionally immortalized neural stem cell lines as candidates for clinical development that has so far led to the identification of two cell line candidates, one of which is in pre-clinical development for the treatment of stroke (ReN001) and the other (ReN005) is under evaluation for HD. Progressing individual cell lines to the clinic using the c-mycER[TAM] technology is covered in three distinct phases up to a regulatory submission for clinical trials approval:

(i) An initial discovery phase where primary cells are transduced with retrovirus and clones taken to cell lines selected with the required biological profile.
(ii) A non-GMP cell banking phase for process development, pre-clinical testing and establishment of regulatory assays.
(iii) A GMP banking phase for manufacturing from Master Cell Bank to Drug Substance lots (Investigational Medicinal Product) and final Drug Product.

6.3.2.1 Cell Line Discovery Process

For clinical programs at ReNeuron, cell lines were generated through retroviral transduction of freshly dispersed cells from first trimester fetal brain tissue, either cortex or striatum, from which approximately 100 individual cell lines were selected, ring cloned and individually expanded. In the absence of identifiable selection markers predictive of functional outcome, a rational screen was required to select promising candidates to progress towards leads for testing using in vivo models. Factors considered to be important in vivo included growth rates, freeze-thaw viability, clonality, genetic stability, transgene-induced conditionality, molecular phenotype and differentiation into all three neural cell types after removal of mitogen growth factors and 4-OHT. We used a combination of these assays to select 16 lines for in vivo screening using histological endpoints. Karyotype analysis using G-banding was conducted on each of these lines and only 1 cell line of the 16 had an abnormal feature, a stable translocation, which resulted in rejection. Clonality of lead candidates was assessed by Southern blot analysis. These data for the cortex derived cell line CTX0E03 used in the ReN001 lead product are reported in [70]. A sample set of key features is shown in Fig. 6.3 where normal diploid karyotype and activation of telomerase reverse transcriptase (hTERT) are shown. Similar data have been compiled with the striatal-derived cell line, STR0C05, which has also shown a normal stable karyotype, has good growth characteristics and is clonal.

Screening in vivo was designed to reduce the 16 lines, 8 from cortex, 8 from striatum, to a number (4–6 lines) that could reasonably be investigated in studies using different animal models of neurological disorder. We chose a histological

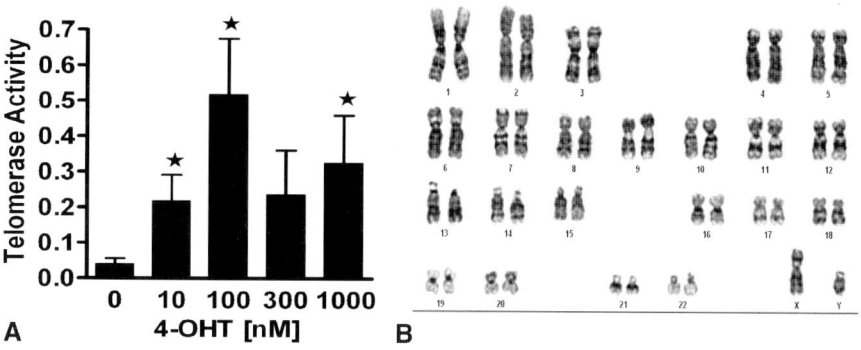

A   4-OHT [nM]   B

Fig. 6.3 c-mycER[TAM] functionality. In Fig. 6.3A, CTX0E03 cells immortalized with c-mycER[TAM] were grown in the presence or absence of 4-OHT and the activity of telomerase activity measured by PCR ELISA. Similar cells grown in the presence of 4-OHT were arrested in metaphase and analyzed for karyotype. As seen in Fig. 6.3B, CTX0E03 display a normal male karyotype which persists all the way to clinical lot production

screening study to investigate the capacity for survival and differentiation of the cells when injected into a lesioned brain. For this study, rats received unilateral quinolinic acid lesions (1.0 µl of a 0.08M solution in sodium phosphate buffered saline) in the right striatum. After recovery, the rats were implanted with cells at two sites in the intact and lesioned striatum, and in the dorsal hippocampus in the non-lesioned hemisphere (total 6 µl, 50,000 cells/µl). Rats were taken for histology at 2 and 5 weeks survival. From this study, cell lines were selected for testing in behavioral recovery models in vivo.

The choice of models for pre-clinical testing of stem cell lines needs careful consideration because models should be relevant to clinical conditions and reasonably consistent to allow comparisons across experiments. Lesion models generally reflect the consequences, not the processes or causes of disease, but are useful as screens because they are reproducible. Ischemic models in rats, for example middle cerebral artery occlusion (MCAo) for stroke and four vessel occlusion (4VO) for global ischemia, more accurately reflect the cascade of processes initiated by interruption of cerebral blood flow that are common to rats and people, and behavioral outcomes have been reasonably well-characterized.

Different models require different types of functional assessment, for example global ischemic damage results in damage to the hippocampal circuitry, which results in impaired cognitive performance, measurable by impaired spatial learning in the water maze. Stroke damage induced by MCAo disrupts both motor and cognitive performance, depending on whether the infarct is predominantly striatal or cortical. For these conditions a battery of tests is often used to asses cognitive and motor function including removal of sticky tape from forepaws to detect sensory-motor deficits, amphetamine-induced rotation bias, the whisker reflex test and the body sway test for gross motor asymmetry, the staircase test for skilled paw reaching using fine motor control, and spatial learning in the water maze for cognitive function.

Behavioral recovery and cell survival results with c-mycER^{TAM} cells were variable across the different cell lines, but positive indications of efficacy emerged for the CTX0E03 cell line across at least two lesion models. For example, CTX0E03 grafts improved spatial learning in rats with 4VO damage, but just failing to achieve statistical significance. CTX0E03 cell implants significantly improved paw reaching and body sway bias in rats with striatal lesions (unpublished data). The most striking behavioral improvements however were seen following left-hemisphere stroke as previously described [70, 71]. Similarly STR0C05 has shown efficacy in the quinolinic acid lesion rat model of HD [72] and as shown in Fig. 6.4. Establishing early proof of concept is a key milestone in product development. Triggering a development program requires a large financial commitment ($3–5 million) to take a cell line through a pre-clinical manufacturing and testing program. The CTX0E03 cell line was progressed at this point from research phase into a development program ReN001. At the end of the research phase, a non-GMP lot of cells was laid down at ReNeuron at an early passage, <20, that would serve as the common source of material for all future cell bank manufacturing, either non-GMP

CTX0E03
STROKE MODEL STICKY TAPE CONTACT

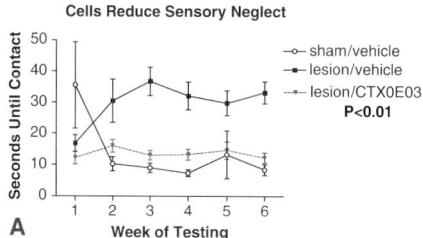

CTX0E03
STROKE MODEL STICKY TAPE REMOVAL

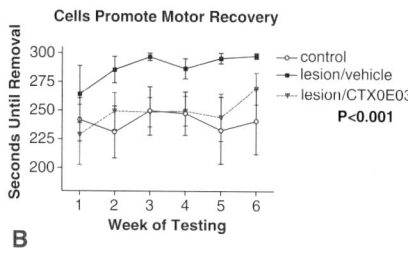

STR0C05
HUNTINGTONS MODEL: BODY SWAY TEST

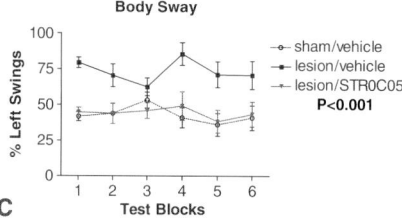

STR0C05
HUNTINGTONS MODEL : STAIRCASE TEST

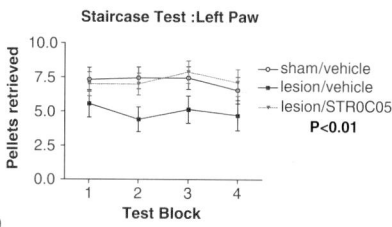

Fig. 6.4 Behavioral recovery with mycER^{TAM} cell lines. Cells were directly implanted into the CNS of rats that were given a stroke (panels **A** & **B**) or were treated with quinolinic acid (panels **C** & **D**) to emulate Huntington's disease. The ability of cells (red triangles) to normalize lesioned behavior (blue squares) back towards normal, sham (open circles) behavior, was monitored over time. A clear recovery effect with CTX0E03 is seen in both the sticky tape contact (**A**) and removal (**B**) tests in stroke. Similarly a clear recovery effect is seen with STR0C05 in the body sway test (**C**) and in the staircase test (**D**) (*See Color Plates*)

under quality assured clean room (class 10,000) conditions as operates at ReNeuron, or under full cGMP conditions. The standard manufacturing process for the CTX0E03 cell line is expansion in T175 cells with passaging by trypsinization every 3–4 days. On average, a cell bank is generated from a single vial expanded over six to seven passages to generate 50–100 vials, each containing 5×10^6 cells which are then stored in vapor phase liquid nitrogen. This parallel cell banking approach allows for any manufacturing development work to be carried out in advance of GMP manufacturing. The standard sequence of cell banking requirements for biologicals is Master Cell Bank (MCB), Working Cell Bank (WCB) and Drug Substance (DS) from which drug product is made (Fig. 6.1). An End of Production Cell Bank can also be established beyond the point of manufacture of any clinical product to verify long term biological and genetic stability of the product.

6.3.2.2   Non-GMP Manufacturing/Process Development

As described earlier, non-GMP cell banks were manufactured at ReNeuron up to the point of drug substance and drug product manufacture. This enabled the cell manufacturing process to be validated and the process for formulation and release testing of drug product to be developed. For example, formulation of cells at the required concentration and delivery of cells through the clinical implantation device has been verified. Assays for cell line identity (molecular assays using qRTPCR and cellular phenotype using immunocytochemistry) have been developed and a number of safety aspects of the c-mycER technology have been confirmed in vitro to rule out the possibility of reactivation of cells by re-exposure to 4-OHT, tamoxifen or endogenous steroid hormones. One particular assay has been established to monitor the expression by quantitative RTPCR of down stream targets of the myc gene including hTERT, histone deacetylase and CCND2, that serve as markers for c-mycER[TAM] activation [73]. These genes are selectively up-regulated by 4-OHT but not by other endogenous steroid hormones. Critical quality attributes for individual lot production of cells include the need for equivalence testing. Again we have established an assay based on qRTPCR that has set the range of expression of a number of genes specific for individual cell lines. Any manufactured batch of cells might be required to conform to this expression profile. More routine cell bank release specifications are also applied to non-GMP lots of drug substance in line with regulatory requirements including mycoplasma and sterility (purity), nestin expression by immunocytochemistry and full sequencing of the integrated transgene as part of a regulatory package This cell bank equivalence and release testing has enabled the use of non-GMP material in a range of GLP pre-clinical safety testing involving intracranial implantation of CTX0E03 in suitable animal models. At time of writing, long term safety studies with CTX0E03 are on going. In addition to GLP safety studies, in house studies with clinical lot equivalent drug product have confirmed efficacy of CTX0E03 in the MCAo rat model of stroke. This dose response study mimicked the proposed clinical implantation procedure with a single site implantation and confirmed the ability of CTX0E03 to restore sensori-motor function in an animal model of stroke [74].

6.3.2.3   GMP Manufacturing for Clinical Use

Manufacturing cell banks for medicinal products to cGMP standard is a formal regulatory requirement. Having identified a cell line suitable for progressing into development, a strategy must be developed for GMP manufacture and release testing. This is normally carried out by contract manufacturer following technical transfer of the manufacturing process or it can be carried out internally with the appropriate manufacturing licensing approval. Testing requirements for cell bank release of cell products leading to investigational medicinal product manufacture cover three main issues safety, purity and identity. These tests must be validated and carried out to a recognized quality standard such as US or European Pharmacopeia. For cell therapy products including ReNeuron's MCB, release tests include those for sterility and mycoplasma, retroviruses, adventitious virus agents, human viruses and species-specific viruses. General guidelines on microbiological tests for release of cell banks for cell therapy products are documented by the FDA [75]. In addition to general microbiological tests, other safety tests, including in vivo tumorigenicity, are run at this point. Identity and stability of a cell line are monitored using karyology and product specific phenotypic assays, nestin expression for example. As would be the case for any genetically modified cell line, ReNeuron's cell lines are captured by gene therapy regulations; hence the integration site of the transgene has been identified, the integrated pro-virus has been fully sequenced and assays for integrated gene copy number established. Beyond the MCB, a reduced level of testing can be applied to WCBs and release of drug substance lots. For cell therapy products, the manufacture of drug product from drug substance may involve additional cell culture processing. From a quality perspective it is imperative that sterility be assured through direct testing of materials prior to use and establishment of validated aseptic processing. For ReNeuron cell lines, in common with other neurological treatments, cells are formulated at point of use with a limited shelf life (several hours). Rapid release testing can be carried out including gram stain, rapid endotoxin and mycoplasma. In this situation sterility is assured through in process testing up to and beyond the time of implantation. As such, an action plan must be available within the clinical protocol to deal with any adverse sterility event following implantation in the patient. Beyond Phase 1 there are additional challenges to product manufacture and release of cell based medicinal products including the requirement of a validated potency assay prior to initiating Phase III studies.

Progressing neural stem cell lines to the clinic requires a combination of biological know-how and regulatory compliance to manufacture genuine novel medicinal products suitable for clinical trials. As discussed, there are a few products including ReN001 heading towards Phase 1 studies using both native and genetically modified human stem cell lines. However, the advantages of using the c-mycER technology for the production of conditionally immortalized cell lines lie in enabling large scale GMP manufacturing that allows multiple clinical lot production while retaining the product stability and reproducibility required of a medicinal product. Having come through a full cGMP banking campaign, ReN001 has verified this approach with the c-mycER technology, and other cell lines for neural and non-neural indications will follow. The STROC05 cell line discussed earlier has progressed to cGMP manufacture of a master cell bank with the possibility of progressing this line for HD and midbrain-derived dopaminergic cell lines are currently under evaluation in pre-clinical models of PD.

References

1. McMurrey CT. (2001) Huntington's disease: new hope for therapeutics. *TINS* 24, S32–S38.
2. Bjorklund A & Lindvall O. (2000) Self-repair in the brain. *Nature* 405, 892–895.
3. Kenea NL & Mehmet H. (2002) Neural stem cells. *J. Pathol.* 197, 536–550.

4. Halme DG & Kessler DA. (2006) FDA regulation of stem-cell-based therapies. *NEJM* 355, 1730–1735.
5. FDA *21 CFR Part 1271* (2005).
6. Directive 2006/17/EC (2006) Implementing 2004/23/EC on setting standards of quality and safety for donation, procurement, testing, processing, preservation, storage and distribution of human tissues and cells
7. Kondziolka D, Steinberg GK, Cullen SB & McGrogan M. (2004) Evaluation of surgical techniques for neuronal cell transplantation used in patients with stroke. *Cell Transplant.* 13, 740–754.
8. Vendrame M, Cassady I, Newcomb J, et al. (2004) Infusion of human Umbilical cord blood cells in a rat model of stroke dose dependently rescues behavioural deficits and reduces infarct volume. *Stroke* 35, 2390–2395.
9. Jin K, Sun Y, Xie L, et al. (2005) Comparison of ischemia-directed migration of neural precursor cells after intrastriatal, intraventricular or intravenous transplantation in the rat. *Neurobiol. Dis.* 18, 366–374.
10. Björklund A, Dunnett SB & Nikkah G. (1994) Nigral transplants in the rat Parkinson model. In: Dunnett SB & Bjorklund A. (Eds), *Functional Neural Transplantation.* New York: Raven, pp. 47–69.
11. Björklund LM, Sanchez-Pernaute R, Chung S, et al. (2002) Embryonic stem cells develop into functional dopaminergic neurons after transplantation in a Parkinson rat model. *PNAS* 19, 2344–2349.
12. Hodges H, Allen Y, Kershaw T, et al. (1991) Effects of cholinergic-rich neural grafts on radial maze performance after excitotoxic lesions of the forebrain cholinergic projection system-1: amelioration of cognitive deficits by transplants into cortex and hippocampus, but not basal forebrain. *Neuroscience* 45, 587–607.
13. Björklund A, Campbell K, Sirinathsinghji DJ, et al. (1994) Functional capacity of striatal transplants in the rat Huntington model. In: Dunnett SB & Björklund A. (Eds), *Functional Neural Transplantation.* New York: Raven.
14. Sinden JD, Hodges H & Gray JA. (1995) Neural transplantation and recovery of cognitive function. *Behav. Brain Sci.* 18, 10–35
15. Netto CA, Hodges H, Sinden JD et al. (1993) Effects of fetal hippocampal grafts on ischaemic-induced deficits in spatial navigation in the water maze. *Neuroscience* 54, 69–92.
16. Nunn JA & Hodges H. (1994) Cognitive deficits induced by global cerebral ischaemia: relationship to brain damage and reversal by transplants. *Behav. Brain Res.* 65, 1–31.
17. Lindvall O. (2000) Neural transplantation in Parkinson's disease. In: Chadwick DJ & Goode JA. (Eds), *Neural Transplantation in Neurodegenerative Disease: Current Status and New Directions.* John Wiley, Chichester; New York, pp. 110–128.
18. Freeman TB, Cicchetti F, Hauser O, et al. (2000). Transplanted fetal striatum in Huntington's disease: phenotypic development and lack of pathology. *PNAS* 97, 13877–13882
19. Bachoud-Levi AC, Remy P, Nguyen JP et al. (2000) Motor and cognitive improvements in patients with Huntington's disease after neural transplantation. *Lancet* 356, 1975–1979.
20. Peschanski M, Bachoud-Levi AC & Hantraye P. (2004) Integrating fetal neural transplants into a therapeutic strategy: the example of Huntington's disease. *Brain* 127, 1219–1228.
21. Olanow CW, Goetz CG, Kordower JH, et al. (2003) A double-blind controlled trial of bilateral fetal nigral transplantation in Parkinson's disease. *Ann. Neurol.* 54, 403–414.
22. Freed CR, Greene PE, Breeze RE, et al. (2001) Transplantation of dopamine neurons for severe Parkinson's disease. *NEJM* 344, 701–709.
23. Hodges H, Watts H & Reuter I. (2003) Stem cells: prospects for functional repair of brain damage. *Transplantat. Proc.* 35, 1250–1255.
24. Savitz SI, Rosenbaum DM, Dinsmore JH, et al. (2002) Cell transplantation for stroke. *Annal Neurol.* 52, 266–275.
25. Fink JS, Schumacher JM, Ellias SL, et al. (2000) Porcine Xenografts in Parkinson's disease and Huntington's disease patients: preliminary results. *Cell Transplant.* 9, 273–278.
26. Schumacher JM, Ellias SL, Palmer EP, et al. (2000) Transplantation of embryonic porcine mesencephalic tissue in patients with PD. *Neurology* 54, 1042–1050.

27. Savitz SI, Dinsmore JH, Wu J, et al. (2005) Neurotransplantation of fetal porcine cells in patients with basal ganglia infarcts: a preliminary safety and feasibility study. *Cerebrovasc. Dis.* 20, 101–107.

28. Ritzhaupt A, vander Laan LJW, Solomen DR, et al. (2002) Porcine Endogenous retrovirus infects but does not replicate in non-human primate primary cells and cell lines. *J. Virol.* 76, 11312–11320.

29. Lee SH, Lumelsky N, Studer L, et al. (2000) Efficient generation of midbrain and hindbrain neurons from mouse embryonic stem cells. *Nat. Biotechnol.* 18, 675–679.

30. Schulz TC, Noggle SA, Palmarini, et al. (2004) Differentiation of human embryonic stem cells to dopaminergic neurons in serum-free suspension culture. *Stem Cells* 22, 1218–1238.

31. Kim J-H, Auerbach JM, Rodriguez-Gomez JA, et al. (2002) Dopamine neurons derived from embryonic stem cells in an animal model of Parkinson's disease. *Nature* 418, 50–56.

32. Takagi Y, Takahashi J, Saiki H, et al. (2005) Dopaminergic neurons generated from monkey embryonic stem cells function in a Parkinson primate model. *J. Clin. Invest.* 115, 102–109.

33. Brundin P, Karlsson J, Emgard M, et al. (2000) Improving the survival of grafted dopaminergic neurons: a review over current approaches. *Cell Transp.* 9, 179–195.

34. Carpenter MK, Cui X, Hu ZY, et al. (1999) In vitro expansion of a multipotent population of human neural progenitor cells. *Exp. Neurol.* 158, 265–278.

35. Caldwell MA, He X, Wilkin N, et al. (2001) Growth factors regulate the survival and fate of cells derived from human neurospheres. *Nat. Biotech.* 19, 475–479.

36. www.Geron.com.

37. Vescovi AL, Parati EA, Gritti A, et al. (1999) Isolation and cloning of multipotential stem cells from the embryonic human CNS and establishment of transplantable human neural stem cell lines by epigenetic stimulation. *Exp. Neurol.* 156, 71–83.

38. Villa A, Snyder EY, Vescovi A & Martinez-Serano A. (2000) Establishment and properties of a growth factor dependent, perpetual neural stem cell line from the human CNS. *Exp. Neurol.* 161, 67–84.

39. Wu P, Tarasenko YI & Gu Y. (2002) Region specific generation of cholinergic neurons from fetal human neural stem cells grafted in adult rat. *Nat. Neurosci.* 5(12), 1271–1278.

40. Uchida N, Buck DW, He D, et al. (2000) Direct isolation of human central nervous system stem cells. *PNAS* 97, 14720–14725.

41. Kelly S, Bliss TM, Shah AK, et al. (2004) Transplanted human fetal neural stem cells survive, migrate, and differentiate in ischaemic rat cerebral cortex. *PNAS* 101, 11839–11844.

42. Cummings BJ, Uchida N, Tamaki SJ, et al. (2005) Human neural stem cells differentiate and promote locomotor recovery in spinal-cord injured mice. *Proc. Nat. Acad. Sci. USA* 102, 14069–14074.

43. www.StemCellsInc.com.

44. Jiang Y, Jahagirdar BN, Reinhardt RL, et al. (2002) Pluripotency of mesenchymal stem cells derived from adult marrow. *Nature* 418, 41–49.

45. Chen J, Li Y, Wang L, et al. (2001) Therapeutic benefit of intravenous administration of bone marrow stromal cells after cerebral ischemia in rats. *Stroke* 32, 1005–1011.

46. Chen J, Sanberg PR, Li Y, et al. (2001) Intravenous administration of human umbilical cord blood reduces behavioural deficits after stroke in rats. *Stroke* 32, 2682–2688.

47. Gage FH, Coates PW, Palmer TD, et al. (1995) Survival and differentiation of adult neuronal progenitor cells transplanted to the adult brain. *PNAS* 92, 11879–11883.

48. Bliss T, Guzman R, Daadi M., et al. (2007) Cell transplantation therapy for stroke. *Stroke* 38, 817–826.

49. Borlongan CV, Tajima Y, Trojanowski JQ, et al. (1998) Transplantation of cryopreserved human embryonal carcinoma-deived neurons (NT2N cells) promotes functional recovery in ischemic rats. *Exp. Neurol.* 149, 310–321.

50. Kondziolka D, Wechsler L, Goldstein S, et al. (2000) Transplantation of cultured human neuronal cells for patients with stroke. *Neurol.* 55, 565–569.

51. Flax JD, Aurora S, Yang CH, et al. (1998) Engraftable human neural stem cells respond to developmental cues and express foreign genes. *Nat. Biotech.* 16, 1033–1039.

52. Harley C, Futcher A & Greider C. (1990) Telomeres shorten during aging of human fibroblasts. *Nature* 345, 458–460.
53. Roy NS, Nakano T, Keyoung HM, et al. (2004) Telomerase immortalization of neuronally restricted progenitor cells derived from human fetal spinal cord. *Nat. Biotechnol.* 22, 297–305.
54. Martinez-Serrano A & Bjorkland A. (1997) Immortalized neural progenitor cells for CNS gene transfer and repair. *TINS* 94, 14809–14814.
55. Jat, PS, Noble MD, Ataliotis P, et al. (1991) Direct derivation of conditionally immortal cell lines from an H-2Kb-tsA58 transgenic mouse. *PNAS* 88. 5096–5100.
56. Mellodew K, Suhr R, Uwanogho D, et al. (2004) Nestin expression is lost in a neural stem cell line through a mechanism involving the proteasome and Notch signalling. *Dev. Brain Res.* 151, 13–23.
57. Sinden J, Rashid–Doubell F, Kershaw T, et al. (1997) Recovery of spatial learning by grafts of a conditionally-immortalised hippocampal neuroepithelial cell line into the ischaemia-lesioned hippocampus. *Neuroscience* 81, 599–608.
58. Hoshimura M, Ray J, Sah DWW & Gage F. (1996) Differentiation of the immortalized neuronal progenitor cell line HC2S2 into neurons by regulatable suppression of the v-myc oncogene. *PNAS* 93, 1518–1523.
59. Sah DW, Ray J, Gage F. (1997) Bipotent progenitor cell lines from the human CNS. *Nat. Biotechnol.* 5(6), 574–580.
60. Cerni C. (2000) Telomeres, telomerase and myc: an update. *Mutat. Res.* 462, 31–47.
61. Patel S, Hicks C, Sowinski P, et al. (2004) Influence of immortalisation strategy on the engraftment of human foetal neural stem cells in brains of ischaemic rats. *FENS* Paris, P13868.
62. Villa A, Navarro-Galve B, Bueno C, et al. (2004) Long term molecular and cellular stability of human neural stem cell lines. *Exp. Cell Res.* 294(2), 559–570.
63. Liste I, Garcia E & Martinez-Serano A. (2004) The generation of dopaminergic neurons by human neural stem cells is enhanced by Bcl-X$_L$ both in vitro and in vivo. *J. Neurosci.* 24(48), 10786–10795.
64. Donato R, Miljan EA, Hines SJ, et al. (2007) Differential development of neuronal physiological responsiveness in two human neural stem cell lines *BMC Neurosci.* 8, 36.
65. Gossen M & Bujard H. (1992) Tight control of gene expression in mammalian cells by tetra-cycline-responsive promoters. *PNAS* 89, 5547–5551.
66. Lotharius J, Barg S, Wiekop P, et al. (2002) Effect of mutant α-synuclein on dopamine home-ostasis in a new human mesencephalic cell line. *J. Biol. Chem.* 277, 38884–38894.
67. Kim SU. (2004) Human neural stem cells genetically modified for brain repair in neurological disorders. *Neuropathology* 24, 159–171.
68. Danielian PS, White R, Hoare SA, et al. (1993) Identification of residues in the estrogen receptor that confer differential sensitivity to estrogen and hydroxytamoxifen. *Mol. Endocrinol.* 7, 232–240.
69. Littlewood TD, Hancock DC, Danielian PS, et al. (1995) A modified oestrogen receptor-ligand binding domain as an improved switch for the regulation of heterologous proteins. *Nuc. Acids Res.* 23, 1686–1690.
70. Pollock K, Stroemer P, Patel S, et al. (2006) A conditionally immortal clonal stem cell line from human cortical neuroepithelium for the treatment of ischaemic stroke. *Exp. Neurol.* 199, 143–155.
71. Stroemer P, Pollock K, Patel S, et al. (2004) Transplanted MycER™ human neural stem cell line improves functional recovery in a rat model of stroke. *Am. Neurol. Assoc.* Toronto meeting.
72. Pollock K, Patel S, Stevanato L et al. (2004) Transplanted MycER™ immortalised human neural stem cell lines support functional recovery in rat models of neurodegenerative disease. *Soc. Neurosci.* San Diego meeting.
73. Hope AD, Oliveira CA, Blakemore WE, Pollock K, Sinden JD (2006) Specificity of the mycERTAM transgene to 4-OHT confers conditional proliferation and genetic stability in CTX0E03 stem cells. In: 4th International Society for Stem Cell Research, p. 271. Toronto meeting.
74. Stroemer RP, et al., manuscript in preparation.
75. FDA Guidances for reviewers (2003) Instructions and templates for CMC reviewers of human somatic cell therapy investigational new drug applications.

Chapter 7
Human Neural Stem Cells for Biopharmaceutical Applications

Lilian Hook[1]*, **Norma Fulton**[1], **Gregor Russell**[1], and **Timothy Allsopp**[2]

Abstract Neural stem cells, cells which have the ability to self-renew and to differentiate into three neural lineages, hold great potential for many applications in biomedical research, cellular therapy and drug discovery. However, the use of neural stem cells for these applications has been hampered by the lack of availability of stable, pure cell lines. In this review we describe the recent generation of homogenous, pluripotent, stable mouse and human neural stem (NS) cell lines. These cell lines, which can be generated from both foetal and adult tissue and ES cells, possess many attributes which make them amenable to use in the biopharmaceutical industry, such as ease of scale-up, purity and a stable phenotype over extended passage. These characteristics are discussed, along with the technical, safety and ethical issues associated with the use of NS cells in therapeutic and drug discovery applications.

Keywords Neural stem (NS) cell; cell therapy; drug screening; manufacture; ethics; safety

7.1 Introduction

Neural stem cells (NSC) are self-renewing, multipotent cells restricted to generate the three neural lineages – neurons, astrocytes and oligodendrocytes. NSCs are present in mammals throughout embryogenesis, persisting into adulthood, although it is believed they change their potential and become more restricted during development [1]. NSCs have been derived and propagated *in vitro* from the fetal and adult central nervous system (CNS) of many species. In general, these cells have been grown in

---

[1] Stem Cell Sciences UK Ltd., Roger Land Building, Kings Buildings, West Mains Road, Edinburgh, EH9 3JQ, UK

[2] Stem Cell Sciences UK Ltd., Minerva Building 250, Babraham Research Campus, Cambridge, CB22 3AT, UK

*Corresponding Author:
e-mail: lilian.hook@stemcellsciences.com

Y. Shi, D.O. Clegg (eds.) *Stem Cell Research and Therapeutics*,
© Springer Science+Business Media B.V. 2008

floating spheres which are heterogeneous in nature, consisting of NSCs, committed progenitors and differentiated cells. It has not been possible to propagate them for any length of time without loss of, in particular, their neurogenic potential. Prolonged adherent propagation of NSCs normally requires transformation [2]. Neural stem and progenitor cells have also been derived from mouse and human embryonic stem (ES) cells, although typically again cells capable of propagation are cultured as floating neurospheres and are heterogeneous in nature.

Recently however, neural stem cells have been derived from mouse ES cells, CNS and human fetal CNS that can be expanded indefinitely in monolayer conditions without loss of neurogenic potential [3]. These cells have been termed NS cells due to their similarity in many attributes to embryonic stem (ES) cells, principally, homogeneous symmetrical division *in vitro* under appropriate culture conditions.

NS cells are continuously growing, self-renewing, non-immortalised neural stem cell lines, thought to be similar in phenotype to neural stem cells found *in vivo*. They can be readily derived from embryonic stem cells and fetal or adult brain, and are grown in monolayer, serum free conditions in the presence of the growth factors fibroblast growth factor (FGF-2) and epidermal growth factor (EGF) whereby they self renew indefinitely as a homogenous culture. NS cells are characterised by a bi-polar morphology, expression of neural stem cell markers such as nestin and BLBP, lack of expression of differentiated cell markers and the ability to differentiate *in vitro* and *in vivo* to mature neurons, astrocytes and oligodendrocytes. In comparison to reagents derived previously, NS cell lines clearly represent a major advance in neural stem cell technology.

Due to their homogenous nature and relative ease of derivation, NS cells offer enormous potential in many areas of biomedical research. Their homogeneity means they will be useful for elucidating the molecular mechanisms by which neural stem cells develop, self renew and differentiate and for studying disease phenotypes. Additionally, their suitability for scale up processes makes them an attractive candidate for *in vitro* drug screening assays, and as they are easily transfected, for large scale genetic screens. Equally, since NS cells can differentiate to neurons and glia *in vitro* and *in vivo*, they offer a limitless source of cells for cellular therapy in conditions such as Parkinson's disease and epilepsy. NS cell lines therefore have potential in many areas of stem cell technology, and it is anticipated that they will be of enormous benefit to pharmaceutical and clinical programs.

In this chapter we will review the characteristics and potential applications of NS cells, in particular human NS cells, and the practical and ethical issues associated with such uses.

7.2   NS Cell Properties

7.2.1   *Derivation and Propagation of NS Cells*

In 2005, Conti et al. [3] reported the derivation of NS cell lines from both embryonic stem (ES) cells and from fetal forebrain of mouse and human. These NS cells were derived under serum and feeder-free conditions and propagated without the requirement for floating neurospheres which have previously been shown to support the maintenance and isolation of neural stem-like cells [4].

The protocols for derivation of mouse and human NS cells are very similar and consequently will be discussed together. NS cells were initially isolated from differentiating cultures of mouse ES cells. Neuroectodermal precursors can be generated from mouse ES cells in a serum-free and adherent culture system [5]. Conti et al. [3] showed by isolating these neuroectodermal precursors and culturing them as floating aggregates, NS cells could subsequently be isolated and maintained under adherent conditions in expansion media (NS-A basal media + N2 supplement) that critically included both exogenous EGF and FGF-2.

The generation of NS cells from established hES cell lines has not yet been reported. However, Conti et al. [3] were able to transfer spontaneously differentiated neuroepithelial precursors that arose during the early stages of an hES cell derivation into a feeder-free environment, and culture these cells in NS cell expansion media. After four weeks, an adherent and homogenous NS cell like population emerged that displayed the morphology and some of the markers characteristic of mouse ES cell derived NS cells.

There exist distinct similarities both in morphology and marker identification between NS cells and the *in vivo* population of neurogenic radial glia. Both cell types undergo dynamic morphological change, including nuclear migration, and display a distinct bipolar morphology. In addition, NS cells express neural stem/progenitor cell markers such as nestin which was initially characteristic as a marker of radial glia in developing rat brain [6]. Traditionally, it was thought that radial glia function as a substrate/guide upon which newly generated immature neurons migrate. However, views of radial glia function have recently been extended to include their acting as neural progenitors based on their shared characteristic markers, morphology and ability to generate neurons [7, 8]. It was therefore investigated whether NS cells could be isolated and maintained from fetal neural tissue and it was found that NS cells could be derived from primary CNS of embryonic day (E) 16.5 mouse fetal forebrain and Carnegie stage 19–20 human fetal cortex. NS cells could be isolated via an initial floating aggregate stage and subsequently transferred and maintained in the continued presence of EGF and FGF-2 on gelatin coated tissue culture plastic (Fig. 7.1). Subsequently, it has been shown that laminin is a preferable substrate for derivation and propagation of human NS cells. The derivation of NS cells from fetal cortex does not absolutely rely on the formation of neurospheres. Disassociated primary cortex from E12.5 mouse has been plated directly onto laminin in the presence of EGF and FGF-2 whereby the cells attach and rapidly adopt a homogenous morphology. These cells share the characteristics of previously established NS cell lines cultured on laminin as well as retaining the ability to differentiate into neurons and astrocytes [9].

NS cells have been isolated from many regions of the embryonic CNS, including the spinal cord, indicating their ubiquitous presence throughout early development. Previous studies in mouse have shown that neural stem-like cells could be isolated from both embryonic striatal primordia and the neural crest or peripheral nervous system [10, 11]. In culture these cells proliferated from explanted tissue in the presence of the mitogens EGF and FGF-2. Isolation of NS cells from fore-, mid-, hindbrain and spinal cord from fetal tissue may yield populations that possess subtle or

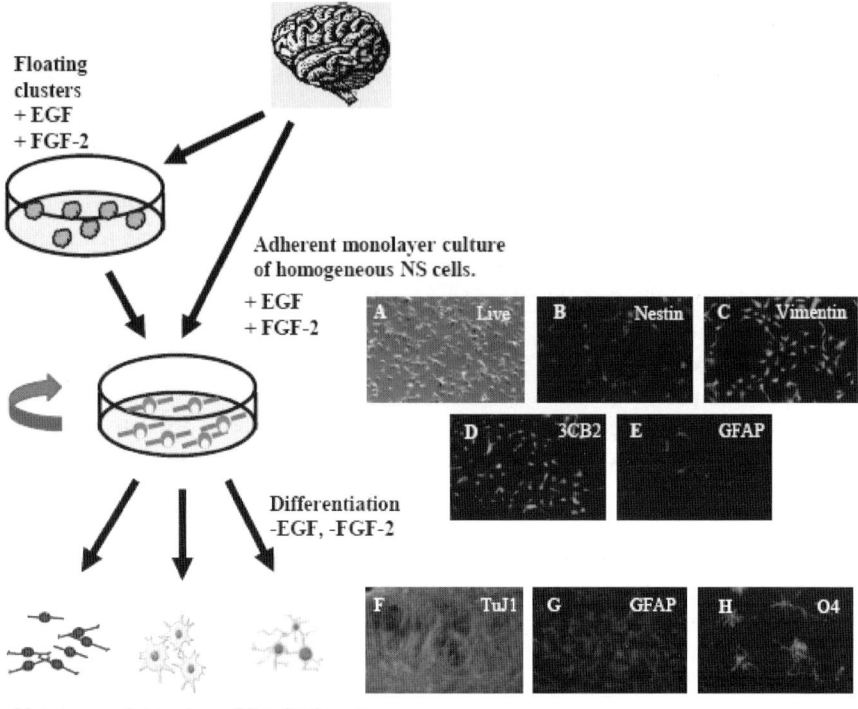

Fig. 7.1 Derivation, propagation and differentiation of human NS cells. NS cells can be derived from various regions of the fetal brain. Through the actions of EGF and FGF-2 NS cells can be expanded in monolayer conditions either from floating clusters (green) or directly in an adherent monolayer culture. (**A**) Passage 21 human NS cells in expansion media and (**B–E**) immunostained for human NS cell/radial glia markers. hNS cells can differentiate to form neurons, astrocytes and oligodendrocytes. (**F–H**) Differentiated hNS immunostained for neural (Tuj1), astrocyte (GFAP) and oligodendrocyte (O4) markers (Oligodendrocyte image courtesy of Y. Sun) (*See Color Plates*)

inherent properties that differentiate them from other regionally isolated NS cells. This may be useful in the generation of specific neural subtypes that may be relevant to future clinical application and/or drug screening. However, it remains to be seen whether cell lines isolated from different regions can maintain their regional identity after prolonged *in vitro* propagation and whether they do indeed generate neuronal subtypes particular to the region of origin.

In the adult brain, ongoing neurogenesis has been convincingly shown within regions of the subventricular zone (SVZ) and subgranular layer of the hippocampus [12, 13], and cells extracted from the adult nervous system have previously been expanded *in vitro* [4, 10, 14]. Pollard et al. [9] reported the isolation and propagation of NS cell lines from adult mouse brain following the same isolation and propagation techniques employed previously for fetal tissues.

NS cells are cultured as an adherent, homogenous population dependent on the presence of exogenous FGF-2 and EGF. Under these conditions, they undergo continued symmetrical cell division (self-renewal) while retaining the ability to generate functional neurons, astrocytes and oligodendrocytes both *in vitro* and upon transplantation into adult rodent brain. NS cells can also be successfully cryopreserved and recovered using standard techniques, retaining their characteristics.

The presence of FGF-2 and/or EGF has previously been shown to play an important role in the *in vitro* culture of mammalian neural precursors [4, 14, 15]. It seems that EGF is critical in maintaining NS cell identity as its removal results in extensive cell death with remaining cells adopting a differentiated morphology [3]. However it isn't absolutely required in the derivation process, although accompanying differentiation is observed in its absence [9]. The presence of FGF-2 appears necessary during derivation, however in established NS cell lines it is not strictly required. Upon its removal NS cells retain their homogenous morphology, the capacity for differentiation and their ability for clonal growth. In the presence of a pharmacological inhibitor of the FGF-2 receptor (SU5402), NS cell colonies appear slightly smaller with slower doubling times indicating that autocrine FGF-2 signaling can contribute to NS cell propagation [9]. It may be that FGF-2 exposure during derivation induces EGF receptor expression in NS cells. It is currently unclear how prolonged exposure to these factors affects NS cells, particularly in terms of their regional identity.

7.2.2 NS Cell Characteristics

NS cells in their undifferentiated state are characterised by a unique bipolar morphology that can help identify them from the heterogeneity associated with early culture. Derivation from human fetal material gives rise to a seemingly mixed population of NS cells, exhibiting both classic bipolar NS cell morphology and other cell morphologies. It has been shown however, via time-lapse monitoring, that these cell morphologies are plastic and interconvertible [3]. NS cells also display interkinetic nuclear migration along the cell process, a feature which is characteristic of neuroepithelial and radial glia cells *in vivo* [16], strengthening the idea that NS cells may be closely related to the radial glia lineage.

Under adherent culture conditions and in the presence of FGF-2 and EGF, NS cells are capable of symmetrical self-renewal [3]. Mouse ES derived NS cells still proliferate after 115 passages and retain a normal diploid karyotype at late passage. Importantly, these cells also retain their neurogenic potential after such extensive passaging. This is in contrast to other long-term passaged NSCs that tend to become more gliogenic after prolonged culture periods, often losing the ability to generate neurons at all [17]. However, similar studies need to be carried out on human NS cells to determine whether they too are stable over many passages. This is particularly important if NS cell lines are to be used for clinical applications. Human NS (hNS) cells proliferate more slowly than mouse NS (mNS) cells, with doubling times of 3–5 days compared to 24 h for mouse. The culture conditions adapted from mNS cell derivation and propagation may warrant further refinements for application to the human system to establish optimal growth and differentiation. To date, human fetal derived NS cells have been maintained for up to 35 passages, retaining a normal karyotype and the ability to generate neurons. This constitutes over six months in continuous culture.

NS cells are immunoreactive for a range of neural precursor/radial glia markers such as Nestin, Vimentin, RC2, 3CB2, Sox-2 and brain lipid-binding protein (BLBP). However, subtle differences exist between mouse and human NS cells. For example, hNS cells exhibit moderate levels of glial fibrillary acidic protein (GFAP) expression unlike mouse NS cells [3], reflecting the differences between the species *in vivo* [8, 18]. More detailed study of mouse NS cells via Genechip analysis and RT-PCR showed they are negative for the pluripotency markers Oct-4, Nanog and Eras and markers of mesoderm and endoderm lineages. They also express the neural precursor markers Sox3, Emx2 and Pax6 and the bHLH transcription factors Olig2 and Mash1. A particular set of transcription factors may confer the capacity for self-renewal; however this combination of transcription factor expression may not exist *in vivo* but rather reflect *in vitro* culture conditions, particularly the combination of EGF and FGF-2 [9]. Despite this, these markers are consistent with neurogenic radial glia present during the development of the nervous system.

NS cells are competent for both glial and neuronal differentiation. A mixed population of predominantly neurons (Tuj-1+, Map-2+) and astrocytes (GFAP+) is generated upon plating of NS cells onto a poly-ornithin/laminin substrate with removal of FGF-2 and EGF (Fig. 7.1). Neuronal maturation can be further enhanced by switching the media to differing ratios of neurobasal:NSA and supplementing with B27, brain derived neurotrophic factor (BDNF) and nerve growth factor (NGF) [3]. mNS cells generate predominantly GABAergic neurons which also express mature markers such as synaptophysin and voltage-gated ion channels. After several weeks of maturation these neurons are electrophysiologically active, exhibiting voltage-gated Na^+, K^+ and Ca^{2+} currents similar to those observed in primary neurons [3]. Further study is required to determine whether hNS derived neurons are also functionally active. Exposure of differentiating cultures to serum or BMP4 results in the generation of nearly pure populations of astrocytes expressing GFAP. Under standard differentiation conditions only very few oligodendrocytes are generated. However, Glaser et al. [19] reported that upon proliferation with FGF-2, platelet derived growth factor (PDGF) and forskolin, followed by differentiation in the presence of thyroid hormone (T3) and ascorbic acid, NS cells could effectively generate oligodendrocytes (~20%) which express the oligodendrocytic specific markers O4, CNPase and myelin proteolipid protein.

Another important characteristic of NS cells is their amenability to genetic alteration. Cells can be transfected by electroporation, nucleofection and lentiviral transduction. This has important implications for the use of NS cells in disease modeling and drug screening. The ability to carry out gene targeting in NS cells by homologous recombination is currently under investigation.

7.3 Biopharmaceutical Applications

Many of the characteristics of NS cells described above make them suitable candidates for applications in the biopharmaceutical industry such as drug screening, disease modelling and cell replacement therapies. The utility of NS cells for these applications is described below.

7.3.1 Drug Screening

Current methods of drug screening rely largely on the use of recombinant transformed cell lines that express the target of interest, e.g., the NMDA receptor [20], but otherwise are not directly relevant to the disease being studied. The use of primary cells is desirable since they are physiologically relevant, containing all the endogenous signalling pathways and factors that are expressed *in vivo*. However, primary cells are relatively difficult to obtain and since they can typically only be passaged a few times before senescence or death it is time consuming and technically challenging to obtain cells in sufficient numbers for high throughput screening applications. Additionally, variability between donors and in preparation of cell batches can lead to inconsistent results. Stem cells offer an attractive alternative to primary cells and recombinant cell lines in that they can generate physiologically relevant cell types but can be propagated for prolonged periods of time and cryopreserved, while maintaining their differentiation potential. Therefore large batches of undifferentiated or differentiated cells can be generated that could be used in a series of experiments or screens.

In particular, the adherent, homogenous nature of NS cells lends them to drug screening applications and with their direct physiological relevance they are more attractive than conventional recombinant cell lines. It will be necessary however to validate the functional attributes of the progeny generated and their similarity to cells derived *ex vivo*. One particular problem could be that differentiated cultures generated *in vitro* may not contain the same mixture of cell types that is required to replicate *in vivo* function.

It is predicted that stem cells could be used throughout the process of high throughput drug screening from target validation through to medicinal chemistry [21]. The understanding of gene function is paramount to identifying and validating drug targets. In this respect the homogenous nature and ease of genetic modification of NS cells will be beneficial in gene profiling and loss/gain of function experiments. The transfection of cDNA or RNAi, either of known targets or through library screening, will enable elucidation of gene function [22]. The ability to achieve gene targeting and knock outs by homologous recombination in NS cells is currently being explored. However, the ability to generate NS cells from modified ES cells or CNS of modified mice offers an alternative to generating knockout NS cells. The genetic modification of NS cells also allows the generation of reporter lines for primary and secondary screens. In addition, the use of hNS cells in particular could reduce the need for extensive *in vivo* animal testing and offer the additional benefit of being able to study the effects of genetic diversity on drug efficacy.

In addition to using NS cells and their derivatives for more traditional drug screening they also have potential to be useful for discovering novel drugs or factors which could promote endogenous cells to replace lost or diseased cells in conditions such as stroke. Screening may also be used to identify new molecules that improve the differentiation of NS cells to particular subtypes of neurons that could then be used to improve production of cells for cell replacement therapies, e.g., ventral mesencephalic dopaminergic neurons for Parkinson's disease (c.f. section 7.3.3).

7.3.2 Disease Models

The ability to genetically modify NS cells and also the ability to generate them from modified ES cells and mouse models make them attractive candidates for disease modelling whereby genes are knocked out, or point mutations engineered to recapitulate diseases with a known genetic basis. In addition, techniques such as nuclear transfer make the possibility of generating NS cells from "diseased" hES cells a possibility [23, 24]. For example, skin cells taken from a patient suffering from a genetically based disease such as Huntingdon's could be used to generate a blastocyst via nuclear transfer. This blastocyst could be used to generate a hES cell line, which in turn could be used to generate a line of hNS cells that bears the genetic mutation. Such cells could be used as an *in vitro* model of the disease for both understanding its molecular basis and for drug screening. Similarly, recent advances in development of ES-like cells from somatic cells via transduction of a simple set of transcription factors could enable generation of many disease specific hES cell derived hNS cell lines [25–27]. The true potential of such disease modelling techniques have yet to be demonstrated and it is likely that that they will be limited by the ability to generate *in vitro* all the cell types in the correct proportions to truly model the disease. However, stem cells generated from patients that carry disease specific mutations, in particular, will at least comprise the complete genetic basis of the disease, leading to enhanced understanding, as compared to the modelling of disease by introducing mutations into existing cell lines.

The homogenous nature and direct physiological relevance of hNS cells also offers the potential for discovery of novel biomarkers for monitoring endogenous stem cell proliferation and differentiation or for tracking the integration and function of transplanted stem cells [28, 29]. Such biomarkers would be useful as non-invasive methods for diagnosis, monitoring of disease progression and assessment of response to drugs and injury. The identification of markers that are upregulated in response to drugs with known mechanisms of action and neurotoxic substances would be beneficial for *in vitro* drug discovery and toxicology screening. The ability to differentiate hNS cells to pure populations of neuronal and glial cells could lead to the discovery of biomarkers for various different stages of neurogenesis and potentially for specific neuronal subtypes that are compromised in certain diseases. Additionally, the use of disease specific NS cells as described above could identify biomarkers for diagnosis or monitoring progression of the disease in question.

7.3.3 Cell Replacement Therapies

Neurodegenerative diseases such as Parkinson's, Huntingdon's and multiple sclerosis, have become the focus of interest for potential cell replacement therapies. Such treatments have several advantages over conventional drug therapies, primarily the potential to provide long-term benefits of a physiological nature.

Previous studies using cell replacement therapies for such disorders have focused on using primary human fetal material with minimal expansion in culture before implantation [30–32]. These have shown some success but suffer from obvious limitations in adequate provision of material and standardization between different samples. hNS cells derived from hES cells or fetal tissue have the potential to generate unlimited supplies of neural cells for replacement therapies since they have the advantage that they can be grown for prolonged periods of time without loss of their neurogenic and homogenous properties, i.e., for long enough to bank sufficient cells to treat multiple patients. Importantly since they can also be cryopreserved, different batches of cells can be quality controlled before release to clinic.

To date only mouse NS cells have been transplanted into test animals to assess survival and integration [3]. Both ES cell derived and CNS derived mNS cells were able to integrate into the striatum or hippocampus of fetal and adult rat brains. The cells differentiated into neurons and glia but did not migrate extensively from the injection site. Cells survived for up to six weeks and importantly no tumors were observed at least six months after transplant. It has subsequently been demonstrated that pre-differentiating the cells to a stage in between that of NS cells and mature neurons greatly enhances the generation of neurons *in vivo*. Similarly, NS cell derived oligodendrocytes have been transplanted into a myelin-deficient rat model where they successfully ensheathed host axons in the brain [19].

The restricted potential of NS cells offers advantages over the use of hES derived cells for cell therapy. Although hES cells can be grown indefinitely and theoretically to large scale they have some disadvantages over tissue specific stem cells. Firstly, since they are pluripotent it is harder to obtain the specific lineage of cells required for a particular therapy. It may be necessary to use genetic manipulation of the cells to implement lineage selection strategies or to direct differentiation down a particular pathway, e.g., by overexpression of a particular transcription factor. In addition, there is the possibility that differentiated cultures of hES cells would still contain some undifferentiated cells which could form tumors upon transplantation. However, the generation of hES cells via nuclear transfer from, or transfection of, a patient's somatic cells does offer the potential of generating patient specific hNS cells for the treatment of neurological disorders [23, 24].

Several other important questions need to be answered before hNS cells could be used for therapeutic purposes, such as mode of delivery and ability to reach the target area; longevity of survival and functionality; optimal differentiation status of the cells; need for administration of additional agents and the mode of action of transplanted cells. It may be that cells themselves differentiate into functional, integrated cells of the desired type. However, it may be that they would secrete factors that promote endogenous stem or progenitor cells to propagate and differentiate. Most likely, it would be a combination of both mechanisms. Safety issues are also of paramount importance and are discussed in the following sections.

7.4 Technical and Safety Issues for Biopharmaceutical Applications

In order to realize the potential of using stem cells for drug discovery or cell replacement therapies it will be necessary to manufacture cells in sufficient quantities under GMP conditions in a consistent manner. For clinical applications, the safety of cells in both manufacture and performance is particularly critical.

7.4.1 Cell Culture Conditions

When considering the derivation, expansion and differentiation of NS cells *in vitro* for clinical applications an important factor is the cell culture medium used. Any such medium should be manufactured to GMP quality, be reproducible, standardized and, most importantly, safe. It must maintain cells in a consistent, reproducible way, while preserving a normal karyotype, growth characteristics and undifferentiated status. Ideally this would mean products are serum free, animal component free and fully defined.

Serum is an undefined mix of components that can influence the growth characteristics of cells. As such, different batches can vary significantly and therefore extensive testing of different lots is required. Additionally, there is a risk that serum will contain pathogens of either animal or human origin depending on its source [33]. Therefore the complete removal of serum related products from the culture system is the optimal way to ensure the safety and reproducibility of cell cultures.

The propagation of human cells in conditions containing animal products raises the possibility of transference of animal pathogens but also of inducing an immune response upon transplantation. For example, human cells cultured in animal component containing conditions such as in serum replacement products or on mouse feeders have been shown to express the non-human immunogenic sialic acid Neu5Gc. Circulating antibodies to this molecule are present in humans and could compromise successful transplantation processes using such cells [34, 35]. The replacement of animal components with human or recombinant counterparts would negate such safety issues. However, human derived products also carry a risk of transmitting human pathogens and therefore, ideally, medium supplements would be comprised entirely of recombinant products. This would also ensure that different media batches are more reproducible.

Serum free and animal component free medium has been designed that supports the derivation, propagation and differentiation of hNS cells. Work is ongoing to further develop this medium to be fully recombinant.

NS cells are propagated in a feeder-free environment, which is beneficial not only as a simpler method of culture but also results in a more controlled environment. However, NS cells do require tissue culture plastic to be coated with a substrate for efficient propagation and differentiation. In the case of hNS cells, the substrates used are laminin and poly-ornithin/laminin for propagation and differentiation, respectively. The source, or replacement, of such substrates needs to be considered carefully if cells are to be used for clinical purposes both from a consistency and safety point of view.

7.4.2   Scale-Up

Provision of the pharmaceutical industry with an unlimited supply of stem cells for drug discovery or clinical application requires the production of cells on a large scale, preferably in batches that could treat many patients or be sufficient for several drug screens. As described above, the manual culture of NS cells is well understood, with established and robust methods. However, traditional manual or stationary culture methods are not suitable for the generation of large numbers of cells, proving too expensive and labor intensive [36].

There are two main approaches for the efficient large-scale production of cells (Fig. 7.2):

(i) Bioreactors allow the growth of cells in suspension culture thereby increasing the surface area to volume ratio. Cells can either be cultured as floating aggregates or be innoculated onto microcarriers whereby cells attach to microspheres coated with a substrate such as gelatin, collagen or laminin [37–39]. In such a system it is possible to control pH, oxygen, osmolality and temperature

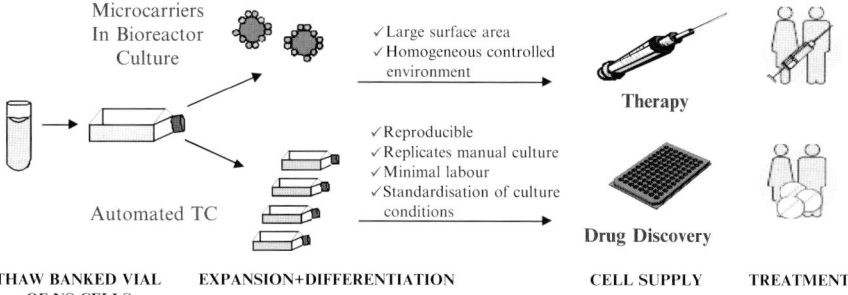

Fig. 7.2 Overview of bioprocessing of human NS cells for drug discovery and therapy. Human NS cells could be expanded and differentiated either by bioreactor culture or automated tissue culture techniques. Bioreactor culture could provide large batches of cells for transplant therapies, whereas automated tissue culture may be more suited to the generation of batches of cells in an assay ready configuration for drug discovery (*See Color Plates*)

as well as nutrient delivery, cell density and inoculation efficiency [36]. However, it is necessary to strictly control the size of the aggregates and the effects of shearing on the cells due to continuous stirring [36, 40, 41].

(ii) The second approach to cell culture scale-up is the use of automated cell culture platforms such as the Select T (The Automation Partnership). Such systems have the advantage of being more reproducible than manual culture approaches and less labor intensive. Cell culture conditions can be standardized, contamination reduced significantly and the system can count cells and check viability before passaging or plating into small well format for screening assays. Additionally, each flask can be processed with its own unique set of parameters.

These two different methods of scaling up cell production have different advantages and may be suited to different applications. The advantages of using a suspension bioreactor are the large surface area to volume ratio enabling a large number of cells to be grown under the same conditions at the same time. This may be more suited to the generation of batches of cells for clinical use. The use of automated cell culture machines may be more suited to the production of cells in small well format for drug screening applications where the whole process from scale-up, plating out of cells and screening can be automated.

mNS cells have been successfully cultured on microcarriers in bioreactors and on the automated SelecT machine. Cells retained undifferentiated markers and the capacity to differentiate. The large-scale culture of human NS cells is currently being explored and more work is required to understand how these cells proliferate and differentiate in large-scale culture systems. The scale-up of stem cells in general tends to be more problematic than that of other cells since fundamental characteristics such as their undifferentiated state can be easily unbalanced.

7.4.3 Quality Control and Cell Banking

An important aspect of standardized cell provision is the generation of quality controlled cell banks. This requires both regulatory and technical issues to be addressed.

It is crucial to document and control all aspects of the cell production process through donor selection, collection, processing, cell characterization, cryopreservation, evaluation and release of the final product. Regulatory standards for some of these practices have already been established for cell lines used in the production of viral vaccines and recombinant therapeutic products [42], and any therapies using stem cells require a combination of these regulations and the guidelines for human tissue transplantation. The European Human Tissue Directive, 2004, sets the standards of quality and safety for the donation, procurement, testing, processing, preservation and distribution of human tissues and cells (Directive 2004/23/EC of The European Parliament and of the Council). A very important aspect is the generation of quality control (QC) and quality assurance (QA) assays whereby a minimum data set of functional and phenotypic attributes is set, leading to criteria for release and tolerance to batch variability [43]. In particular, it is essential to document the molecular signature of each cell line so that it is possible to determine if cells become contaminated with other cell lines at any point in the process.

The establishment of cell banks also requires the resolution of technical issues. For example, it must be possible to scale-up and efficiently and simply freeze and thaw cell lines without compromising their functional attributes. In addition, for clinical use, the optimal differentiation status of the cells prior to transplantation needs to be identified and incorporated into the design such that both a master cell bank and a bank of transplant ready cells is generated. By banking cell lines ready for transplant, cell distribution to clinics will be simplified, along with minimizing the manipulations that are required before cells can be transplanted, therefore minimizing the variation in cell populations transplanted in different locations. The shelf-life of cell lines in terms of their efficacy and the stability of genetic factors and differentiation potential is also important as this will determine the time window for scaling up and banking cells. mNS cells have been shown to have remarkable functional and genetic stability over multiple passages and therefore are very amenable to cell banking [3]. Whether human NS cells are similarly stable is currently under investigation.

7.4.4 Tumorigenicity and Immunogenicity

Amongst the significant problems to be considered for any potential cell replacement therapy is the immunological status of the cells to be transplanted and of the recipient tissue. Upon tissue grafting, the majority of problems arise when the recipient produces antibodies to specific endogenous polymorphic peptides in the donor tissue. Major Histocompatibility Complex antigens (Class I and II) and HLA antigens are involved, along with T lymphocytes and microglial cells [44, 45]. These responses are cellular in nature and commonly occur when there are similarities between the host and the donor. A more severe form of rejection can occur when there is very little phylogenic relationship between the host and donor which involves the complement system and natural killer cells [45].

The brain has traditionally been thought of as an immune privileged site [46] as grafts appear to survive well without being attacked by the host immune system. This is thought to be largely due to the inability of molecules to cross the blood brain barrier, the absence of antigen presenting cells and sparse lymphatic drainage [46]. There is also some evidence that cells derived from the CNS are non-immunogenic [47–50]. This leads to the possibility that hNS cell grafts may not incur the same degree of immune reaction as other transplants, particularly if cells are to be transplanted directly into the brain. However, this would need to be tested extensively in animal models to see if this was indeed the case.

One way to minimize the immunological barriers between host and donor is to create stem cell banks whereby donors can be matched to recipients as is done for organ transplantation. Alternatively, the generation of patient specific hNS cells as described in section 7.3.3 would eliminate the issue of immune rejection.

Another of the barriers associated with any potential cell therapy is the possibility that transplanted cells might proliferate in a disorganised and erratic manner causing the formation of a tumor [51]. It has been widely demonstrated that embryonic stem cell lines generate teratomas when injected into mice and this is a potential problem in using hES derived somatic cells as it would be necessary to ensure that cultures contained no residual undifferentiated ES cells [52, 53]. The transplant of mNS cells into recipient rodent brains did not result in any tumorigenic effects up to six months after transplant, and cell cycle analysis after four weeks showed that only 1% of cells expressed the marker of proliferation Ki67. In addition, injection of mNS cells under the kidney capsule of mice did not result in the formation of teratomas as is observed with ES cells [3]. This data suggests that hNS cells may not be tumorigenic *in vivo*. However, there has been a report that transplant of a purified dopaminergic neuron population derived from hES cells that contained no detectable residual hES cells resulted in a high incidence of uncontrolled proliferation of neural epithelial like cells [54]. Therefore, the transplantation of hNS cells could have a similar effect. There is evidence from mNS cells that pre-differentiation of NS cells prior to transplant increases their survival and integration. Use of such a regime for hNS cells could decrease the chances of transplanted cells proliferating in an unregulated manner.

7.4.5   Ethical Considerations

The source of tissue for the production of stem cells and their use in medical research and potential clinical application in human disease is a widely discussed and controversial ethical topic. Stem cells can be derived from embryonic, fetal and adult sources, each of which raises different issues. In addition, the legal and ethical considerations surrounding human derived stem cell lines are conflicting in different jurisdictions concerning what is permitted regarding research, sourcing and use.

Embryonic stem cells are the most controversial of stem cells and work on these cells is severely restricted in many countries. Human embryonic stem cells are most commonly derived from surplus IVF embryos that have been donated from patients once they have concluded their treatment. However, blastocysts can also be specifically created for hES derivation from donated eggs and spermatozoa or by Somatic Cell Nuclear Transfer (SCNT), also known as therapeutic cloning [23, 24]. Creation of blastocysts specifically for hES cell derivation is a highly controversial topic, and therapeutic cloning is only allowed in certain countries where it is tightly regulated and a licence required to perform such work. The use of fetal tissue is similarly controversial to using IVF embryos, although the issues here are primarily concerned with the morality of abortion. The potential benefits of using such material must be weighed up with the ethical and moral reasoning for and against abortion when considering the use of foetal derived stem cells.

The ethics of stem cell procurement are also of fundamental importance to the use of fetal and embryonic stem cells for research and transplantation. It is important that patient confidentiality is respected and that fully informed consent is obtained when acquiring supernumerary embryos and oocytes or aborted foetuses. Such informed consent should include information on whether the subsequent use of the samples will involve any commercial work. The generation of SCNT embryos for derivation of patient specific or disease specific hES cells and their derivatives requires the use of donated oocytes. This raises difficult questions, as the procedure to obtain oocytes is invasive and painful and donors participate for purely altruistic reasons and not as part of other ongoing treatment such as IVF [55]. There is much debate as to whether such donors should be offered financial incentives or whether this could lead to undue inducement and commodification of human body parts. Currently, it is permitted to compensate donors only for their time and discomfort meaning technically the oocytes themselves have not been bought. Arguments surrounding the payment or not of donors are also linked to the use of the resultant stem cell lines. If they are only to be used for pure research, then one could argue that donation should be free. However, when cells are to be used by commercial organizations for profit driven activity such as drug screening, the argument becomes more complicated regarding whether the donors should receive some share of that profit. Additionally, the question of ownership of the cell lines is raised.

It has been argued that the ethical concerns surrounding the use of blastocyst or fetal derived stem cells could be resolved by the use of adult derived tissue specific stem cells. There is evidence that neural stem cells persist in the adult CNS and also that some adult mesenchymal stem cells have neurogenic potential *in vitro* and upon transplantation [56]. In this case autologous cells or those obtained from donors similarly to current organ transplant practices could be used for transplantation. However, due to various efficacy and technical issues, many consider that at present, embryonic or fetal stem cells provide the best potential resource for neuronal stem cell biopharmaceutical applications.

In addition to the ethical issues surrounding the origin and procurement of stem cells, the ethics of novel treatments need to be considered when developing new therapies. This is especially pertinent when dealing with cell based therapies where efficacy, mode of delivery and dosage are difficult to test in animal models. A balance has to be reached between the potential benefits of such a novel treatment and the current best placed treatment.

7.5 Summary

Neural stem cells hold great promise for various biopharmaceutical applications. In particular, the recently isolated fetal and ES cell derived NS cells described above have several attributes which make them more amenable to these applications than previously available resources. They can be propagated as a homogeneous, adherent population, maintaining differentiation potential and genetic stability over extended culture. In addition, they can be grown and differentiated at scale, in small well format and can be genetically modified. They therefore represent a stable physiological cell resource that holds potential for use in drug screening, diagnostics, toxicology and cell replacement therapies.

References

1. Merkle F, Alvarez-Buylla A (2006) Neural stem cells in mammalian development. Curr Opin Biol 18: 704–709
2. Pollock K, Stroemer P, Patel S, Stevanato L, Hope A, Miljan E, Dong Z, Hodges H, Price J, Sinden JD (2006) A conditionally immortal clonal stem cell line from human cortical neuroepithelium for the treatment of ischemic stroke. Exp Neurol 199 (1): 143–155
3. Conti L, Pollard SM, Gorba T, Reitano E, Toselli M, Biella G, Sun Y, Sanzone S, Ying Q-L, Cattaneo E, Smith A (2005) Niche-independent symmetrical self-renewal of a mammalian tissue stem cell. PLoS Biol 3: e283
4. Reynolds BA, Weiss S (1992) Generation of neurons and astrocytes from isolated cells of the adult mammalian central nervous system. Science 255 (5052): 1707–1710
5. Ying Q-L, Stavridis M, Griffiths D, Li M, Smith A (2003) Conversion of embryonic stem cells into neuroectodermal precursors in adherent monoculture. Nat Biotechnol 21: 183–186
6. Hockfield S, McKay RD (1985) Identification of major cell classes in the developing mammalian nervous system. J Neurosci 5: 3310–3328
7. Kriegstein AR (2005) Constructing circuits: neurogenesis and migration in the developing neocortex. Epilepsia 46 (Suppl 7): 15–21
8. Malatesta P, Hartfuss E, Gotz M (2000) Isolation of radial glial cells by fluorescent-activated cell sorting reveals a neuronal lineage. Development 127: 5253–5263
9. Pollard SM, Conti L, Sun Y, Goffredo G, Smith A (2006) Adherent neural stem (NS) cells from fetal and adult forebrain. Cereb Cortex 16: i112–i120
10. Reynolds BA, Tetzlaff W, Weiss S (1992) A multipotent EGF-responsive striatal embryonic progenitor cell produces neurons and astrocytes. J Neurosci 12 (11): 4565–4574
11. Stemple DL, Andderson DJ (1992) Isolation of a stem cell for neurons and glia from the mammalian neural crest. Cell 71: 973–985
12. Gage FH, Kempermann G, Palmer TD, Peterson DA, Ray J (1998) Multipotent progenitors cells in the dentate gyrus. J Neurobiol 36 (2): 249–266
13. Doetsch F, Caillé I, Lim DA, García-Verdugo, Alvarez-Buylla A (1999) Subventricular zone astrocytes are neural stem cells in the adult mammalian brain. Cell 97: 703–716
14. Cattaneo E, McKay R (1990) Proliferation and differentiation of neuronal stem cells regulated by nerve growth factor. Nature 347: 762–765
15. Gage FH (2000) Mammalian neural stem cells. Science 287: 1433–1438
16. Pinto L, Gotz M (2007) Radial glial heterogeneity – the source of diverse progeny in the CNS. Prog Neurobiol 83 (1): 2–23
17. Anderson L, Burnstein RM, He X, Luce R, Furlong R, Foltynie T, Sykacek P, Menon DK, Caldwell MA (2007) Gene expression changes in long term expanded human neural progenitor cells passaged by chopping lead to loss of neurogenic potential in vivo. Exp Neurol 204 (2): 512–524
18. Rakic P (2003) Elusive radial glia cells: historical and evolutionary perspective. Glia 43: 19–32
19. Glaser T, Pollard SM, Smith A, Brüstle O (2007) Tripotential differentiation of adherently expandable neural stem (NS) cells. PLoS ONE 2 (3): e298. doi:10.1371/journal. pone.0000298

20. Kemp J, McKernan R (2002) NMDA receptor pathways as drug targets. Nat Neurosci 5: 1039–1042
21. McNeish J (2004) Embryonic stem cells in drug discovery. Nat Rev Drug Discov 3: 70–80
22. Ivanova N, Dobrin R, Lu R, Kotenko I, Levorse J, deCoste C, Schafer X, Lun Y, Lemischka I (2006) dissecting self-renewal in stem cells with RNA interference. Nature 442: 533–538
23. Munsie M, Michalska C, O'Brien C, Trounson, M, Pera M, Mountford P (2000) Isolation of pluripotent embryonic stem cells from reprogrammed adult mouse somatic cell nuclei. Curr Biol 10: 989–992
24. Wakayama T, Tabar V, Rodriguez I, Perry A, Studer L, Mombaerts P (2001) Differentiation of embryonic stem cell lines generated from adult somatic cells by nuclear transfer. Science 292: 740–743
25. Okita K, Ichisaka T, Yamanaka S (2007) Generation of germline-competent induced pluripotent stem cells. Nature 448 (7151): 313–317
26. Takahashi K, Tanabe K, Ohnuki M, Narita M, Ichisaka T, Tomoda K, Yamanaka S (2007) Induction of pluripotent stem cells from adult human fibroblasts by defined factors. Cell 131 (5): 861–872
27. Yu J, Vodyanik MA, Smuga-Otto K, Antosiewicz-Bourget J, Frane JL, Tian S, Nie J, Jonsdottir GA, Ruotti V, Stewart R, Slukvin II, Thomson JA (2007) Induced pluripotent stem cell lines derived from human somatic cells. Science 318: 1917–1920.
28. Manganas L, Zhang X, Li Y, Hazel R, Smith S, Wagshul M, Henn F, Benveniste H, Djuric P, Enikolopov G, Maletic-Savtic M (2007) Magnetic resonance spectroscopy identifies neural progenitor cells in the live human brain. Science 318: 980–985
29. Cezar GG, Quam JA, Smith AM, Guilherme J, Rosa M, Piekarczyk MS, Brown JF, Gage FH, Muotri AR (2007) Identification of small molecules from human embryonic stem cells using metabolomics. Stem Cells Dev 16 (6): 869–882.
30. Lindvall O, Bjorkland A (2004) Cell therapy in Parkinson's disease. NeuroRx 1 (4): 382–393
31. Bachoud-Lévi A, Gaura V, Brugières P, Lefaucheur J, Boissé M, Maison P, Baudic S, Ribeiro M, Bourdet C, Remy P, Cesaro P, Hantraye P, Peschanski M (2006) Effect of fetal neural transplants in patients with Huntington's disease 6 years after surgery: a long-term follow-up study. Lancet Neurol 5 (4): 303–309
32. Kelly S, Bliss TM, Shah AK, Sun GH, Ma M, Foo WC, Masel J, Yenari MA, Weissman IL, Uchida N, Palmer T, Steinberg GK (2004) Transplanted human fetal neural stem cells survive, migrate, and differentiate in ischemic rat cerebral cortex. Proc Natl Acad Sci USA 101 (32): 11839–11844
33. Mallon BS, Park KY, Chen KG, Hamilton RS, McKay RDG (2006) Toward xeno-free culture of human embryonic stem cells. Int J Biochem Cell Biol 38 (7): 1063–1075
34. Nasonkin IO, Koliatsos VE (2006) Nonhuman sialic acid Neu5Gc is very low in human embryonic stem cell-derived neural precursors differentiated with B27/N2 and noggin: implications for transplantation. Exp Neurol 20: 525–529
35. Martin MJ, Muotri A, Gage F, Varki A (2005) Human embryonic stem cells express an immunogenic nonhuman sialic acid. Nat Med 11 (2): 228–232
36. Kallos MS, Sen A, Behie LA (2003) Large-scale expansion of mammalian neural stem cells: a review. Med Biol Eng Comp 14 (3): 271–282
37. Thomson H (2007) Bioprocessing of embryonic stem cells for drug discovery. Trends Biotechnol 25 (5): 224–230
38. Draper JS, Moore HD, Ruban LN, Gokhale PJ, Andrews PW (2004) Culture and characterization of human embryonic stem cells. Stem Cells Dev 13 (4): 325–336.
39. Maitra A, Arking DE, Shivapurkar N, et al. (2005) Genomic alterations in cultured human embryonic stem cells. Nat Genet 37 (10): 1099–1103
40. Carpenter MK, Cui X, Hu ZY, Jackson J, Sherman S, Seiger A, Wahlberg LU (1999) In vitro expansion of a multipotent population of human neural progenitor cells. Exp Neurol 158 (2): 265–278

41. Fricker RA, Carpenter MK, Winkler C, Greco C, Gates MA, Bjorklund A (1999) Site-specific migration and neuronal differentiation of human neural progenitor cells after transplantation in the adult rat brain. J Neurosci 19 (14): 5990–6005

42. Stacey G (2004) Validation of cell culture media components. Hum Fertil (Camb) 7 (2): 113–118

43. Stacey G, Auerbach JM (2007) Quality Control Procedures for Stem Cell Lines In: Freshney I (ed) Culture of Human Stem Cells. Wiley-Liss, New York

44. Bradley JA, Bolton EM, Pederson RA (2002) Stem cell medicine encounters the immune system. Nat Rev Immunol 2: 859–871

45. Barker RA (2004) Immune problems in central nervous system cell therapy. J Am Soc Exp Neurother 1: 472–481

46. Medawar P (1948) Immunity to homologous grafted skin. I. The suppression of cell division in skin grafts transplanted to immunized animals, II. The relationship between the antigens of blood and skin. Br J Exp Pathol 29: 58–69

47. Wenkel H (2000) Systemic immune deviation in the brain that does not depend on the integrity of the blood-brain barrier. J Immunol 164: 5125–5131

48. Young MJ, Ray J, Whiteley SJ, Klassen H, Gage FH (2000) Neuronal differentiation and morphological integration of hippocampal progenitor cells transplanted to the retina of immature and mature dystrophic rats. Mol Cell Neurosci 16 (3): 197–205

49. Hori J, Ng TF, Shatos M, Klassen H, Streilein JW, Young MJ (2003) Neural progenitor cells lack immunogenicity and resist destruction as allografts. Stem Cells 21: 405–416

50. Henderson BT, Clough CG, Hughes RC, Hitchcock ER, Kenny BG (1991) Implantation of human fetal ventral mesencephalon to the right caudate nucleus in advanced Parkinson's disease. Arch Neurol 48 (8): 822–827

51. Mitjavila-Garcia MT, Simonin C, Peschanski M (2005) Embryonic stem cells: meeting the needs for cell therapy. Adv Drug Del Rev 12; 57 (13): 1935–1943

52. Amit M, Carpenter MK, Inokuma MS, Chiu CP, Harris CP, Waknitz MA, Itskovitz-Eldor J, Thomson JA (2000) Clonally derived human embryonic stem cell lines maintain pluripotency and proliferative potential for prolonged periods of culture. Dev Biol 227 (2): 271–278

53. Martin GR (1981) Isolation of a pluripotent cell line from early mouse embryos cultured in medium conditioned by teratocarcinoma stem cells. Proc Natl Acad Sci USA 78 (12): 7634–7638

54. Roy S, Cleren C, Singh S, Yang L, Beal M, Goldman S (2006) Functional engraftment of human ES cell–derived dopaminergic neurons enriched by coculture with telomerase-immortalized midbrain astrocytes. Nat Med 12 (11): 1259–1268

55. Mertes H, Pennings G (2007) Oocyte donation for stem cell research. Hum Reprod 22 (3): 629–634

56. Zietlow R, Lane E, Dunnett S, Rosser A (2008) Human stem cells for CNS repair. Cell Tissue Res 331 (1): 301–322

Chapter 8
The Analysis of MicroRNAs in Stem Cells

Loyal A. Goff[1], Uma Lakshmipathy[2], and Ronald P. Hart[1]*

Abstract MicroRNAs represent a newly-discovered class of regulatory molecules that has been demonstrated to be required for stem cell function. Methods for measuring unique microRNAs are particularly useful in classifying stem cells or for studying mechanisms underlying their differentiation. Furthermore, straightforward bioinformatic and statistical methods are useful in investigating large sets of data to formulate hypotheses or identify microRNAs associated with a specific effect or phenotype. We present an overview of microRNA biology, detection techniques including microarrays, as well as methods for analyzing the resulting data in the context of stem cell function.

Keywords: microRNA, small RNA, Stem cell, microarray, deep sequencing, sample preparation, data analysis, biclustering.

8.1 Background

No current discussion of stem cell maintenance, regulation or differentiation can be complete without mention of the largest class of tiny regulators of gene expression, microRNAs. The relatively recent discovery of this class of small non-coding RNAs has turned many common assumptions regarding cellular networks on end. Various types of small, non-coding RNAs exist as modulators of gene expression, affecting transcription rate [50, 85], heterochromatin formation [107, 130], transposon silencing [133], mRNA stability [13, 46, 160], and mRNA translation into functional proteins [101, 102, 120]. MicroRNAs represent a class of endogenous

[1] W.M. Keck Center for Collaborative Neuroscience, and the Rutgers Stem Cell Research Center, Rutgers University, Piscataway, NJ, USA

[2] Regenerative Medicine, Invitrogen, Inc., Carlsbad, CA, USA

*Corresponding Author:
604 Allison Rd Rm D251, Piscataway, NJ 08854, USA
e-mail: rhart@rci.rutgers.edu

Y. Shi, D.O. Clegg (eds.) *Stem Cell Research and Therapeutics*,
© Springer Science+Business Media B.V. 2008

genes whose primary role appears to be post-translational regulation of specific target mRNAs [3, 11]. MicroRNA genes are encoded both as intergenic transcripts as well within intronic sequences. The concept of intronic microRNAs alone demonstrates that there is a greater compression of genetic information contained within our genomes than previously understood, and the identification of over 1,000 human microRNA sequences to date suggests that there is indeed more regulatory complexity than previously appreciated.

What exactly are microRNAs? While a mature microRNA can arise from an independent transcript, a poly-cistronic cluster, or an intronic sequence, each of these produces a stem-loop RNA precursor sequence consisting of ~100 paired bases. These stem loops then become the substrate for the multi-protein "Microprocessor" complex [37, 51]. Association with this complex confers binding by the dsRNA binding enzyme Pasha and enzymatic cleavage of the hairpin from the primary transcript by the nuclear RNase III enzyme Drosha [37, 55, 56, 91, 168, 169]. The cleaved hairpins are then exported from the nucleus via Exportin-5 and, once in the cytoplasm, associate with the miRNP (microribonucleoprotein) complex. The proteins within this complex include Dicer, a second RNase III enzyme that removes that loop from the hairpin sequence, and a helicase to separate the resulting duplex and remove the microRNA* strand (the strand complementary to the mature microRNA). The result is a 'primed' ribonuclear complex capable of targeting a specific sequence. This specificity is conferred by the presentation of the now single-stranded ~21mer mature microRNA, which will recognize the 3′ untranslated region (3′ UTR) of a target mRNA. At our present level of understanding, there are several mechanisms of action that might occur at this point. A bound miRNP complex demonstrating a high degree of complementarity is capable of activating its "Slicer" activity resulting in the cleavage of the mRNA transcript at the site of miRNP binding [100, 163]. This ultimately results in the degradation of the transcript. Additionally, mRNA degradation has been observed through 5′ de-capping mechanisms [13, 127] as well as rapid de-adenylation [46, 160]. More commonly with respect to mammalian microRNAs, the interaction of a primed miRNP and its specific target results not in the degradation of the mRNA but rather in the repression of translation. Again, several different mechanisms for translational repression have been observed. Bound microRNAs are capable of directing target mRNAs to specific sub-cellular locations known as P-bodies [13, 95, 101, 102, 120, 127], or simply stalling protein production through direct hindrance of ribosomes [80, 118] or interfering with translation initiation [68, 121]. Estimates suggest there are ~400 microRNA genes in each invertebrate species, and ~1,000–1,500 genes in mammals [93, 97], with some groups predicting as many as 10,000–20,000 microRNA genes per genome [109]. The widespread impact of this new layer of gene regulation is also becoming more apparent in that several groups estimate anywhere from ~30% to 95% of the genome may be targets for microRNAs [93, 109]. This type of gene control represents a novel regulatory mechanism, and is predicted to affect many crucial cellular processes and developmental programs, including neurogenesis.

Only a few validated target mRNAs have been identified in animals. This information, combined with correlated tissue expression data and functional analyses, highlights some of the important roles for microRNAs. microRNAs have been shown to play a role in numerous cancers [1, 23, 25, 26, 38, 42, 52, 59–61, 64, 70, 81, 84, 129, 131, 142, 149], cardiac hypertrophy/failure [149], and several other disorders. Additionally, cellular processes such as fat metabolism [40, 161], insulin regulation [122, 123], apoptosis [7, 29, 34, 162], cell cycle regulation [58, 95, 135], maternal-zygotic transition [46, 110, 156], viral defense [35, 90], axis specification/patterning [45, 57, 63, 71, 104], tissue formation [32, 43, 115, 164], as well as stem cell specification and differentiation [4, 16, 21, 32, 39, 58, 65, 66, 79, 92, 115, 126, 135, 137, 138, 140, 159, 171] have all been associated with microRNA activity.

Shortly after the identification of microRNAs, tissue surveys were conducted to assess the potential impact of these small inhibitors [6, 8, 83, 117, 145]. It became immediately apparent that most microRNAs are highly tissue restricted, with only a slight overlap between tissues for any given microRNA. A few microRNAs, such as the let-7 family, appear to be ubiquitously expressed in all tissue types [8, 117, 145], suggesting a role in regulating the more basal, and therefore more prevalent processes within the cell, such as cell-cycle regulation [70]. More commonly, a set of tissue specific microRNAs are associated with specific cellular functions. This correlation, while only predictive of a microRNA's role, is strengthened by associated functional analysis of microRNA activity via over-expression [70, 123, 148] and inhibition studies [39]. For example, antisense targeting of miR-122, a liver specific microRNA, led to dysregulation of lipid metabolism in the liver [40]. Using similar approaches of combining tissue-specific expression data with functional assays has led to a greater understanding of the impact of microRNAs in the cell, without the need for specifically identifying valid mRNA targets. Using this approach, groups have ascribed general functions for given microRNAs in context, such as the requirement for miR-125b for the proliferation of differentiated cells [92], miR-143 for the regulation of adipocyte differentiation [39], and numerous others [79, 146]. It would be shortsighted at this point to restrict the potential roles that microRNAs may be performing in the cell as new roles are being unraveled at an accelerated rate. The diversity in the already established roles for microRNAs demonstrates that this class of small regulatory RNA molecules plays an integral role in numerous biological pathways and suggests that they will play an important role in other cellular processes including differentiation.

One of the more interesting roles suggested for these small inhibitors of translation is the regulation and specification of stem cells. Several studies have attempted to determine the global role of microRNAs in development by selective knockdown of required components of the microRNA/RNAi pathway [17, 73]. A few groups have determined that Dicer, the RNase III enzyme responsible for processing microRNAs, and therefore required for microRNA activity, is required for murine cell differentiation and specification [17, 73, 114]. Evidence shows that a Dicer-1 null mutant mouse was embryonic lethal due to a depletion of stem cells [17], as well as demonstrating a failure of existing stem cells to adequately differentiate [73].

Interestingly, a similar study was conducted in zebrafish where it was shown that embryos with a maternal-zygotic Dicer mutant are capable of stem cell maintenance and differentiation but are defective in patterning, morphogenesis, and organogensis, suggesting that the role of microRNAs in stem cell regulation may have changed dramatically during the course of evolution [45]. A mouse knockout of the DGCR8 (Pasha) gene, required for the recognition and accurate processing of microRNA precursors, demonstrated the requirement of functional mature microRNAs for appropriate differentiation of ES cells. It was shown that ES cells lacking a functional DGCR8 gene failed to completely differentiate and retained the pluripotency markers Oct4 and Nanog, despite the onset of selected differentiation markers as well [151]. Furthermore, knockout mice lacking Argonaute2 (Ago2), the catalytic component of the RISC complex, exhibited severe defects in neural development, including the failure to close neural tube [100]. These experiments highlight the critical, if not yet well understood role that microRNAs play during stem cell development.

Early on, it was noted that stem cells express unique populations of microRNAs that were not present in any adult tissues [46, 65, 66, 110, 138], some of which additionally appear to be species specific. A conserved eutherian microRNA cluster is expressed exclusively in undifferentiated stem cells and is immediately downregulated upon induction of differentiation [65, 66]. Since microRNAs are hypothesized to have a predominately repressive role, it is reasonable to speculate that these microRNAs are responsible for maintaining a stem-like state through repression of pro-differentiation factors. A similar group of microRNAs, although with distinctly unique sequences and genomic locations, is evident in differentiating human embryonic stem cells [138]. The presence of these embryonic stem cell-specific microRNAs, and their clearance during differentiation, suggests a role in restricting cell differentiation. In contrast, new populations of tissue specific microRNAs are coordinately induced during differentiation and specification of stem cells [31, 32, 45, 74, 79, 83, 86, 89, 111, 140, 157]. Conserved microRNAs miR-1 and miR-206 are both induced during, and are required for, muscle cell differentiation and specification in mammals [32, 116] or birds [140]. Expression of miR-181 in hematopoietic stem cells is associated with an increase in B-cell specification [31], while other hematopoietic microRNAs (miR-142, and miR-155) are also induced during blood cell maturation [31, 125, 137]. Finally, subsets of microRNAs can be used to classify, for example, differences between embryonic stem cells, embryoid bodies, and embryonic carcinoma [89]. The requirement for microRNA activity during development and the influence that specific microRNAs have upon differentiation strengthen the argument that microRNAs are required for establishing and perhaps maintaining a differentiated state.

Without a doubt, microRNAs are present and active in both stem cell maintenance and differentiation. But before we are able to fully comprehend the roles of these small molecules, we must be familiar with the current methods for detection, analysis, and contextual interpretation of microRNAs. We present here an overview of current techniques in microRNA expression profiling, and suggest several possible workflows for analysis and interpretation of microRNA expression data.

8.2   Available Tools for Detecting MicroRNAs

Shortly after the realization that microRNAs were both abundant and ubiquitous regulators within the cell, many standard techniques were adapted to accommodate these new molecules. The first microRNAs identified were visualized by standard Northern blotting. A commonly-used and reliable technique, the Northern blot was easily deployed and required little adaptation to detect microRNAs. It unfortunately suffered from the short-comings of being fairly low throughput and time-consuming. Shortly after this, standard and quantitative real-time PCR (qPCR) were modified for identification and detection of microRNAs [30]. In general, qPCR techniques have been shown to yield the greatest dynamic range, improved specificity, and increased sensitivity in microRNA detection assays. In one case, qPCR allowed detection of microRNAs from single cultured neurons or laser captured somatodendritic compartments [87]. qPCR is a moderately high-throughput assay allowing rapid validation of a broader number of microRNAs than, for example, Northerns.

With the appearance of microRNA microarrays [6, 8, 48, 96, 111, 117, 145], however, a large number of microRNA genes could be assayed in parallel and true surveys or expression analyses could be conducted [6, 8, 83, 88, 117, 134, 145]. Several platforms emerged in rapid fashion [5, 8, 12, 18, 23, 24, 39, 47, 82, 96, 97, 99, 111, 139], and many commercial sources of microRNA arrays are readily available (Table 8.1); each with their own advantages and disadvantages. Most of these are based on the public list of microRNAs found in the miRBase database maintained at the Sanger Institute (http://microrna.sanger.ac.uk) [53]. A select few include probes for predicted microRNA genes or additional microRNAs that have not yet been indexed by the Sanger registry. Most of the commercial microRNA arrays are relatively quick to release updated probe sets as novel microRNAs are released in miRBase. Early considerations in probe design for microRNA microarrays focused mainly on the problem of variable melting temperatures (T_m) across microRNAs. To ensure an adequate and consistent signal during an array experiment, it is ideal for the probes to have a relatively narrow T_m range. With fairly short sequences from which to design probes, limited strategies are available to accomplish this goal. Solutions included logical sequence truncation or increasing the stringency of hybridization in one of several ways. With most of the array-based methods, it is difficult to claim resolution of specific microRNAs within 1 nt of the probe sequence since the melting temperatures are quite low compared with the longer probes often used for mRNA detection [48]. However, higher specificity can be achieved using direct labeling of microRNAs to obtain RNA:DNA hybridization (Ncode™) or by LNA oligo probes (mirCURY™), which enhance base stacking and phosphate-backbone reorganization, resulting in an increased thermal stability. Other detection techniques include ELISA-like or bead-anchored hybridizations using probes and labeling similar to array methods to perform high-throughput analyses on robotic liquid handling systems [114]. We focus this chapter on the use of any of the available microRNA microarray platforms for high-throughput analysis of microRNA expression.

Table 8.1 Commercial sources of microRNA microarrays

Product name	Source	References
Human miRNA Microarray	Agilent	[150]
mirVana™	Ambion/Applied Biosystems	[36, 170]
Species Specific MicroRNA Arrays	CombiMatrix	
MirCURY™	Exiqon, Inc.	[28, 112]
GenoExplorer™	GenoSensor Corp.	[9, 33, 154]
NCode™	Invitrogen, Inc.	[47, 72]
Human microRNA Microarray	LC Sciences	[67, 144]

Validation of microarray results originally depended on Northern blots but recently qPCR has become the method of choice. However, while qPCR may be a more convenient method for validation of a small to moderate number of micro RNAs, the microarray quality control project (MAQC) [136] determined that the best validation of an array experiment is to repeat the experiment on a separate array platform. Attention should be given in the project design phase to adequately prepare for some basic form of validation (i.e., ensure adequate material is available and that an acceptable method for validation has been considered).

8.3 Experimental Design Considerations

A microarray study is only as good as its experimental design. The amount of time spent planning and preparing an assay will pay off in the form of easily interpretable data, better quality results, and, ideally, straightforward answers to the experimental question. Consider what it is that you are interested in uncovering with an array study. A general survey alone to merely identify microRNAs present in a tissue sample will probably yield too little information and will most likely not produce results acceptable for publication. Conversely, a complex, broad, and unguided assay can be very confusing and cloud meaningful results in a sea of data.

A differential expression study can suggest whether or not microRNAs are being regulated (via any number of mechanisms) between two or more conditions. The number of conditions of interest will most likely determine the design of an experiment. A simple comparison of two conditions, for example, treated vs. control, can be conducted most effectively with a series of replicate two-color arrays. A more complex experimental design, such as a time course, multiple treatment conditions, or a multivariate study will require more careful design considerations.

Regardless of the scale of your experiment, replicate samples should be employed to capture and account for biological variability. Obviously, the more replicates that are used, the more statistical power is gained and the more confidence can be expressed in reporting results. The trade-off has traditionally been that more replicates require a significantly larger cost. This should not be so limiting since the relative cost per sample has decreased substantially in the past few years, and will continue to decrease as new technology and new competition emerges. True biological replicates should be balanced with respect to arrays and dyes. We recommend an absolute minimum of three replicates per sample, but encourage the investigator to sample as many as is economically feasible for any given experiment.

8.4   MicroRNA Preparation and Handling

As with any RNA work, care and consideration must be given to ensure a clean, sterile, and nuclease-free environment. RNA is considerably more susceptible to degradation than DNA, and we find that degradation of the smaller microRNA generally is associated with degradation of higher molecular weight cellular RNAs such as ribosomal RNAs. Care should be taken to wear gloves when handling isolated RNA to protect your sample from RNAses found on the skin. RNA work should be conducted in a dedicated and clean space that is routinely treated with a nuclease inhibitor (e.g. RNaseZap, Ambion Cat #0611001A). If you begin to notice increased degradation of your isolated RNA, or generally reduced signal intensities in consecutive experiments, a thorough cleaning of your workspace is recommended.

An early realization was that the majority of labs involved in RNA work were commonly discarding RNA comprising less than ~100 bases in length. This was assumed to be primarily degradation products resulting from the RNA isolation techniques themselves. A widespread technique involved the ethanol-mediated binding of RNA to silica gel cartridges (for example, Qiagen RNeasy™). This allowed for the retention of large RNA molecules and the exclusion of anything passing through the cartridge, including weakly binding smaller RNA molecules. This method was easily modified by the manufacturer for retention of microRNA sequences by increasing the concentration of ethanol to drive a stronger affinity for the silica. While this did increase the yield of microRNAs, the increase in ethanol concentration often carried over to downstream applications potentially affecting reaction efficiencies. After much trial and error, we recommend a standard Trizol (Invitrogen Cat # 15596-018) RNA isolation followed by ammonium acetate/ethanol precipitation. If required, a carrier such as linear acrylamide (Ambion Cat #AM9520) can be used to increase yield and help precipitate the RNA. The result is an ultra-pure total RNA preparation that contains RNA of all sizes including microRNAs. Downstream applications may require that the microRNAs be isolated from the total RNA population. Several commercial products, including the miR-Vana™ Kit (Ambion, Austin, TX) or the PureLink™ miRNA Isolation Kit (Invitrogen, Carlsbad, CA), have been developed that will allow size fractionation based on selective column binding affinities or gel electrophoresis. We propose a simpler method of size fractionation via filtration. Centrifuge filter devices are a relatively inexpensive method for size selection and have demonstrated good isolation and separation properties. Begin by passing a sample of total RNA preparation through a ~100,000 molecular weight cutoff (MWCO) filter (Microcon YM-100 Cat# 42412). The microRNAs and any other small RNA (≤100bp) will pass through the filter and the larger RNA (mRNA, rRNA) will remain as retentate. The flow-through contains microRNA. The mRNA may be recovered by inverting and centrifuging the filter. Since the microRNA will co-purify with any low molecular weight contaminants, an additional clean-up procedure step is to concentrate the sample on a 3,000 MWCO filter (YM-3) to remove salts, phenol, or other impurities.

There are several rapid and simple assays that can be conducted on isolated microRNA that will test the quality and quantity of the total RNA or microRNA. A common technique to quantify an RNA preparation is to measure the absorbance at 260 nm (A_{260}) with a low-volume spectrophotometer, such as the Nanodrop ND-1000, which requires only 1–2 μl of sample. Typically, the absorbance is measured, corrected for dilution, and multiplied by a constant conversion factor to determine the concentration. The conversion factor for RNA is typically 40 μg/ml per A_{260} unit. This constant is derived from both the average molecular weight of RNA and the extinction coefficient. Since microRNAs have a significantly shorter sequence than the average RNA, this coefficient is insufficient. The approximation of the constant for microRNA that should be used to calculate concentration is 33 μg/ml per A_{260} unit. This is an important consideration only when microRNAs are isolated separately from total RNA.

In addition to microRNA quantity, quality of the preparation can be inferred by measuring the A_{230} and A_{280}. Since typical contaminating components absorb light at these two wavelengths (e.g., proteins at ~280 nm, ethanol at ~230 nm) the standard ratios A_{260}/A_{280} and A_{260}/A_{230} can be used as a measure of RNA purity. A "clean" preparation typically produces A_{260}/A_{280} and A_{260}/A_{230} ratios ≥ 2.0 (when measured at pH 8). If your sample produces values in either of these ratios < 1.8, we recommend additional cleanup steps to remove contaminants carried over from the RNA isolation.

While the spectrophotometer is a useful device to quantify RNA samples and determine their purity, it cannot determine the quality of the RNA itself (i.e., how intact is the RNA). High molecular weight RNA or total RNA fractions are typically assessed by gel electrophoresis. This is not realistic for microRNA samples, which regularly do not have enough mass to spare for a gel analysis. A practical solution is capillary electrophoresis. We recommend the Agilent Bioanalyzer 2100 system (Agilent, Santa Clara, CA) for several reasons. There are two available RNA quality assays that each measure different concentrations of input RNA material, although the quantity measurements are listed by the manufacturer as accurate ±50%. Additionally, the small RNA bioanalyzer kit enables the characterization of microRNA down to the picogram/microliter level [105]. The calculated RNA Integrity Number (RIN) provides a consistent and standard metric for the evaluation of total RNA quality. In the absence of this system, we recommend traditional agarose gel electrophoresis of the high molecular weight RNA fraction, or unfractionated total RNA, as a proxy for the assessment of microRNA quality within the same sample.

8.5 Probe-Level Interpretation of MicroRNA Array Data

Most commercial microRNA microarray platforms focus exclusively on the micro-RNAs derived from the most common model organisms; human, mouse, and rat. At the time of writing this chapter, the NCode™ platform from Invitrogen was designed to include probes for the above named species and additionally, probes for zebrafish, *Drosophila*, and the nematode *C. elegans* [48]. Since multiple microRNAs appear to share strong evolutionary origins and are highly conserved across multiple lineages, we can use the information content available to expand both the applications of these arrays, as well as our understanding of the expression of microRNAs across multiple species.

The high level of interspecies conservation of a large set of microRNAs means that the probes designed against human microRNAs, for example, may be useful for identifying novel microRNAs from similar vertebrate species. Furthermore, since most of the microRNA array platforms cannot distinguish between two molecules with 1 bp difference between them, those microRNAs that have diverged ≤1 bp should be detected by that probe. Through the course of our array design, we have been able to successfully map all known microRNAs from human, mouse, rat, zebrafish, *Drosophila*, and *C. elegans* to ~90% of the remaining known metazoan microRNA sequences. While this will not include the microRNAs which have been observed to be species-specific, a good deal of information from other model organisms is made available using an existing platform. This advantage has been useful as well in confirming the existence of novel microRNAs in one species that are homologous to known microRNAs. For example, the illumination of a probe for hsa-miR-519a from a labeled rat microRNA sample suggests the presence of a rat homolog for miR-519a. While this is at best circumstantial evidence, a list of potential homologs to be tested further could readily be obtained by hybridization to the existing platforms. It would be short-sighted to limit interpretation of microRNA array data to the given probes from one species.

Once a probe sequence is available to the public, a standard BLAST search against all known microRNAs will effectively "re-annotate" that specific probe. For the NCode™ microRNA array platform, this has already been conducted. A web tool is available (http://cord.rutgers.edu/gal_generator/) into which a blank array map can be input, and any number of available species can be selected. Probe identifiers are indexed and compared to previous BLAST results across all known microRNAs from all available species, identifying those probes designed for human microRNAs that are, for example, exact matches to gorilla. Probes found to vary by one or two nucleotides from a perfect match for a given species are labeled as negative controls to determine hybridization specificity. The output is a custom array layout file specifically annotated for any given species or combination of species, allowing the use of a single array to detect most microRNAs in all species found in miRBase. Take advantage of these highly conserved sequences when designing experiments. The lack of availability of a specific species microRNA microarray should not hinder the use of commercially available microRNA arrays.

8.6   Common Data Analysis Workflows for MicroRNA Microarrays

Much thought has been put into analysis of gene expression data over the past several years. Increasing use of microarray technology has highlighted the need for robust and accurate workflows for dealing with massive amounts of gene expression data. Many novel algorithms have emerged to deal with multivariate microarray data. For the most part, microRNA expression data can be treated with exactly the same methods as mRNA data. qPCR and array platforms have had to change very little to adapt to these smaller molecules and therefore standard workflows continue to apply. However, several of the traditional normalization methods are based on assumptions that do not hold true for current microRNA expression data.

As with most data analysis, the appropriate workflow is the one that makes the most sense in the context of the specific biological question being asked. In most cases, multiple arrays are used in a single experiment. This requires scaling and/or normalization methods to make the arrays comparable and compensate for artifacts or effects between arrays. Readily available techniques include a list of model-fitting approaches. Most model-fitting algorithms such as locally-weighted linear regression (loess), spline fitting (gspline), or linear modeling assume that there are a relatively large number (>1,000) of detectable measurements upon which to base interpretations. Additionally, most of these normalization methods assume that the majority of measurements will remain unchanged across the majority of the arrays (or conditions).

For smaller microRNA array experiments these assumptions may not be met. Since there are currently slightly less than 1,000 human microRNAs known, it is quite possible that a smaller microRNA dataset will not have a minimum number of measurements to meet this assumption. Reported measurements of microRNA expression levels are quite dynamic as well. The majority of microRNAs are expressed in a highly tissue-specific manner. This again would violate the assumption that genes remain relatively unchanged across arrays. For these otherwise limited datasets, we propose that a more appropriate choice for a normalization technique is a non-parametric method such as quantile normalization. Speed and colleagues were the first to apply quantile normalization to microarray datasets [19] and this was done originally on single-channel Affymetrix™ arrays. The only assumption is that the distribution of gene abundances is *nearly* the same in all samples. This is true for low abundance genes, and to a fairly good approximation, for genes of moderate abundance, but does not necessarily hold true for the few high-abundance genes, whose typical levels vary noticeably from sample to sample. In this normalization scheme, a gene X channel matrix is constructed from the dataset using background-subtracted intensity values. The matrix is then sorted by column into "quantiles" and the mean intensity value is taken across each row. This mean value then replaces the value in the original matrix order effectively forcing an identical distribution across all of the arrays. This brute-force normalization is an effective, rank-based method for reducing the effects of array and dye bias by re-scaling the entire dataset. This can be accomplished easily in the R environment (http://www.r-project.org) using portions of the limma [155] package contained within Bioconductor [44] (http://www.bioconductor.org) (Panel 8.1).

Once the dataset has been normalized and corrected, you must now examine your experimental question. In most cases this is the identification of differentially expressed microRNAs. There are a wide variety of analyses from which to choose. For a simple two parameter comparison, the standard Student's t-test is often appropriate. We recommend SAM (Significance Analysis of Microarrays; http://www-stat.stanford.edu/~tibs/SAM/), a widely-used test similar to a t-test but including an estimate of false discovery error and designed specifically for microarray data. Standard ANOVA methods can also be used to explore the variance across more than two conditions. Regardless of the statistical test chosen, P-values must be corrected for multiple testing. With the high number of statistical tests (one for each gene), the likelihood of satisfying the null hypothesis (all means are equal across conditions) by chance alone increases. To take this into consideration, we must correct for performing multiple tests. The preferred method in microarray studies is to control the false discovery rate (FDR), or the expected proportion of incorrectly rejected null hypotheses. Benjamini-Hochberg [14], Bonferroni [62], and Westfall-Young [152, 153] are three commonly used types of multiple testing corrections; each is available from within R. The result will be a list of significantly regulated microRNAs that have passed the stringency test for multiple testing.

While this workflow is appropriate for small microRNA datasets, a more powerful and suitable approach is available for robust, multivariate expression datasets. Linear models have tremendous power to describe data, but have only recently become popular for microarray data analysis. Modeling a dataset entails the construction of a linear equation that "describes" the data based on a series of pre-defined parameters. The goal then is to be able to re-create the dataset with a minimal amount of parameters, while accounting for random errors. This is best

Panel 8.1 Quantile normalization in R. Quantile normalization can be performed fairly easily within the R environment. Begin by starting a session in the directory containing a comma-separated file containing a "gene x array" of background subtracted values. The following code and comments will describe the workflow within R:

```
#Load required library
library('limma')
#read file "file.csv" into object 'raw'
raw < -read.csv("file.csv", header = T)
#generate a box-whiskers plot for raw data to #determine variability across arrays
boxplot(log2(raw), main = "Raw")
#convert to matrix and normalize quantiles
norm < -normalizeQuantiles(as.matrix(raw))
norm < -as.data.frame(norm)
#generate box-whiskers plot for normalized data to confirm normalization
boxplot(log2(norm), main = "Normalized")
#write normalized values to new file
write.csv(norm,file = "norm.csv")
quit()
```

described by Kerr and Churchill [75–78], who describe a "minimal model" for two-color microarray data analysis that incorporates array, dye, gene, and sample effects (Panel 8.2). In addition to these parameters, combinatorial effects are also incorporated into their model to describe spot effects (array X gene), labeling effects (dye X gene), and gene-specific sample effects (sample X gene). It is this last effect that is most important as it describes the differential expression of a given gene across each sample. Care should be taken to balance the design when laying out an experiment for linear model analysis. Spreading your samples across multiple independent arrays and labeling the replicates with alternating dyes will help to estimate the technical errors produced by hybridization of individual arrays and dye labeling effects. Poor experimental balance can result in confounded parameters that cannot be estimated. Once the linear model has been described and fit to the dataset, F-tests are conducted on a per-gene basis comparing the model with and without the 'sample X gene' effects. This determines whether or not this effect contributes to a significant portion of the observed intensity value for the given gene, given the

Panel 8.2 Linear modeling of microarray data. The linear model concept attempts to mathematically define a dataset based on a given set of defined parameters. In essence, the experimenter describes the characteristics of the samples that are most important to a specific experiment. The "design" file is used to outline the parameters in an experiment and may be as simple as a "condition" parameter categorizing a sample as control or experimental, or significantly more complex. RNA source, sample preparation, technician name, or date of assay, are a small fraction of the parameters that can be included in a larger experiment. Each can be tested to determine if there is a significant "effect" on the resulting dataset. Once the parameters have been defined and associated with particular samples, a "comparison" matrix is used to describe the comparisons of interest among the many parameters. This is a fairly straightforward process for single-channel array data, but can become significantly more involved when dealing with two-color array data. To address this class of microarray data, Kerr and Churchill [75, 76, 78] proposed a standard linear model that attempts to describe some common sources of error in two-color microarray experiments. The model:

$$Y_{ijkg} = \mu + A_i + D_j + V_k + G_g + AG_{ig} + DG_{jg} + VG_{kg} + \varepsilon_{ijkg}$$

Where:

Y_{ijkg} = the observed values from the array experiment for the ith array, jth dye, kth sample, and gth gene.

μ = the estimated mean of the dataset.

A_i = the effect of being on the ith array.

D_j = the effect of being on the jth dye.

V_k = the effect of being on the kth sample.

G_g = the effect of being on the gth gene.

AG_{ig} = the combinatorial effect describing the spotting effect.

DG_{jg} = the combinatorial effect describing the gene-specific labeling effect.

VG_{kg} = the combinatorial effect describing the effect of being a given gene in a specific sample.

ε_{ijkg} = random error.

This model will take each of these parameters into consideration when fit to microarray data. The effect that is usually the most interesting is the VG_{kg} effect. This model can be fit with or without this specific effect and a per-gene F-test between the two fits will identify any genes with a considerable variance across any of the samples. P-values can be either tabulated from an F-distribution or, more appropriately, bootstrapped by finding the probability that a randomly permuted dataset will produce F-values greater than that observed with the original dataset. These P-values should be subject to the same multiple testing corrections used for standard array analysis.

distribution of the existing data. At this point, p-values can be bootstrapped by randomly permuting the dataset and conducting the same F-test. The probability of randomly obtaining a higher F-value will be determined empirically. P-values are adjusted for multiple comparisons using a standard 5% FDR cutoff.

The advantages of this data analysis approach are that few assumptions about the data are required *a priori*. The data themselves are used to drive the analysis. Ideally, linear modeling can be used to examine any number of parameters simultaneously (i.e., cell line, phenotype, differentiation state, etc.), and the more parameters that are included, the more accurate the resulting estimates of effect. The primary drawback is the rather large number of samples required to maintain sufficient degrees of freedom required for the estimation of each parameter. For each estimated value, a degree of freedom must be sacrificed. Since there are a large number of parameters involved (Array, Dye, Sample, Gene, etc.) this requires a robust dataset to make these estimates possible. The more replicates that are conducted, the more degrees of freedom available, yet experiment cost is a very common limiting factor inhibiting large numbers of replicates. This balance must be considered prior to accepting an experimental design, as the benefit of using linear modeling of microarray data is lost when you have to begin to sacrifice parameters to measure due to insufficient degrees of freedom. Linear modeling can be conducted using one of several freely available packages from the R/Bioconductor [44] environment. Limma [155] is a flexible and powerful linear modeling package that has extensive documentation, and is easily adaptable for both two-color as well as single-channel arrays. There is an accompanying graphical user interface (limmaGUI) that makes data input and analysis more streamlined and accessible. We routinely use the R/MAANOVA package [75, 76, 78] to analyze our microRNA data. This package provides detailed instructions for preparing your dataset and outlining the parameters for your experiment. In addition, MAANOVA provides a host of post-modeling features that help to streamline the analysis and interpretation of your significant genes.

8.7 Biclustering

The expression profiling of microRNAs is an important step in understanding the roles these molecules may play in regulating different cellular processes. However, what little we know about microRNAs suggests that these RNAs act exclusively through regulation of other genes. With this in mind, it then becomes prudent to examine the expression of the targets of these microRNAs under the same conditions, so as to (A) identify the pool of available targets under a given condition and (B) identify/predict specific targets for a subset of regulated microRNA based on the differential expression of target mRNAs. By directly comparing microRNA expression data to data obtained from other assays such as mRNA profiles, additional information can be gleaned as well. mRNAs known to have a role in transcriptional regulation have been shown to exert pressures on the promoter regions of intergenic microRNAs (LAG, 2007, unpublished results). These interactions, as well as those satisfying other hypotheses, begin to emerge as underlying patterns in this combinatorial dataset.

The concept of biclustering has been used frequently to reveal relationships between genes based on their associations across numerous treatments or conditions [94, 103, 124, 147]. Logically, the tighter the association across multiple stressors, knockouts, treatments, or other conditions, the more confidence one would have that two genes are associated with similar biological processes and/or networks. The simplest approach to a biclustering analysis would be a cross-correlation study (Fig. 8.1). Basic hierarchical clustering across both genes and conditions would begin to unravel these relationships. This approach has been adapted by several groups to begin to reveal networks of relationships between microRNAs and their target mRNAs. One begins by constructing a matrix of correlations for all possible microRNA:mRNA pairs within a dataset. The cross-correlation, or correlation across these correlations, is then determined and used to relate neighboring microRNAs to each other based solely on their relationships across all observed mRNAs. The inverse is applied to mRNAs as well resulting in a two-dimensional hierarchical clustering matrix describing the relationships both within and between molecule types. We previously used cross-correlation clustering to investigate

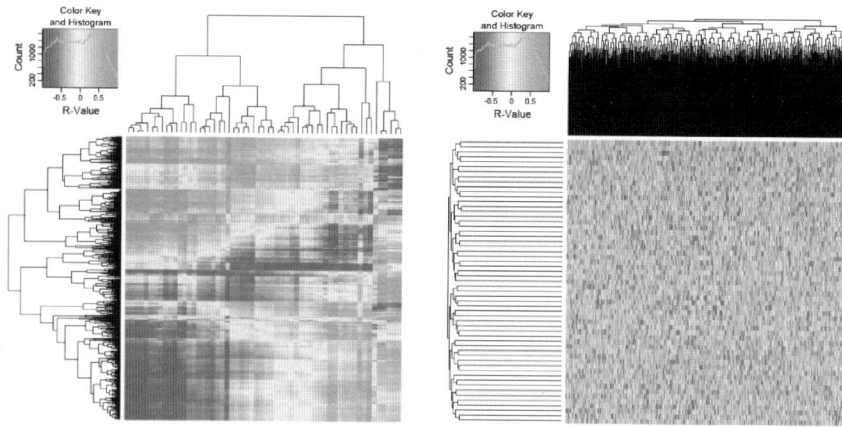

Fig. 8.1 The cross correlation matrix. Using a heatmap-like visualization technique, the correlations between microRNAs and mRNAs can be easily and readily visualized. In this experiment comparing human embryonic stem cells with embryoid bodies or embryonic carcinoma cells, regulated microRNAs (columns) are correlated to significant mRNAs (rows), and the resulting R-values are used to color the component blocks. Hierarchical clustering in both dimensions groups molecules based on their correlation across the opposing molecule type. Subclusters that are negatively correlated (red) may represent potential microRNA:mRNA target interactions resulting in degradation of the target mRNA. Regions showing strong positive correlation (green) may help to identify microRNAs and mRNAs that may have a shared functional pathway or transcriptional regulatory mechanism. The value of the biological information is seen when the connections between microRNA and mRNA are severed by randomly permuting the cross correlation matrix using the identical dataset, resulting in the complete abolition of subclusters (*See Color Plates*)

mRNAs and microRNAs differentially expressed between human embryonic stem cells, embryoid bodies, and embryonic carcinoma.

By focusing on subclusters of the cross-correlation matrix, several different interactions between microRNAs and mRNAs can be inferred. Since microRNAs have been shown to mediate mRNA degradation in certain conditions, it is reasonable to suggest that this activity could be identified in a subset, or bicluster, of the cross-correlation matrix demonstrating strong negative correlations across multiple conditions (actually, mRNA targeting would represent only one of two possible models of negative correlation). More specifically, if we can focus on a bicluster that contains mRNA that are downregulated as corresponding microRNA increase in abundance, we find the ideal subcluster to test putative interactions. A quick scan of a now more limited subset of mRNA may reveal a conserved microRNA binding motif amongst the candidate mRNA 3′UTRs. This approach is logical when we realize that our focus is on those mRNAs that are actively degraded as a result of microRNA binding activity. The extent of this mechanism in mammals is believed to be relatively little compared to translational repression or sequestration. The majority of microRNA:mRNA targets in mammals then, would probably not be identified in this manner. Interestingly, in apparent contrast to this challenge, a few groups have demonstrated an abundance of regulatory motifs in the 3′UTR of microRNAs downregulated during treatment with a specific microRNA [97]. The regulatory sequence contains a region of complementarity to the microRNA used. It may be that with the overexpression of a microRNA there is a detectable increase in the amount of target degradation that occurs. This suggests that targets can in fact be identified through their negative correlation to an enriched microRNA, but perhaps only in the context of extra-ordinary expression levels.

8.8 Revealing Regulation

While little is known about the functions of expressed microRNAs, even less is known about the mechanisms governing the regulation of microRNAs themselves. MicroRNAs are derived from both spliced intronic regions of mRNAs [98, 165, 166], as well as from unique transcripts located in intergenic regions [54, 88, 167]. Since no specific regulatory mechanism for microRNA processing has yet been identified, it is assumed that the expression of intronic microRNAs is regulated by the same mechanisms that regulate the abundance of the host transcript, as well as mechanisms governing intron splicing. Intergenic microRNAs have been shown to be transcribed by either Pol II [138] or in some cases by Pol III [20]. The Pol II transcripts are 5′-capped and poly(A)-tailed [22, 138] in a similar fashion to known mRNAs. A large number of intergenic microRNAs exist as poly-cistronic clusters. These clusters are often transcribed as a single unit and summarily processed into individual microRNA precursors after nuclear export [2, 59, 61, 65, 83, 138, 143]. Interestingly, early sequence analysis of upstream regions of intergenic microRNAs failed to identify common Pol II minimal promoter elements or similarities to known mRNA promoter elements [22, 66, 138]. A few groups, including our lab, have since cloned and validated promoter regions for a small number of microRNAs, and demonstrated that similar regulatory mechanisms do in fact exist to control the transcription rates of intergenic microRNA. These mechanisms include conserved and occupied transcription factor binding sites as well as chromatin modifications, both of which have been shown to exert a regulatory pressure on the cloned promoters [41, 122, 131, 133, 141]. The inverse of the microRNA target analysis of a bicluster would be the determination of common regulatory mechanisms governing the expression levels of both microRNAs and mRNAs. Those transcripts sharing similar transcriptional regulatory mechanisms may be identified as microRNA: mRNA pairs demonstrating a positive correlation, and in most cases appropriate correlations with transcription factors that may be acting on these networks (i.e., positive correlation with activating transcription factors and negative correlation with transcriptional repressors).

Another approach that can be adopted to help unravel the regulatory mechanisms of microRNAs involves that bioinformatic prediction of a response to a specific transcription factor or factors based on upstream sequence analysis. We have recently applied this approach to study a specific pathway in differentiating mesenchymal stem cells (MSC) [49]. Upon identification of a specific pathway inhibitor (in this case, Tyrphostin AG-370) that significantly alters the ability of MSC to differentiate into osteocytes [120], we hypothesized that this effect may be mediated in part by regulated microRNA activity. Since AG-370 specifically inhibits the PDGF pathway, we conducted a literature search to identify transcription factors directly downstream of the PDGF receptors. Position weight matrices for each of these transcription factors were obtained from the TRANSFAC database [106, 158] and used to scan the 5 Kb upstream sequences of microRNAs that had been previously identified as significantly regulated during osteogenic differentiation of human MSCs. A comparison of the number of positive hits among the significant microRNAs to the number obtained from a sample of expressed but not regulated microRNA upstream sequences confirmed that these microRNAs were enriched for putative PDGF pathway binding sites ($p < 0.05$). A z-score analysis of individual microRNA upstream sequence hits vs. the average number of hits for all regulated and non-regulated upstream sequences was unable to identify individual microRNAs significantly enriched for binding sites after a multiple testing correction. However, the resulting p-value-rank-ordered list provided a confidence list that allowed us to rank microRNA regulatory sequences based on their predicted responses. Subsequent testing of regulated microRNA activity via qPCR during osteogenic differentiation in the presence of the inhibitor demonstrated that those microRNAs ranking higher in our confidence list showed a greater likelihood of being modulated by AG-370 treatment [49]. This workflow enables the prediction of microRNAs that may be responsive to a particular pathway or treatment, and the validation of these predictions via drug-targeting. This moderately high-throughput assay is just one example of a workflow that can be readily adapted to a wide variety of experimental questions pertinent to both microRNAs and stem cells.

8.9 Future Technologies

Current trends in technology will enable a fuller understanding of both the number and extent of microRNAs regulating stem cell function. Ultra high-throughput, deep sequencing technologies are beginning to emerge and re-define how nucleic acid sequences are identified, quantified, and regulated. Three competing yet similar technologies have emerged as the fore-runners in the field of deep sequencing. Each requires the preparation of a cDNA library, sequence amplification by PCR, high-density display of amplified sequences, and direct sequencing by either synthesis [15] or ligation methods [27]. With the ability to read, in parallel, upwards of 40 million ~35–50 bp sequences, the challenges of complexity and size of genetic information are readily addressed and ultra high-throughput assays become feasible for most investigators [10, 15, 69, 108, 128]. The application of these technologies to small RNAs is not lost, and in fact represents some of the first uses for deep sequencing. Direct sequencing of small RNAs requires no *a priori* knowledge of the microRNA sequence, which provides an immediate advantage for discovery over microarray technologies requiring the construction of complementary probes. However, access to a nearly-complete genome sequence is an important requirement since, in our experience, only ~50% of deep-sequencing microRNA tags can be aligned to genome, limiting the collection of valid data (LAG, 2008, unpublished results). However, by counting the frequencies of each unique ~35mer sequenced and validated by genome alignment, one can begin to examine the expression of specific sequences without the common complications of cross-hybridization, dye bias, microarray sensitivity, or saturation that plague microarray analyses. Counted data for each unique read can be interpreted as a direct measure of expression for use in differential expression studies.

As we begin to delve deeper into the genome in search of microRNAs and their targets, stem cells become an important piece of the puzzle. The previously described requirement of Dicer, DGCR8, and other members of the microRNA biogenesis pathway for both differentiation and maintenance of stem cells, combined with bioinformatic predictions of 10,000 microRNA genes, suggest that unknown numbers of novel sequences remain to be discovered in stem cells. A better appreciation of the mechanisms of stem cell regulation and the players involved will advance our understanding of the these crucial cells, and foster innovations in therapeutic applications of stem cells as well. The use of these next-generation techniques, however, must be accompanied by rigorous and novel statistical interpretations, as well as accommodations for the dimensions of the resulting data. Few biologists have had to deal with the volumes of data that will be generated in the near future, and even fewer have experience with mining and interpreting such large datasets. Collaborations with statisticians and computer scientists, and a focus on developing the next generation of biologists with strong working knowledge of both computer programming and statistical interpretation will be essential in discovering and interpreting microRNA regulatory mechanisms in differentiating stem cells.

Acknowledgements We thank Brad Love (Invitrogen) and Rebecka Jörnsten (Department of Statistics, Rutgers University) for patiently instructing us in statistical concepts and methods. LAG and RPH were supported by grants from NIH, the New Jersey Commission on Spinal Cord Research, the New Jersey Commission on Science and Technology, and Invitrogen, Inc.

References

1. Akao, Y., Y. Nakagawa, and T. Naoe, MicroRNAs 143 and 145 are possible common onco-microRNAs in human cancers. Oncol Rep, 2006. **16**(4): 845–50.
2. Altuvia, Y., P. Landgraf, G. Lithwick, N. Elefant, S. Pfeffer, A. Aravin, M.J. Brownstein, T. Tuschl, and H. Margalit, Clustering and conservation patterns of human microRNAs. Nucleic Acids Res, 2005. **33**(8): 2697–706.
3. Ambros, V., microRNAs: tiny regulators with great potential. Cell, 2001. **107**(7): 823–6.
4. Anderson, C., H. Catoe, and R. Werner, MIR-206 regulates connexin43 expression during skeletal muscle development. Nucleic Acids Res, 2006. **34**(20): 5863–71.
5. Babak, T., W. Zhang, Q. Morris, B.J. Blencowe, and T.R. Hughes, Probing microRNAs with microarrays: tissue specificity and functional inference. RNA, 2004. **10**(11): 1813.
6. Babak, T., W. Zhang, Q. Morris, B.J. Blencowe, and T.R. Hughes, Probing microRNAs with microarrays: tissue specificity and functional inference. RNA, 2004. **10**(11): 1813–9.
7. Baehrecke, E.H., miRNAs: micro managers of programmed cell death. Curr Biol, 2003. **13**(12): R473–5.
8. Barad, O., E. Meiri, A. Avniel, R. Aharonov, A. Barzilai, I. Bentwich, U. Einav, S. Gilad, P. Hurban, Y. Karov, E.K. Lobenhofer, E. Sharon, Y.M. Shiboleth, M. Shtutman, Z. Bentwich, and P. Einat, MicroRNA expression detected by oligonucleotide microarrays: system establishment and expression profiling in human tissues. Genome Res, 2004. **14**(12): 2486–94.
9. Baroukh, N., M.A. Ravier, M.K. Loder, E.V. Hill, A. Bounacer, R. Scharfmann, G.A. Rutter, and E. Van Obberghen, MicroRNA-124a regulates Foxa2 expression and intracellular signaling in pancreatic beta-cell lines. J Biol Chem, 2007. **282**(27): 19575–88.
10. Barski, A., S. Cuddapah, K. Cui, T.Y. Roh, D.E. Schones, Z. Wang, G. Wei, I. Chepelev, and K. Zhao, High-resolution profiling of histone methylations in the human genome. Cell, 2007. **129**(4): 823–37.
11. Bartel, D.P., MicroRNAs: genomics, biogenesis, mechanism, and function. Cell, 2004. **116**(2): 281–97.
12. Baskerville, S. and D.P. Bartel, Microarray profiling of microRNAs reveals frequent coexpression with neighboring miRNAs and host genes. RNA, 2005. **11**(3): 241–7.
13. Behm-Ansmant, I., J. Rehwinkel, T. Doerks, A. Stark, P. Bork, and E. Izaurralde, mRNA degradation by miRNAs and GW182 requires both CCR4:NOT deadenylase and DCP1: DCP2 decapping complexes. Genes Dev, 2006. **20**(14): 1885–98.
14. Benjamini, Y. and Y. Hochberg, Controlling the false discovery rate: a practical and powerful approach to multiple testing. J Roy Stat Soc B, 1995. **57**: 289–300.
15. Bentley, D.R., Whole-genome re-sequencing. Curr Opin Genet Dev, 2006. **16**(6): 545–52.
16. Bentwich, I., A postulated role for microRNA in cellular differentiation. Faseb J, 2005. **19**(8): 875–9.
17. Bernstein, E., S.Y. Kim, M.A. Carmell, E.P. Murchison, H. Alcorn, M.Z. Li, A.A. Mills, S.J. Elledge, K.V. Anderson, and G.J. Hannon, Dicer is essential for mouse development. Nat Genet, 2003. **35**(3): 215–7.
18. Beuvink, I., F.A. Kolb, W. Budach, A. Garnier, J. Lange, F. Natt, U. Dengler, J. Hall, W. Filipowicz, and J. Weiler, A novel microarray approach reveals new tissue-specific signatures of known and predicted mammalian microRNAs. Nucleic Acids Res, 2007. **35**(7): e52.
19. Bolstad, B.M., R.A. Irizarry, M. Astrand, and T.P. Speed, A comparison of normalization methods for high density oligonucleotide array data based on variance and bias. Bioinformatics, 2003. **19**(2): 185–93.

20. Borchert, G.M., W. Lanier, and B.L. Davidson, RNA polymerase III transcribes human microRNAs. Nat Struct Mol Biol, 2006. 13(12): 1097–101.

21. Brennecke, J., A. Stark, and S.M. Cohen, Not miR-ly muscular: microRNAs and muscle development. Genes Dev, 2005. 19(19): 2261–4.

22. Cai, X., C.H. Hagedorn, and B.R. Cullen, Human microRNAs are processed from capped, polyadenylated transcripts that can also function as mRNAs. RNA, 2004. 10(12): 1957–66.

23. Calin, G.A., C.D. Dumitru, M. Shimizu, R. Bichi, S. Zupo, E. Noch, H. Aldler, S. Rattan, M. Keating, K. Rai, L. Rassenti, T. Kipps, M. Negrini, F. Bullrich, and C.M. Croce, Frequent deletions and down-regulation of micro- RNA genes miR15 and miR16 at 13q14 in chronic lymphocytic leukemia. Proc Natl Acad Sci U S A, 2002. 99(24): 15524–9.

24. Calin, G.A., C.G. Liu, C. Sevignani, M. Ferracin, N. Felli, C.D. Dumitru, M. Shimizu, A. Cimmino, S. Zupo, M. Dono, M.L. Dell'Aquila, H. Alder, L. Rassenti, T.J. Kipps, F. Bullrich, M. Negrini, and C.M. Croce, MicroRNA profiling reveals distinct signatures in B cell chronic lymphocytic leukemias. Proc Natl Acad Sci U S A, 2004. 101(32): 11755.

25. Calin, G.A., C. Sevignani, C.D. Dumitru, T. Hyslop, E. Noch, S. Yendamuri, M. Shimizu, S. Rattan, F. Bullrich, M. Negrini, and C.M. Croce, Human microRNA genes are frequently located at fragile sites and genomic regions involved in cancers. Proc Natl Acad Sci U S A, 2004. 101(9): 2999–3004.

26. Calin, G.A., M. Ferracin, A. Cimmino, G. Di Leva, M. Shimizu, S.E. Wojcik, M.V. Iorio, R. Visone, N.I. Sever, M. Fabbri, R. Iuliano, T. Palumbo, F. Pichiorri, C. Roldo, R. Garzon, C. Sevignani, L. Rassenti, H. Alder, S. Volinia, C.G. Liu, T.J. Kipps, M. Negrini, and C.M. Croce, A MicroRNA signature associated with prognosis and progression in chronic lymphocytic leukemia. N Engl J Med, 2005. 353(17): 1793–801.

27. Carninci, P., T. Kasukawa, S. Katayama, J. Gough, M.C. Frith, N. Maeda, R. Oyama, T. Ravasi, B. Lenhard, C. Wells, R. Kodzius, K. Shimokawa, V.B. Bajic, S.E. Brenner, S. Batalov, A.R. Forrest, M. Zavolan, M.J. Davis, L.G. Wilming, V. Aidinis, J.E. Allen, A. Ambesi-Impiombato, R. Apweiler, R.N. Aturaliya, T.L. Bailey, M. Bansal, L. Baxter, K.W. Beisel, T. Bersano, H. Bono, A.M. Chalk, K.P. Chiu, V. Choudhary, A. Christoffels, D.R. Clutterbuck, M.L. Crowe, E. Dalla, B.P. Dalrymple, B. de Bono, G. Della Gatta, D. di Bernardo, T. Down, P. Engstrom, M. Fagiolini, G. Faulkner, C.F. Fletcher, T. Fukushima, M. Furuno, S. Futaki, M. Gariboldi, P. Georgii-Hemming, T.R. Gingeras, T. Gojobori, R.E. Green, S. Gustincich, M. Harbers, Y. Hayashi, T.K. Hensch, N. Hirokawa, D. Hill, L. Huminiecki, M. Iacono, K. Ikeo, A. Iwama, T. Ishikawa, M. Jakt, A. Kanapin, M. Katoh, Y. Kawasawa, J. Kelso, H. Kitamura, H. Kitano, G. Kollias, S.P. Krishnan, A. Kruger, S.K. Kummerfeld, I.V. Kurochkin, L.F. Lareau, D. Lazarevic, L. Lipovich, J. Liu, S. Liuni, S. McWilliam, M. Madan Babu, M. Madera, L. Marchionni, H. Matsuda, S. Matsuzawa, H. Miki, F. Mignone, S. Miyake, K. Morris, S. Mottagui-Tabar, N. Mulder, N. Nakano, H. Nakauchi, P. Ng, R. Nilsson, S. Nishiguchi, S. Nishikawa, F. Nori, O. Ohara, Y. Okazaki, V. Orlando, K.C. Pang, W.J. Pavan, G. Pavesi, G. Pesole, N. Petrovsky, S. Piazza, J. Reed, J.F. Reid, B.Z. Ring, M. Ringwald, B. Rost, Y. Ruan, S.L. Salzberg, A. Sandelin, C. Schneider, C. Schonbach, K. Sekiguchi, C.A. Semple, S. Seno, L. Sessa, Y. Sheng, Y. Shibata, H. Shimada, K. Shimada, D. Silva, B. Sinclair, S. Sperling, E. Stupka, K. Sugiura, R. Sultana, Y. Takenaka, K. Taki, K. Tammoja, S.L. Tan, S. Tang, M.S. Taylor, J. Tegner, S.A. Teichmann, H.R. Ueda, E. van Nimwegen, R. Verardo, C.L. Wei, K. Yagi, H. Yamanishi, E. Zabarovsky, S. Zhu, A. Zimmer, W. Hide, C. Bult, S.M. Grimmond, R.D. Teasdale, E.T. Liu, V. Brusic, J. Quackenbush, C. Wahlestedt, J.S. Mattick, D.A. Hume, C. Kai, D. Sasaki, Y. Tomaru, S. Fukuda, M. Kanamori-Katayama, M. Suzuki, J. Aoki, T. Arakawa, J. Iida, K. Imamura, M. Itoh, T. Kato, H. Kawaji, N. Kawagashira, T. Kawashima, M. Kojima, S. Kondo, H. Konno, K. Nakano, N. Ninomiya, T. Nishio, M. Okada, C. Plessy, K. Shibata, T. Shiraki, S. Suzuki, M. Tagami, K. Waki, A. Watahiki, Y. Okamura-Oho, H. Suzuki, J. Kawai and Y. Hayashizaki, The transcriptional landscape of the mammalian genome. Science, 2005. 309(5740): 1559–63.

28. Castoldi, M., S. Schmidt, V. Benes, M. Noerholm, A.E. Kulozik, M.W. Hentze, and M.U. Muckenthaler, A sensitive array for microRNA expression profiling (miChip) based on locked nucleic acids (LNA). RNA, 2006. 12(5): 913–20.

29. Chan, J.A., A.M. Krichevsky, and K.S. Kosik, MicroRNA-21 is an antiapoptotic factor in human glioblastoma cells. Cancer Res, 2005. **65**(14): 6029–33.

30. Chen, C., D.A. Ridzon, A.J. Broomer, Z. Zhou, D.H. Lee, J.T. Nguyen, M. Barbisin, N.L. Xu, V.R. Mahuvakar, M.R. Andersen, K.Q. Lao, K.J. Livak, and K.J. Guegler, Real-time quantification of microRNAs by stem-loop RT-PCR. Nucleic Acids Res, 2005. **33**(20): e179.

31. Chen, C.Z. and H.F. Lodish, MicroRNAs as regulators of mammalian hematopoiesis. Semin Immunol, 2005. **17**(2): 155–65.

32. Chen, J.F., E.M. Mandel, J.M. Thomson, Q. Wu, T.E. Callis, S.M. Hammond, F.L. Conlon, and D.Z. Wang, The role of microRNA-1 and microRNA-133 in skeletal muscle proliferation and differentiation. Nat Genet, 2006. **38**(2): 228–33.

33. Chen, X.M., P.L. Splinter, P. O'Hara S, and N.F. Larusso, A cellular micro-RNA, let-7i, regulates toll-like receptor 4 expression and contributes to cholangiocyte immune responses against cryptosporidium parvum Infection. J Biol Chem, 2007. **282**(39): 28929–38.

34. Cimmino, A., G.A. Calin, M. Fabbri, M.V. Iorio, M. Ferracin, M. Shimizu, S.E. Wojcik, R.I. Aqeilan, S. Zupo, M. Dono, L. Rassenti, H. Alder, S. Volinia, C.G. Liu, T.J. Kipps, M. Negrini, and C.M. Croce, miR-15 and miR-16 induce apoptosis by targeting BCL2. Proc Natl Acad Sci U S A, 2005. **102**(39): 13944–9.

35. Cullen, B.R., Derivation and function of small interfering RNAs and microRNAs. Virus Res, 2004. **102**(1): 3–9.

36. Davison, T.S., C.D. Johnson, and B.F. Andruss, Analyzing micro-RNA expression using microarrays. Methods Enzymol, 2006. **411**: 14–34.

37. Denli, A.M., B.B. Tops, R.H. Plasterk, R.F. Ketting, and G.J. Hannon, Processing of primary microRNAs by the Microprocessor complex. Nature, 2004. **432**(7014): 231–5.

38. Eder, M. and M. Scherr, MicroRNA and lung cancer. N Engl J Med, 2005. **352**(23): 2446–8.

39. Esau, C., X. Kang, E. Peralta, E. Hanson, E.G. Marcusson, L.V. Ravichandran, Y. Sun, S. Koo, R.J. Perera, R. Jain, N.M. Dean, S.M. Freier, C.F. Bennett, B. Lollo, and R. Griffey, MicroRNA-143 regulates adipocyte differentiation. J Biol Chem, 2004. **279**(50): 52361–5.

40. Esau, C., S. Davis, S.F. Murray, X.X. Yu, S.K. Pandey, M. Pear, L. Watts, S.L. Booten, M. Graham, R. McKay, A. Subramaniam, S. Propp, B.A. Lollo, S. Freier, C.F. Bennett, S. Bhanot, and B.P. Monia, miR-122 regulation of lipid metabolism revealed by in vivo antisense targeting. Cell Metab, 2006. **3**(2): 87–98.

41. Fazi, F., A. Rosa, A. Fatica, V. Gelmetti, M.L. De Marchis, C. Nervi, and I. Bozzoni, A minicircuitry comprised of microRNA-223 and transcription factors NFI-A and C/EBPalpha regulates human granulopoiesis. Cell, 2005. **123**(5): 819–31.

42. Felli, N., L. Fontana, E. Pelosi, R. Botta, D. Bonci, F. Facchiano, F. Liuzzi, V. Lulli, O. Morsilli, S. Santoro, M. Valtieri, G.A. Calin, C.G. Liu, A. Sorrentino, C.M. Croce, and C. Peschle, MicroRNAs 221 and 222 inhibit normal erythropoiesis and erythroleukemic cell growth via kit receptor down-modulation. Proc Natl Acad Sci U S A, 2005. **102**(50): 18081–6.

43. Frederikse, P.H., R. Donnelly, and L.M. Partyka, miRNA and Dicer in the mammalian lens: expression of brain-specific miRNAs in the lens. Histochem Cell Biol, 2006. **126**(1): 1–8.

44. Gentleman, R.C., V.J. Carey, D.M. Bates, B. Bolstad, M. Dettling, S. Dudoit, B. Ellis, L. Gautier, Y. Ge, J. Gentry, K. Hornik, T. Hothorn, W. Huber, S. Iacus, R. Irizarry, F. Leisch, C. Li, M. Maechler, A.J. Rossini, G. Sawitzki, C. Smith, G. Smyth, L. Tierney, J.Y. Yang, and J. Zhang, Bioconductor: open software development for computational biology and bioinformatics. Genome Biol, 2004. **5**(10): R80.

45. Giraldez, A.J., R.M. Cinalli, M.E. Glasner, A.J. Enright, J.M. Thomson, S. Baskerville, S.M. Hammond, D.P. Bartel, and A.F. Schier, MicroRNAs regulate brain morphogenesis in zebrafish. Science, 2005. **308**(5723): 833–8.

46. Giraldez, A.J., Y. Mishima, J. Rihel, R.J. Grocock, S. Van Dongen, K. Inoue, A.J. Enright, and A.F. Schier, Zebrafish MiR-430 promotes deadenylation and clearance of maternal mRNAs. Science, 2006. **312**(5770): 75–9.

47. Goff, L.A., M. Yang, J. Bowers, R.C. Getts, R.W. Padgett, and R.P. Hart, Rational probe optimization and enhanced detection strategy for microRNAs using microarrays. RNA Biology, 2005. **2**(3): e9–e16.
48. Goff, L.A., M. Yang, J. Bowers, R.C. Getts, R.W. Padgett, and R.P. Hart, Rational probe optimization and enhanced detection strategy for microRNAs using microarrays. RNA Biol, 2005. **2**(3): 93–100.
49. Goff, L.A., S. Boucher, C. Ricupero, S. Fenstermacher, M. Swerdel, L. Chase, C. Adams, J.D. Chesnut, U. Lakshmipathy, and R.P. Hart, Differentiating human multipotent mesenchymal stromal cells regulate microRNAs: prediction of microRNA regulation by PDGF during osteogenesis. Exp Hematol, 2008. In press.
50. Goodrich, J.A. and J.F. Kugel, Non-coding-RNA regulators of RNA polymerase II transcription. Nat Rev Mol Cell Biol, 2006. **7**(8): 612–6.
51. Gregory, R.I., K.P. Yan, G. Amuthan, T. Chendrimada, B. Doratotaj, N. Cooch, and R. Shiekhattar, The Microprocessor complex mediates the genesis of microRNAs. Nature, 2004. **432**(7014): 235–40.
52. Gregory, R.I. and R. Shiekhattar, MicroRNA biogenesis and cancer. Cancer Res, 2005. **65**(9): 3509–12.
53. Griffiths-Jones, S., R.J. Grocock, S. van Dongen, A. Bateman, and A.J. Enright, miRBase: microRNA sequences, targets and gene nomenclature. Nucleic Acids Res, 2006. **34**(Database issue): D140–4.
54. Gu, J., T. He, Y. Pei, F. Li, X. Wang, J. Zhang, X. Zhang, and Y. Li, Primary transcripts and expressions of mammal intergenic microRNAs detected by mapping ESTs to their flanking sequences. Mamm Genome, 2006. **17**(10): 1033–41.
55. Han, J., Y. Lee, K.H. Yeom, Y.K. Kim, H. Jin, and V.N. Kim, The Drosha-DGCR8 complex in primary microRNA processing. Genes Dev, 2004. **18**(24): 3016–27.
56. Han, J., Y. Lee, K.H. Yeom, J.W. Nam, I. Heo, J.K. Rhee, S.Y. Sohn, Y. Cho, B.T. Zhang, and V.N. Kim, Molecular basis for the recognition of primary microRNAs by the Drosha-DGCR8 complex. Cell, 2006. **125**(5): 887–901.
57. Harfe, B.D., M.T. McManus, J.H. Mansfield, E. Hornstein, and C.J. Tabin, The RNaseIII enzyme Dicer is required for morphogenesis but not patterning of the vertebrate limb. Proc Natl Acad Sci U S A, 2005. **102**(31): 10898–903.
58. Hatfield, S.D., H.R. Shcherbata, K.A. Fischer, K. Nakahara, R.W. Carthew, and H. Ruohola-Baker, Stem cell division is regulated by the microRNA pathway. Nature, 2005. **435**(7044): 974–8.
59. Hayashita, Y., H. Osada, Y. Tatematsu, H. Yamada, K. Yanagisawa, S. Tomida, Y. Yatabe, K. Kawahara, Y. Sekido, and T. Takahashi, A polycistronic microRNA cluster, miR-17–92, is overexpressed in human lung cancers and enhances cell proliferation. Cancer Res, 2005. **65**(21): 9628–32.
60. He, H., K. Jazdzewski, W. Li, S. Liyanarachchi, R. Nagy, S. Volinia, G.A. Calin, C.G. Liu, K. Franssila, S. Suster, R.T. Kloos, C.M. Croce, and A. de la Chapelle, The role of microRNA genes in papillary thyroid carcinoma. Proc Natl Acad Sci U S A, 2005. **102**(52): 19075–80.
61. He, L., J.M. Thomson, M.T. Hemann, E. Hernando-Monge, D. Mu, S. Goodson, S. Powers, C. Cordon-Cardo, S.W. Lowe, G.J. Hannon, and S.M. Hammond, A microRNA polycistron as a potential human oncogene. Nature, 2005. **435**(7043): 828–33.
62. Holm, S., A simple sequentially rejective bonferroni test procedure. Scand J Stat, 1979. **6**: 65–70.
63. Hornstein, E., J.H. Mansfield, S. Yekta, J.K. Hu, B.D. Harfe, M.T. McManus, S. Baskerville, D.P. Bartel, and C.J. Tabin, The microRNA miR-196 acts upstream of Hoxb8 and Shh in limb development. Nature, 2005. **438**(7068): 671–4.
64. Hossain, A., M.T. Kuo, and G.F. Saunders, Mir-17-5p regulates breast cancer cell proliferation by inhibiting translation of AIB1 mRNA. Mol Cell Biol, 2006. **26**(21): 8191–201.
65. Houbaviy, H.B., M.F. Murray, and P.A. Sharp, Embryonic stem cell-specific MicroRNAs. Dev Cell, 2003. **5**(2): 351–8.

66. Houbaviy, H.B., L. Dennis, R. Jaenisch, and P.A. Sharp, Characterization of a highly variable eutherian microRNA gene. RNA, 2005. 11(8): 1245–57.

67. Huang, J., F. Wang, E. Argyris, K. Chen, Z. Liang, H. Tian, W. Huang, K. Squires, G. Verlinghieri, and H. Zhang, Cellular microRNAs contribute to HIV-1 latency in resting primary CD4(+) T lymphocytes. Nat Med, 2007. 13(10): 1241–7.

68. Humphreys, D.T., B.J. Westman, D.I. Martin, and T. Preiss, MicroRNAs control translation initiation by inhibiting eukaryotic initiation factor 4E/cap and poly(A) tail function. Proc Natl Acad Sci U S A, 2005. 102(47): 16961–6.

69. Johnson, D.S., A. Mortazavi, R.M. Myers, and B. Wold, Genome-wide mapping of in vivo protein-DNA interactions. Science, 2007. 316(5830): 1497–502.

70. Johnson, S.M., H. Grosshans, J. Shingara, M. Byrom, R. Jarvis, A. Cheng, E. Labourier, K.L. Reinert, D. Brown, and F.J. Slack, RAS is regulated by the let-7 microRNA family. Cell, 2005. 120(5): 635–47.

71. Johnston, R.J. and O. Hobert, A microRNA controlling left/right neuronal asymmetry in Caenorhabditis elegans. Nature, 2003. 426(6968): 845–9.

72. Josephson, R., C.J. Ording, Y. Liu, S. Shin, U. Lakshmipathy, A. Toumadje, B. Love, J.D. Chesnut, P.W. Andrews, M.S. Rao, and J.M. Auerbach, Qualification of embryonal carcinoma 2102Ep as a reference for human embryonic stem cell research. Stem Cells, 2007. 25(2): 437–46.

73. Kanellopoulou, C., S.A. Muljo, A.L. Kung, S. Ganesan, R. Drapkin, T. Jenuwein, D.M. Livingston, and K. Rajewsky, Dicer-deficient mouse embryonic stem cells are defective in differentiation and centromeric silencing. Genes Dev, 2005. 19(4): 489–501.

74. Kawasaki, H. and K. Taira, Functional analysis of microRNAs during the retinoic acid-induced neuronal differentiation of human NT2 cells. Nucleic Acids Res Suppl, 2003. (3): 243–4.

75. Kerr, M.K., M. Martin, and G.A. Churchill, Analysis of variance for gene expression microarray data. J Comput Biol, 2000. 7(6): 819–37.

76. Kerr, M.K. and G.A. Churchill, Experimental design for gene expression microarrays. Biostatistics, 2001. 2(2): 183–201.

77. Kerr, M.K. and G.A. Churchill, Bootstrapping cluster analysis: assessing the reliability of conclusions from microarray experiments. Proc Natl Acad Sci U S A, 2001. 98(16): 8961–5.

78. Kerr, M.K. and G.A. Churchill, Statistical design and the analysis of gene expression microarray data. Genet Res, 2001. 77(2): 123–8.

79. Kim, H.K., Y.S. Lee, U. Sivaprasad, A. Malhotra, and A. Dutta, Muscle-specific microRNA miR-206 promotes muscle differentiation. J Cell Biol, 2006. 174(5): 677–87.

80. Kim, J., A. Krichevsky, Y. Grad, G.D. Hayes, K.S. Kosik, G.M. Church, and G. Ruvkun, Identification of many microRNAs that copurify with polyribosomes in mammalian neurons. Proc Natl Acad Sci U S A, 2004. 101(1): 360–5.

81. Kluiver, J., E. Haralambieva, D. de Jong, T. Blokzijl, S. Jacobs, B.J. Kroesen, S. Poppema, and A. van den Berg, Lack of BIC and microRNA miR-155 expression in primary cases of Burkitt lymphoma. Genes Chromosomes Cancer, 2006. 45(2): 147–53.

82. Krichevsky, A.M., K.S. King, C.P. Donahue, K. Khrapko, and K.S. Kosik, A microRNA array reveals extensive regulation of microRNAs during brain development. RNA, 2003. 9(10): 1274.

83. Krichevsky, A.M., K.S. King, C.P. Donahue, K. Khrapko, and K.S. Kosik, A microRNA array reveals extensive regulation of microRNAs during brain development. RNA, 2003. 9(10): 1274–81.

84. Kutay, H., S. Bai, J. Datta, T. Motiwala, I. Pogribny, W. Frankel, S.T. Jacob, and K. Ghoshal, Downregulation of miR-122 in the rodent and human hepatocellular carcinomas. J Cell Biochem, 2006. 99(3): 671–8.

85. Kuwabara, T., J. Hsieh, K. Nakashima, K. Taira, and F.H. Gage, A small modulatory dsRNA specifies the fate of adult neural stem cells. Cell, 2004. 116(6): 779–93.

86. Kwon, C., Z. Han, E.N. Olson, and D. Srivastava, MicroRNA1 influences cardiac differentiation in Drosophila and regulates Notch signaling. Proc Natl Acad Sci U S A, 2005. **102**(52): 18986–91.

87. Kye, M.J., T. Liu, S.F. Levy, N.L. Xu, B.B. Groves, R. Bonneau, K. Lao, and K.S. Kosik, Somatodendritic microRNAs identified by laser capture and multiplex RT-PCR. RNA, 2007. **13**(8): 1224–34.

88. Lagos-Quintana, M., R. Rauhut, J. Meyer, A. Borkhardt, and T. Tuschl, New microRNAs from mouse and human. RNA, 2003. **9**(2): 175–9.

89. Lakshmipathy, U., B. Love, L.A. Goff, R. Jornsten, R. Graichen, R.P. Hart, and J.D. Chesnut, MicroRNA expression pattern of undifferentiated and differentiated human embryonic stem cells. Stem Cells Dev, 2007. **16**(6): 1003–16.

90. Lecellier, C.H., P. Dunoyer, K. Arar, J. Lehmann-Che, S. Eyquem, C. Himber, A. Saib, and O. Voinnet, A cellular microRNA mediates antiviral defense in human cells. Science, 2005. **308**(5721): 557–60.

91. Lee, Y., C. Ahn, J. Han, H. Choi, J. Kim, J. Yim, J. Lee, P. Provost, O. Radmark, S. Kim, and V.N. Kim, The nuclear RNase III Drosha initiates microRNA processing. Nature, 2003. **425**(6956): 415–9.

92. Lee, Y.S., H.K. Kim, S. Chung, K.S. Kim, and A. Dutta, Depletion of human micro-RNA miR-125b reveals that it is critical for the proliferation of differentiated cells but not for the down-regulation of putative targets during differentiation. J Biol Chem, 2005. **280**(17): 16635–41.

93. Lewis, B.P., C.B. Burge, and D.P. Bartel, Conserved seed pairing, often flanked by adenosines, indicates that thousands of human genes are microRNA targets. Cell, 2005. **120**(1): 15–20.

94. Li, H., X. Chen, K. Zhang, and T. Jiang, A general framework for biclustering gene expression data. J Bioinform Comput Biol, 2006. **4**(4): 911–33.

95. Lian, S., A. Jakymiw, T. Eystathioy, J.C. Hamel, M.J. Fritzler, and E.K. Chan, GW bodies, microRNAs and the cell cycle. Cell Cycle, 2006. **5**(3): 242–5.

96. Liang, R.Q., W. Li, Y. Li, C.Y. Tan, J.X. Li, Y.X. Jin, and K.C. Ruan, An oligonucleotide microarray for microRNA expression analysis based on labeling RNA with quantum dot and nanogold probe. Nucleic Acids Res, 2005. **33**(2): e17.

97. Lim, L.P., N.C. Lau, P. Garrett-Engele, A. Grimson, J.M. Schelter, J. Castle, D.P. Bartel, P.S. Linsley, and J.M. Johnson, Microarray analysis shows that some microRNAs downregulate large numbers of target mRNAs. Nature, 2005. **433**(7027): 769–73.

98. Lin, S.L., J.D. Miller, and S.Y. Ying, Intronic MicroRNA (miRNA). J Biomed Biotechnol, 2006. **2006**(4): 26818.

99. Liu, C.G., G.A. Calin, B. Meloon, N. Gamliel, C. Sevignani, M. Ferracin, C.D. Dumitru, M. Shimizu, S. Zupo, M. Dono, H. Alder, F. Bullrich, M. Negrini, and C.M. Croce, An oligonucleotide microchip for genome-wide microRNA profiling in human and mouse tissues. Proc Natl Acad Sci U S A, 2004. **101**(26): 9740.

100. Liu, J., M.A. Carmell, F.V. Rivas, C.G. Marsden, J.M. Thomson, J.J. Song, S.M. Hammond, L. Joshua-Tor, and G.J. Hannon, Argonaute2 is the catalytic engine of mammalian RNAi. Science, 2004. **305**(5689): 1437–41.

101. Liu, J., F.V. Rivas, J. Wohlschlegel, J.R. Yates, 3rd, R. Parker, and G.J. Hannon, A role for the P-body component GW182 in microRNA function. Nat Cell Biol, 2005. **7**(12): 1261–6.

102. Liu, J., M.A. Valencia-Sanchez, G.J. Hannon, and R. Parker, MicroRNA-dependent localization of targeted mRNAs to mammalian P-bodies. Nat Cell Biol, 2005. **7**(7): 719–23.

103. Madeira, S.C. and A.L. Oliveira, Biclustering algorithms for biological data analysis: a survey. IEEE/ACM Trans Comput Biol Bioinform, 2004. **1**(1): 24–45.

104. Mansfield, J.H., B.D. Harfe, R. Nissen, J. Obenauer, J. Srineel, A. Chaudhuri, R. Farzan-Kashani, M. Zuker, A.E. Pasquinelli, G. Ruvkun, P.A. Sharp, C.J. Tabin, and M.T. McManus, MicroRNA-responsive 'sensor' transgenes uncover Hox-like and other developmentally regulated patterns of vertebrate microRNA expression. Nat Genet, 2004. **36**(10): 1079–83.

105. Masotti, A., Preckel, T., Analysis of small RNAs with the Agilent 2100 Bioanalyzer. Nature Methods, 2006. **3**(8): iii–iv.
106. Matys, V., E. Fricke, R. Geffers, E. Gossling, M. Haubrock, R. Hehl, K. Hornischer, D. Karas, A.E. Kel, O.V. Kel-Margoulis, D.U. Kloos, S. Land, B. Lewicki-Potapov, H. Michael, R. Munch, I. Reuter, S. Rotert, H. Saxel, M. Scheer, S. Thiele, and E. Wingender, TRANSFAC: transcriptional regulation, from patterns to profiles. Nucleic Acids Res, 2003. **31**(1): 374–8.
107. Matzke, M., W. Aufsatz, T. Kanno, L. Daxinger, I. Papp, M.F. Mette, and A.J. Matzke, Genetic analysis of RNA-mediated transcriptional gene silencing. Biochim Biophys Acta, 2004. **1677**(1–3): 129–41.
108. Mikkelsen, T.S., M. Ku, D.B. Jaffe, B. Issac, E. Lieberman, G. Giannoukos, P. Alvarez, W. Brockman, T.K. Kim, R.P. Koche, W. Lee, E. Mendenhall, A. O'Donovan, A. Presser, C. Russ, X. Xie, A. Meissner, M. Wernig, R. Jaenisch, C. Nusbaum, E.S. Lander, and B.E. Bernstein, Genome-wide maps of chromatin state in pluripotent and lineage-committed cells. Nature, 2007. **448**(7153): 553–60.
109. Miranda, K.C., T. Huynh, Y. Tay, Y.S. Ang, W.L. Tam, A.M. Thomson, B. Lim, and I. Rigoutsos, A pattern-based method for the identification of MicroRNA binding sites and their corresponding heteroduplexes. Cell, 2006. **126**(6): 1203–17.
110. Mishima, Y., A.J. Giraldez, Y. Takeda, T. Fujiwara, H. Sakamoto, A.F. Schier, and K. Inoue, Differential regulation of germline mRNAs in soma and germ cells by zebrafish miR-430. Curr Biol, 2006. **16**(21): 2135–42.
111. Miska, E.A., E. Alvarez-Saavedra, M. Townsend, A. Yoshii, N. Sestan, P. Rakic, M. Constantine-Paton, and H.R. Horvitz, Microarray analysis of microRNA expression in the developing mammalian brain. Genome Biol, 2004. **5**(9): R68.
112. Moffat, I.D., P.C. Boutros, T. Celius, J. Linden, R. Pohjanvirta, and A.B. Okey, MicroRNAs in adult rodent liver are refractory to dioxin treatment. Toxicol Sci, 2007. **99**(2): 470–87.
113. Mora, J.R. and R.C. Getts, Enzymatic microRNA detection in microtiter plates with DNA dendrimers. BioTechniques, 2006. **41**(4): 420, 422, 424.
114. Murchison, E.P., J.F. Partridge, O.H. Tam, S. Cheloufi, and G.J. Hannon, Characterization of Dicer-deficient murine embryonic stem cells. Proc Natl Acad Sci U S A, 2005. **102**(34): 12135–40.
115. Naguibneva, I., M. Ameyar-Zazoua, A. Polesskaya, S. Ait-Si-Ali, R. Groisman, M. Souidi, S. Cuvellier, and A. Harel-Bellan, The microRNA miR-181 targets the homeobox protein Hox-A11 during mammalian myoblast differentiation. Nat Cell Biol, 2006. **8**(3): 278–84.
116. Nakajima, N., T. Takahashi, R. Kitamura, K. Isodono, S. Asada, T. Ueyama, H. Matsubara, and H. Oh, MicroRNA-1 facilitates skeletal myogenic differentiation without affecting osteoblastic and adipogenic differentiation. Biochem Biophys Res Commun, 2006. **350**(4): 1006–12.
117. Nelson, P.T., D.A. Baldwin, L.M. Scearce, J.C. Oberholtzer, J.W. Tobias, and Z. Mourelatos, Microarray-based, high-throughput gene expression profiling of microRNAs. Nat Methods, 2004. **1**(2): 155–61.
118. Nelson, P.T., A.G. Hatzigeorgiou, and Z. Mourelatos, miRNP:mRNA association in polyribosomes in a human neuronal cell line. RNA, 2004. **10**(3): 387–94.
119. Ng, F., S. Boucher, S. Koh, K.S. Sastry, L. Chase, U. Lakshmipathy, C. Choong, Z. Yang, M. Vemuri, M.S. Rao, and V. Tanavde, PDGF, TGF-b and FGF signaling is important for differentiation and growth of Mesenchymal Stem Cells (MSCs): transcriptional profiling can identify markers and signaling pathways important in differentiation of MSC into adipogenic, chondrogenic and osteogenic lineages. Blood, 2008 Mar 10 (Epub ahead of print)
120. Pauley, K.M., T. Eystathioy, A. Jakymiw, J.C. Hamel, M.J. Fritzler, and E.K. Chan, Formation of GW bodies is a consequence of microRNA genesis. EMBO Rep, 2006. **7**(9): 904–10.
121. Pillai, R.S., S.N. Bhattacharyya, C.G. Artus, T. Zoller, N. Cougot, E. Basyuk, E. Bertrand, and W. Filipowicz, Inhibition of translational initiation by Let-7 MicroRNA in human cells. Science, 2005. **309**(5740): 1573–6.

122. Plaisance, V., A. Abderrahmani, V. Perret-Menoud, P. Jacquemin, F. Lemaigre, and R. Regazzi, MicroRNA-9 controls the expression of Granuphilin/Slp4 and the secretory response of insulin-producing cells. J Biol Chem, 2006. **281**(37): 26932–42.
123. Poy, M.N., L. Eliasson, J. Krutzfeldt, S. Kuwajima, X. Ma, P.E. Macdonald, S. Pfeffer, T. Tuschl, N. Rajewsky, P. Rorsman, and M. Stoffel, A pancreatic islet-specific microRNA regulates insulin secretion. Nature, 2004. **432**(7014): 226–30.
124. Prelic, A., S. Bleuler, P. Zimmermann, A. Wille, P. Buhlmann, W. Gruissem, L. Hennig, L. Thiele, and E. Zitzler, A systematic comparison and evaluation of biclustering methods for gene expression data. Bioinformatics, 2006. **22**(9): 1122–9.
125. Ramkissoon, S.H., L.A. Mainwaring, Y. Ogasawara, K. Keyvanfar, J.P. McCoy, Jr., E.M. Sloand, S. Kajigaya, and N.S. Young, Hematopoietic-specific microRNA expression in human cells. Leuk Res, 2006. **30**(5): 643–7.
126. Rao, M., Conserved and divergent paths that regulate self-renewal in mouse and human embryonic stem cells. Dev Biol, 2004. **275**(2): 269–86.
127. Rehwinkel, J., I. Behm-Ansmant, D. Gatfield, and E. Izaurralde, A crucial role for GW182 and the DCP1:DCP2 decapping complex in miRNA-mediated gene silencing. RNA, 2005. **11**(11): 1640–7.
128. Robertson, G., M. Hirst, M. Bainbridge, M. Bilenky, Y. Zhao, T. Zeng, G. Euskirchen, B. Bernier, R. Varhol, A. Delaney, N. Thiessen, O.L. Griffith, A. He, M. Marra, M. Snyder, and S. Jones, Genome-wide profiles of STAT1 DNA association using chromatin immunoprecipitation and massively parallel sequencing. Nat Methods, 2007. **4**(8): 651–7.
129. Roldo, C., E. Missiaglia, J.P. Hagan, M. Falconi, P. Capelli, S. Bersani, G.A. Calin, S. Volinia, C.G. Liu, A. Scarpa, and C.M. Croce, MicroRNA expression abnormalities in pancreatic endocrine and acinar tumors are associated with distinctive pathologic features and clinical behavior. J Clin Oncol, 2006. **24**(29): 4677–84.
130. Saito, K., K.M. Nishida, T. Mori, Y. Kawamura, K. Miyoshi, T. Nagami, H. Siomi, and M.C. Siomi, Specific association of Piwi with rasiRNAs derived from retrotransposon and heterochromatic regions in the Drosophila genome. Genes Dev, 2006. **20**(16): 2214–22.
131. Saito, Y., G. Liang, G. Egger, J.M. Friedman, J.C. Chuang, G.A. Coetzee, and P.A. Jones, Specific activation of microRNA-127 with downregulation of the proto-oncogene BCL6 by chromatin-modifying drugs in human cancer cells. Cancer Cell, 2006. **9**(6): 435–43.
132. Schramke, V. and R. Allshire, Hairpin RNAs and retrotransposon LTRs effect RNAi and chromatin-based gene silencing. Science, 2003. **301**(5636): 1069–74.
133. Scott, G.K., M.D. Mattie, C.E. Berger, S.C. Benz, and C.C. Benz, Rapid alteration of microRNA levels by histone deacetylase inhibition. Cancer Res, 2006. **66**(3): 1277–81.
134. Sempere, L.F., S. Freemantle, I. Pitha-Rowe, E. Moss, E. Dmitrovsky, and V. Ambros, Expression profiling of mammalian microRNAs uncovers a subset of brain-expressed microRNAs with possible roles in murine and human neuronal differentiation. Genome Biol, 2004. **5**(3): R13.
135. Shcherbata, H.R., S. Hatfield, E.J. Ward, S. Reynolds, K.A. Fischer, and H. Ruohola-Baker, The MicroRNA pathway plays a regulatory role in stem cell division. Cell Cycle, 2006. **5**(2): 172–5.
136. Shi, L., L.H. Reid, W.D. Jones, R. Shippy, J.A. Warrington, S.C. Baker, P.J. Collins, F. de Longueville, E.S. Kawasaki, K.Y. Lee, Y. Luo, Y.A. Sun, J.C. Willey, R.A. Setterquist, G.M. Fischer, W. Tong, Y.P. Dragan, D.J. Dix, F.W. Frueh, F.M. Goodsaid, D. Herman, R.V. Jensen, C.D. Johnson, E.K. Lobenhofer, R.K. Puri, U. Schrf, J. Thierry-Mieg, C. Wang, M. Wilson, P.K. Wolber, L. Zhang, S. Amur, W. Bao, C.C. Barbacioru, A.B. Lucas, V. Bertholet, C. Boysen, B. Bromley, D. Brown, A. Brunner, R. Canales, X.M. Cao, T.A. Cebula, J.J. Chen, J. Cheng, T.M. Chu, E. Chudin, J. Corson, J.C. Corton, L.J. Croner, C. Davies, T.S. Davison, G. Delenstarr, X. Deng, D. Dorris, A.C. Eklund, X.H. Fan, H. Fang, S. Fulmer-Smentek, J.C. Fuscoe, K. Gallagher, W. Ge, L. Guo, X. Guo, J. Hager, P.K. Haje, J. Han, T. Han, H.C. Harbottle, S.C. Harris, E. Hatchwell, C.A. Hauser, S. Hester, H. Hong, P. Hurban, S.A. Jackson, H. Ji, C.R. Knight, W.P. Kuo, J.E. LeClerc, S. Levy, Q.Z. Li, C. Liu, Y. Liu, M.J. Lombardi, Y. Ma, S.R. Magnuson, B. Maqsodi, T. McDaniel, N. Mei, O. Myklebost, B.

Ning, N. Novoradovskaya, M.S. Orr, T.W. Osborn, A. Papallo, T.A. Patterson, R.G. Perkins, E.H. Peters, R. Peterson, K.L. Philips, P.S. Pine, L. Pusztai, F. Qian, H. Ren, M. Rosen, B.A. Rosenzweig, R.R. Samaha, M. Schena, G.P. Schroth, S. Shchegrova, D.D. Smith, F. Staedtler, Z. Su, H. Sun, Z. Szallasi, Z. Tezak, D. Thierry-Mieg, K.L. Thompson, I. Tikhonova, Y. Turpaz, B. Vallanat, C. Van, S.J. Walker, S.J. Wang, Y. Wang, R. Wolfinger, A. Wong, J. Wu, C. Xiao, Q. Xie, J. Xu, W. Yang, S. Zhong, Y. Zong and W. Slikker, Jr., The MicroArray Quality Control (MAQC) project shows inter- and intraplatform reproducibility of gene expression measurements. Nat Biotechnol, 2006. **24**(9): 1151–61.

137. Song, L. and R.S. Tuan, MicroRNAs and cell differentiation in mammalian development. Birth Defects Res C Embryo Today, 2006. **78**(2): 140–9.

138. Suh, M.R., Y. Lee, J.Y. Kim, S.K. Kim, S.H. Moon, J.Y. Lee, K.Y. Cha, H.M. Chung, H.S. Yoon, S.Y. Moon, V.N. Kim, and K.S. Kim, Human embryonic stem cells express a unique set of microRNAs. Dev Biol, 2004. **270**(2): 488–98.

139. Sun, Y., S. Koo, N. White, E. Peralta, C. Esau, N.M. Dean, and R.J. Perera, Development of a micro-array to detect human and mouse microRNAs and characterization of expression in human organs. Nucleic Acids Res, 2004. **32**(22): e188.

140. Sweetman, D., T. Rathjen, M. Jefferson, G. Wheeler, T.G. Smith, G.N. Wheeler, A. Munsterberg, and T. Dalmay, FGF-4 signaling is involved in mir-206 expression in developing somites of chicken embryos. Dev Dyn, 2006. **235**(8): 2185–91.

141. Taganov, K.D., M.P. Boldin, K.J. Chang, and D. Baltimore, NF-kappaB-dependent induction of microRNA miR-146, an inhibitor targeted to signaling proteins of innate immune responses. Proc Natl Acad Sci U S A, 2006. **103**(33): 12481–6.

142. Tam, W. and J.E. Dahlberg, miR-155/BIC as an oncogenic microRNA. Genes Chromosomes Cancer, 2006. **45**(2): 211–2.

143. Tanzer, A. and P.F. Stadler, Molecular evolution of a microRNA cluster. J Mol Biol, 2004. **339**(2): 327–35.

144. Tay, Y.M., W.L. Tam, Y.S. Ang, P.M. Gaughwin, H. Yang, W. Wang, R. Liu, J. George, H.H. Ng, R.J. Perera, T. Lufkin, I. Rigoutsos, A.M. Thomson, and B. Lim, MicroRNA-134 modulates the differentiation of mouse embryonic stem cells, where it causes post-transcriptional attenuation of Nanog and LRH1. Stem Cells, 2008. **26**(1): 17–29.

145. Thomson, J.M., J. Parker, C.M. Perou, and S.M. Hammond, A custom microarray platform for analysis of microRNA gene expression. Nat Methods, 2004. **1**(1): 47–53.

146. Tsuchiya, Y., M. Nakajima, S. Takagi, T. Taniya, and T. Yokoi, MicroRNA regulates the expression of human cytochrome P450 1B1. Cancer Res, 2006. **66**(18): 9090–8.

147. Turner, H.L., T.C. Bailey, W.J. Krzanowski, and C.A. Hemingway, Biclustering models for structured microarray data. IEEE/ACM Trans Comput Biol Bioinform, 2005. **2**(4): 316–29.

148. van Rooij, E., L.B. Sutherland, N. Liu, A.H. Williams, J. McAnally, R.D. Gerard, J.A. Richardson, and E.N. Olson, A signature pattern of stress-responsive microRNAs that can evoke cardiac hypertrophy and heart failure. Proc Natl Acad Sci U S A, 2006. **103**(48): 18255–60.

149. Voorhoeve, P.M., C. le Sage, M. Schrier, A.J. Gillis, H. Stoop, R. Nagel, Y.P. Liu, J. van Duijse, J. Drost, A. Griekspoor, E. Zlotorynski, N. Yabuta, G. De Vita, H. Nojima, L.H. Looijenga, and R. Agami, A genetic screen implicates miRNA-372 and miRNA-373 as oncogenes in testicular germ cell tumors. Cell, 2006. **124**(6): 1169–81.

150. Wang, H., R.A. Ach, and B. Curry, Direct and sensitive miRNA profiling from low-input total RNA. RNA, 2007. **13**(1): 151–9.

151. Wang, Y., R. Medvid, C. Melton, R. Jaenisch, and R. Blelloch, DGCR8 is essential for microRNA biogenesis and silencing of embryonic stem cell self-renewal. Nat Genet, 2007. **39**(3): 380–5.

152. Westfall, P.H. and S.S. Young, Resampling-Based Multiple Testing. 1993, New York: Wiley.

153. Westfall, P.H., D.V. Zaykin, and S.S. Young, Multiple tests for genetic effects in association studies. Methods Mol Biol, 2002. **184**: 143–68.

154. Weston, M.D., M.L. Pierce, S. Rocha-Sanchez, K.W. Beisel, and G.A. Soukup, MicroRNA gene expression in the mouse inner ear. Brain Res, 2006. **1111**(1): 95–104.

155. Wettenhall, J.M. and G.K. Smyth, limmaGUI: a graphical user interface for linear modeling of microarray data. Bioinformatics, 2004. **20**(18): 3705–6.

156. Wienholds, E., M.J. Koudijs, F.J. van Eeden, E. Cuppen, and R.H. Plasterk, The microRNA-producing enzyme Dicer1 is essential for zebrafish development. Nat Genet, 2003. **35**(3): 217–8.

157. Wienholds, E., W.P. Kloosterman, E. Miska, E. Alvarez-Saavedra, E. Berezikov, E. de Bruijn, H.R. Horvitz, S. Kauppinen, and R.H. Plasterk, MicroRNA expression in zebrafish embryonic development. Science, 2005. **309**(5732): 310–1.

158. Wingender, E., P. Dietze, H. Karas, and R. Knuppel, TRANSFAC: a database on transcription factors and their DNA binding sites. Nucleic Acids Res, 1996. **24**(1): 238–41.

159. Wu, L. and J.G. Belasco, Micro-RNA regulation of the mammalian lin-28 gene during neuronal differentiation of embryonal carcinoma cells. Mol Cell Biol, 2005. **25**(21): 9198–208.

160. Wu, L., J. Fan, and J.G. Belasco, MicroRNAs direct rapid deadenylation of mRNA. Proc Natl Acad Sci U S A, 2006. **103**(11): 4034–9.

161. Xu, P., S.Y. Vernooy, M. Guo, and B.A. Hay, The Drosophila microRNA Mir-14 suppresses cell death and is required for normal fat metabolism. Curr Biol, 2003. **13**(9): 790–5.

162. Xu, P., M. Guo, and B.A. Hay, MicroRNAs and the regulation of cell death. Trends Genet, 2004. **20**(12): 617–24.

163. Yekta, S., I.H. Shih, and D.P. Bartel, MicroRNA-directed cleavage of HOXB8 mRNA. Science, 2004. **304**(5670): 594–6.

164. Yi, R., D. O'Carroll, H.A. Pasolli, Z. Zhang, F.S. Dietrich, A. Tarakhovsky, and E. Fuchs, Morphogenesis in skin is governed by discrete sets of differentially expressed microRNAs. Nat Genet, 2006. **38**(3): 356–62.

165. Ying, S.Y. and S.L. Lin, Intron-derived microRNAs–fine tuning of gene functions. Gene, 2004. **342**(1): 25–8.

166. Ying, S.Y. and S.L. Lin, Intronic microRNAs. Biochem Biophys Res Commun, 2005. **326**(3): 515–20.

167. Ying, S.Y. and S.L. Lin, Current perspectives in intronic micro RNAs (miRNAs). J Biomed Sci, 2006. **13**(1): 5–15.

168. Zeng, Y. and B.R. Cullen, Efficient processing of primary microRNA hairpins by Drosha requires flanking nonstructured RNA sequences. J Biol Chem, 2005. **280**(30): 27595–603.

169. Zeng, Y., R. Yi, and B.R. Cullen, Recognition and cleavage of primary microRNA precursors by the nuclear processing enzyme Drosha. Embo J, 2005. **24**(1): 138–48.

170. Zhang, L., J. Huang, N. Yang, J. Greshock, M.S. Megraw, A. Giannakakis, S. Liang, T.L. Naylor, A. Barchetti, M.R. Ward, G. Yao, A. Medina, A. O'Brien-Jenkins, D. Katsaros, A. Hatzigeorgiou, P.A. Gimotty, B.L. Weber, and G. Coukos, microRNAs exhibit high frequency genomic alterations in human cancer. Proc Natl Acad Sci U S A, 2006. **103**(24): 9136–41.

171. Zhao, J.J., Y.J. Hua, D.G. Sun, X.X. Meng, H.S. Xiao, and X. Ma, Genome-wide microRNA profiling in human fetal nervous tissues by oligonucleotide microarray. Childs Nerv Syst, 2006. **22**(11): 1419–25.

Chapter 9
Optimized Growth of Human Embryonic Stem Cells

Matthew A. Singer[1]*, Jacqui Johnson[2], Paul Bello[2], Robert Kovelman[1], and Michelle Greene[1]

Abstract Human embryonic stem (ES) cells were first derived and cultured approximately 10 years ago, using essentially the same conditions that were used at the time for mouse ES cells. These original culture conditions were clearly not optimal, and since that time, several forces have driven improvements in human ES cell culture. These include the use of human and autologous feeder layers, the use of a serum replacement product, and the identification of basic fibroblast growth factor (bFGF) as a key molecule for pluripotent cell growth *in vitro*. However, despite these advances, additional improvements still need to be made, particularly with an eye towards eventual therapeutic applications for ES cells. Here we describe an optimized system for human ES cell culture that provides serum-free and animal-component-free long-term expansion capability for human ES cells.

Keywords HEScGRO, human embryonic stem cell, serum-free, xeno-free

9.1 Introduction

Human embryonic stem (ES) cells conform to the general definition of the embryonic stem cell: they are derived from a pluripotent cell population (the interstitial cell mass, or ICM), they can replicate indefinitely in the embryonic state, they maintain a normal chromosomal complement (karyotype), and under appropriate conditions can differentiate into cells representative of all three germ layers in teratomas or in vitro [24]. The first isolation and culture of human ES cells had its origins in the successful culture of mouse embryonal carcinoma (EC) cells from teratocarcinomas

[1]Bioscience Division, Millipore Corporation, Temecula, CA, USA

[2]Stem Cell Sciences Pty Ltd., Melbourne, Australia

*Corresponding Author:
28820 Single Oak Drive, Temecula, CA 92590, USA
e-mail: Matt_Singer@millipore.com

Y. Shi, D.O. Clegg (eds.) *Stem Cell Research and Therapeutics*,
© Springer Science+Business Media B.V. 2008

[10]. The culture of mouse EC cells paved the way for the isolation and culture of mouse ES cells [7, 18], and the culture conditions used to achieve these milestones were almost identical to those used to subsequently isolate and culture human ES cells (reviewed in [41]).

The first isolation of undifferentiated cells from the ICM of the human blastocyst was achieved by Bongso and colleagues, although these isolated cells could not be maintained in culture for more than three passages without undergoing death or differentiation [6]. Drawing upon experience from earlier work which produced ES cell lines from two different species of primate [31, 32], Thomson and colleagues were the first to then isolate and maintain human ES cells in culture [33]; this was followed by Bongso and colleagues [27], who had likely failed earlier due to their culture conditions. Since this time, the derivation of literally hundreds of human ES cell lines in at least 20 countries has been reported [8].

9.2   Early Culture Conditions for Human ES Cells

As described above, the first derivations and culture of human ES cells were done using essentially the same conditions as had been used for mouse ES cells. Thus the first human ES cell culture medium was composed of a high-glucose (4,500 mg/l) Dulbecco's Modified Eagle's Medium (DMEM) that contained 20% fetal bovine serum (FBS) with non-essential amino acids, glutamine and 2-mercaptoethanol [27, 33]. ICM and subsequent human ES cells were plated on feeder layers of mitotically-inactivated mouse embryonic fibroblasts (MEFs), which in turn had been plated on gelatin-coated tissue culture plastic. Leukemia inhibitory factor (LIF), known to be critical for the maintenance of pluripotency of mouse ES cells in culture, was also included, although it was shown in these first human ES cell derivations that it was not required [27].

Passaging of the human ES cells in these early works was primarily accomplished by mechanical dissociation, although exposure to either the enzyme dispase or to calcium- and magnesium-free phosphate-buffered saline was sometimes used. This was a departure from the trypsin solutions commonly used for passaging mouse ES cells, and allowed the human ES cells to be passaged in cell clumps containing multiple (10–100 or more) cells; in general, human ES cells (unlike mouse ES cells) cannot be dispersed to single cells without undergoing cell death or differentiation.

9.3   Forces Driving Human ES Cell Culture Optimization

Even with these first successful derivations of human ES cells, it was recognized that numerous improvements needed to be made to make these cells readily amenable for basic research, industrial-scale applications and therapeutic use. At the most basic level, culture conditions had to keep human ES cells pluripotent indefinitely in culture, able to differentiate into all three germ layers, and able to maintain a stable karyotype. The ideal situation would be to provide a controlled environment where all components were known and whose performance would be consistent over time. Early culture conditions could not provide this due to the presence of both the FBS, for which the composition was undefined and the performance would often vary greatly with different lots, and the MEF feeder layers, which were providing unknown necessary factors to the ES cells through signaling pathways as well as through contribution to the extracellular matrix. Thus there has been a constant need in human ES cell culture to create a defined medium where all components are known and which demonstrate consistent performance.

For industrial-type applications, such as high-throughput screening, cell-based assays and toxicity tests, cell populations have to be greatly expanded to provide the necessary source material. This has proven to be a major obstacle for the use of human ES cells in these types of processes. First, human ES cells grow slowly relative to other cell types (with an average doubling time of 36 hours), and thus more time and expense must be invested in their expansion. Second, they must be passaged in clumps rather than as single cells; this not only reduces their ability to be rapidly expanded, but can also introduce cell number variability into an assay. Thus for industrial applications (as well as for eventual needs for clinical applications) there is a need to improve human ES cell culture to allow rapid expansion of cell populations, preferably from single ES cells.

For therapeutic applications, the goal to introduce derivatives of human ES cells into the human body places stringent restrictions upon the culture conditions of the ES cells themselves. This goal encourages that all components of the human ES cell culture system be defined, but requires that the system contain no components derived from non-humans (a "xeno-free" system), in order to prevent infection by nonhuman pathogens upon transplantation. Xeno-free systems can be created with either carefully qualified components derived from humans or from synthetic or recombinant components. Xeno-free culture systems would also eliminate nonhuman antigens that can illicit an immune response upon transplantation, one example being the uptake by human ES cells of the nonhuman sialic acid Neu5Gc from MEFs and from common formulations of human ES cell culture media [19]. Finally, the need for xeno-free systems extends to human ES cell derivation as well, as an ideal human ES cell line from which to derive cells for therapeutic applications would never be exposed to non-human components.

9.4 Advances in Human ES Cell Culture

The goals described above have driven numerous improvements in human ES cell culture since their first successful derivation 10 years ago. For example, while MEFs remain in common use as feeders, the desire to remove nonhuman components from human ES cell culture has led to several alternatives. One of these is the use of feeders derived from human tissue, whether fibroblasts from the fetal or adult skin [2, 9, 28], or other cell types [13]. Another alternative is feeder cells that have been differentiated from human ES cells in culture [30, 40]; these ES-derived feeder cells can be propagated as independent cell lines using the same culture methods as for MEFs or human fibroblasts. Finally, methods for the feeder-free culture of human ES cells have been developed, and these will be further described below.

The substrates upon which human ES cells are cultured have also undergone improvement. Gelatin (derived from animal sources) is still commonly used despite its lack of definition and the fact that it generally cannot be used in a xeno-free system. Another popular substrate is the solubilized basement membrane preparation extracted from the Engelbreth-Holm-Swarm mouse sarcoma [11]. This preparation is rich in extracellular matix (ECM) components, and supports human ES cell culture in both feeder and feeder-free applications. However, this substrate also is not defined, and often exhibits variation in its performance among different lot preparations; in addition, this preparation is not xeno-free. Recently however, progress has been made in producing substrates that are both defined and xeno-free, as several groups have reported the culture of human ES cells with human or recombinant ECM proteins such as laminin and fibronectin [3, 15, 17].

The biggest focus for the optimization of human ES cell culture, however, has been in the area of culture media. An early advancement was the substitution of FBS with a serum-replacer that had originally been formulated for serum-free culture of mouse ES cells [25]. This formulation contains bovine serum albumin rather than whole serum, and proved suitable for serum-free culture of human ES cells as well [1]. In addition, it was shown as early as 2001 that human ES cells could be cultured in media containing this serum replacer without a requirement for MEF feeder layers [37], as long as the culture medium was preconditioned by these same MEFs prior to use. This feeder-free culture allowed human ES cells to be grown as pluripotent stem cells without any other cell type present in the culture dish. This serum-replacer is still in common use for human ES cell culture today; however, this complex formulation still suffers from the drawbacks of being undefined (particularly after conditioning by MEFs, whose contributions to human ES cell pluripotency *in vitro* are still not well understood), and from having non-human components.

Advancements in culture media have also been made in the area of growth factors, cytokines and mitogens that keep human ES cells pluripotent *in vitro* (it is important to note the distinction between factors that are discovered to maintain human ES cell pluripotency *in vitro* and the factors that actually function *in vivo* during embryonic development). Basic fibroblast growth factor (bFGF, also known as FGF2) was found early on to be an essential part of serum-free culture [1]; without its presence in medium containing serum replacer, human ES cells underwent rapid differentiation. Since this time, bFGF has become a critical component of human ES cell culture media. More recently it has been shown that high levels of bFGF can substitute for the conditioning of serum-replacer-based media by MEFs for feeder-free human ES cell culture [14, 38, 39]. However, both the high levels of bFGF used in these studies (either 40, 80 or 100 ng/ml), as well as the fact that bFGF is known to have positive effects upon ectodermal and mesodermal marker expression [29], strongly suggest that additional growth factors and/or cytokines are required for optimal human ES cell culture conditions, particularly in the absence of feeders.

A number of recent publications have begun to identify possible factors for improved pluripotency of human ES cells in feeder-free culture. Activin A, a member of the TGF-b family of signaling molecules, has been shown in several studies to function with or without bFGF to keep human ES cells pluripotent [4, 34, 36]; in the work of Beattie et al., where bFGF was not used, keratinocyte growth factor (KGF) was added. While activin A was presumed in these studies to be inhibiting neuroectoderm differentiation, at least one group has shown that activin A is not critical for human ES cell culture; however, it was unresolved how dependent this result might be upon other components in the medium formulation [16]. Other growth factors that have been reported to allow the successful feeder-free culture of human ES cells (with or without bFGF) are TGFb1 [3, 17], noggin [39], sphingosine-1-phosphate in combination with platelet-derived growth factor [23], flt3 ligand [15, 38], and IFG-II [5], although again, these results may be dependent upon the entire media formulation (e.g., whether serum-replacer is used).

The factors mentioned in the previous paragraph are thought to benefit human ES cell culture by promoting pathways of self-renewal or inhibiting pathways of differentiation. However, other studies have suggested that the addition of antiapoptotic factors to the cell culture environment may also improve human ES cell culture. In particular, blocking apoptosis aids the expansion of human ES cells not only through increased cell numbers in standard culture, but also through increasing the robustness of single cell cloning. For example, addition to the culture media of ligands for the tropomyosin-related kinase (TRK) family of receptors was reported to increase human ES cell cloning efficiency to approximately 30% from a basal level of 6% [26]. Similarly, an inhibitor of the Rho-associated kinase (ROCK) increased cloning efficiency to approximately 27% from about 1% [35]. These results are encouraging for the adaptation of human ES cells to high-throughput applications.

9.5   Xeno-Free, Serum-Free Culture of Human ES Cells

Despite these advances in human ES cell culture, one area that has lacked significant advancement is therapeutic-grade reagents. It is now possible, with the humanization of feeder layers as well as the components of the culture media, to have a culture system without any non-human components. It should be noted that several reports have been made of derivation and/or culture of human ES cells under conditions that can be called xeno-free [15, 17]; however, the media used in these studies generally contained high levels of bFGF (40 ng/ml or higher). This was no doubt because the culture was being done in feeder-free conditions, but this level of stringency may not be necessary, and in fact could be detrimental to the ES cells; each of the two human ES cell lines that were originally derived in feeder-free conditions with the high bFGF levels of Ludwig et al. had an abnormal karyotype [17].

Recently, a novel medium for xeno-free, serum-free culture of human ES cells has been developed. This medium, called HEScGRO™, is a proprietary formulation that contains only humanized or synthetic components, including bFGF that is manufactured under animal-free conditions; in addition, HEScGRO contains human serum albumin rather than its bovine counterpart. HEScGRO was designed for use with human fibroblast feeders and has been validated with two different commercially-available lines, Detroit 551 [12] and WS1; the use of human feeders maintains the xeno-free nature of the culture system and allows the use of low levels of bFGF (20 ng/ml).

HEScGRO has been tested with multiple human ES cell lines, including the H1 (WA01) and H9 (WA09) lines, and the MEL-1, MEL-2 and MEL-4 lines derived at the Australian Stem Cell Centre. These cells grow well in HEScGRO, as judged by the following criteria. First, colony morphology is normal (see Fig. 9.1); colonies have the typical "random" (i.e., non-circular) morphology when human ES cells are grown on human feeders, and the colonies have sharp boundaries without signs of differentiated cells at the edges (Fig. 9.1A). The appearance of individual cells within the colony is also normal; cells are tightly packed, with each cell having a high nuclear-to-cytoplasmic ratio and prominent nucleoli (Fig. 9.1B).

Human ES cells cultured in HEScGRO retain their pluripotency, even after multiple passages in the medium. This is demonstrated not only by expression of pluripotent markers (Figs. 9.2 and 9.3), but also through subsequent differentiation to representatives of all three germ layers (Fig. 9.4). Thus, H1 (Fig. 9.2A, C), H9 (Fig. 9.2E, G) and MEL-4 (Fig. 9.3A, C) cells all continue to express the pluripotent markers OCT4 and TRA-1-60 after more than 15 passages in HEScGRO; the vast majority of cells in a colony express these markers, as can be seen by comparison to the corresponding images of DAPI staining (H1: Fig. 9.2B, D; H9: Fig. 9.2F, H; MEL-4: Fig. 9.3B, D). These cells also retain tissue-specific alkaline phosphatase activity (not shown), another indicator of ES cell pluripotency. Expression

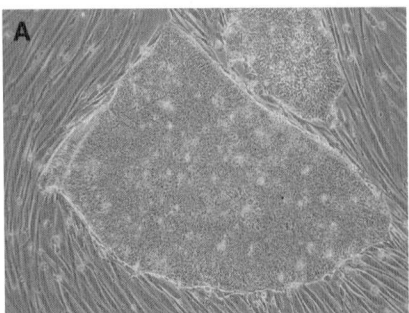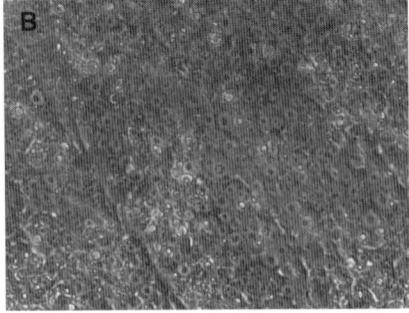

Fig. 9.1 Human ES cells grown in HEScGRO xeno-free, serum-free medium have appearance and morphology typical of human ES cells grown on human feeders. (**A**) H9 (WA09) cells, with well-defined borders and homogenous appearance within the colony. (**B**) MEL-4 cells (shown at higher magnification) display high nuclear-to-cytoplasmic ratio and visible nucleoli (*See Color Plates*)

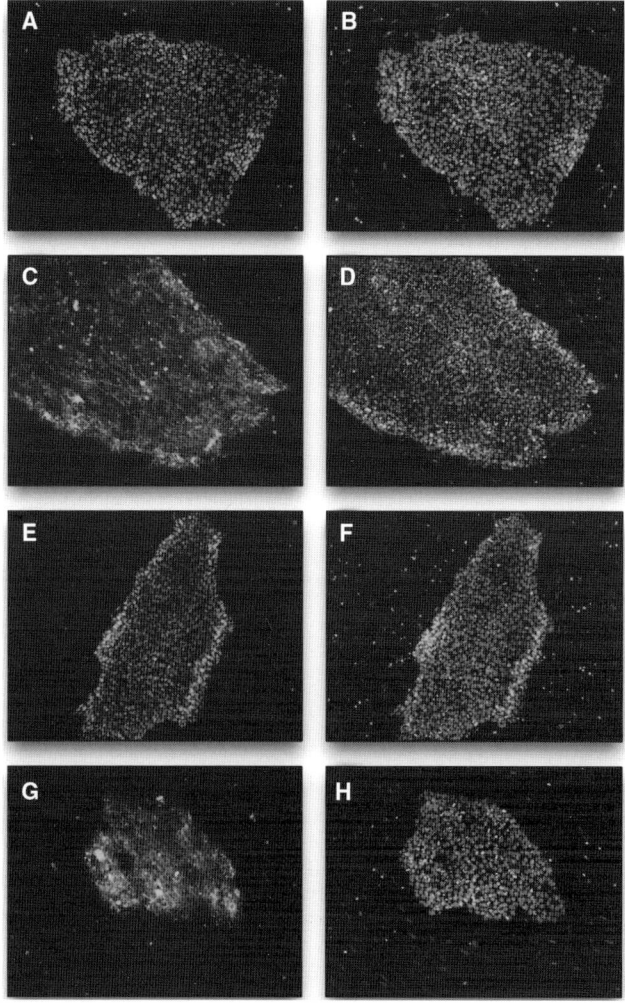

Fig. 9.2 H1 (WA01) and H9 (WA09) cells grown for multiple passages in HEScGRO continue to display markers of pluripotency. (**A–D**) H1 cells after 17 passages in HEScGRO show expression of OCT4 (**A**) and TRA-1-60 (**C**). Cells throughout each colony express these markers, as shown by comparison to the corresponding DAPI staining in **B**, **D**. (**E–H**) H9 cells after 17 passages showing expression of OCT4 (**E**) and TRA-1-60 (**G**), with corresponding DAPI images in **F**, **H** (*See Color Plates*)

of SSEA-1, which in human ES cultures is expressed by differentiated cells, is low or absent (Fig. 9.3E, F). Finally, in each of these experiments, these cells maintained a normal karyotype (not shown).

For differentiation studies, cells grown in HEScGRO were allowed to spontaneously differentiate via embryoid body (EB) formation. Briefly, cells growing in HEScGRO were detached from the cell surface and re-aggregated to form EBs in

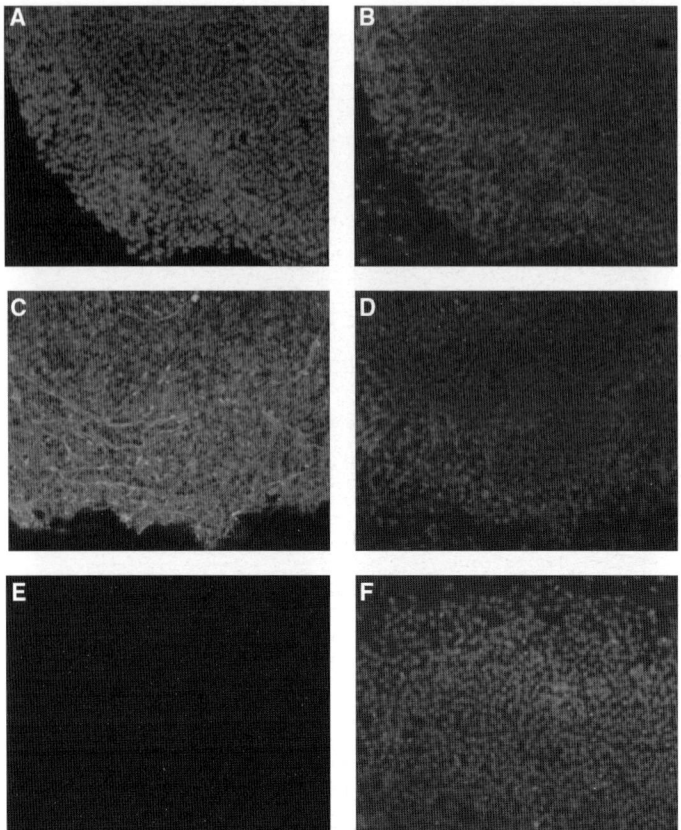

Fig. 9.3 MEL-4 human ES cells grown for 20 passages in HEScGRO have high expression of pluripotency markers and low expression of a differentiation marker. Expression of OCT4 (**A**) and TRA-1-60 (**C**) in passage 20 MEL-4 cells is high, while expression of SSEA-1 (**E**) is low. Corresponding DAPI images are shown in **B**, **D**, and **F** (*See Color Plates*)

suspension [20]. These EBs were subsequently grown in suspension culture in HEScGRO without bFGF as a differentiation medium, and allowed to grow for up to 13 days; each day, samples were removed for analysis by RT-PCR for markers of differentiated lineages. As shown for the MEL-4 line (Fig. 9.4), EBs formed from human ES cells grown in HEScGRO can differentiate cells expressing the following markers for all three embryonic germ layers: alpha-fetoprotein (AFP) and foxA2 (endoderm), nestin and pax6 (ectoderm), and brachyury and flk-1 (mesoderm).

There are some specific attributes to culturing human ES cells in HEScGRO. Colonies of ES cells tend to be flatter in HEScGRO than in serum- or serum-replacer-containing media (although as mentioned, both colony shape and the appearance of individual cells within the colony appear normal).

There are also some specific parameters to which to adhere when using HEScGRO medium. The human feeders (Detroit 551 or WS1, as mentioned above) should be

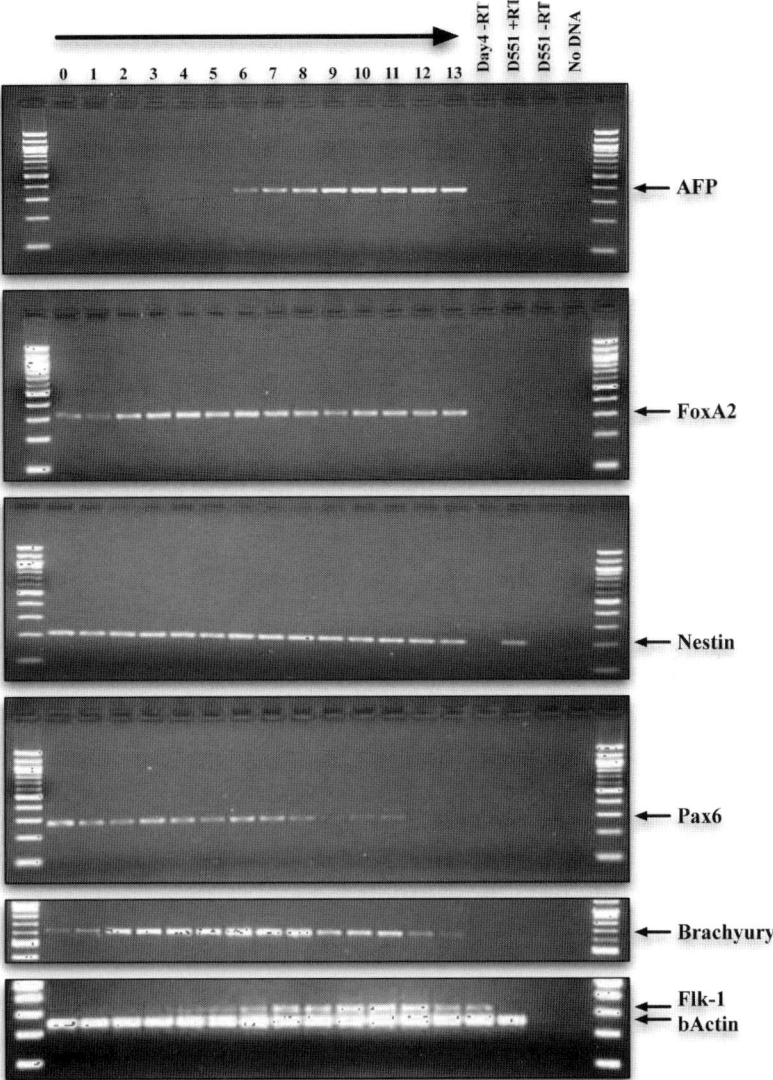

Fig. 9.4 Human ES cells grown in HEScGRO can differentiate to all three germ layers. MEL-4 cells grown in HEScGRO were differentiated via embryoid body (EB) formation in HEScGRO lacking bFGF. Samples were taken every day for 13 days and processed for RT-PCR of the following markers of differentiation: alpha fetoprotein (AFP) and FoxA2 (endoderm), nestin and pax6 (ectoderm), brachyury and flk-1 (mesoderm). Expected products are indicated by the arrows

plated at a density of 60,000 cells per square centimeter at least 1 day prior to plating the ES cells. Once the human ES cells are plated, the media should be changed every day, although every 2 days may be found to be acceptable. For passaging, we have found that manually dissecting colonies grown in HEScGRO culture is best, since this is the gentlest way to handle the cells. As HEScGRO is a serum-free medium, one must be careful when attempting to passage HEScGRO cultures ezymatically. Trypsin should never be used. Of note is that the collagenase type IV commonly used for passaging cells in medium containing serum-replacer will cause cells in HEScGRO to readily differentiate, so its use is also discouraged.

We have found that HEScGRO cultures can be successfully passaged with the collagenase preparation Accumax™, according to the following protocol: first, the medium is removed from the culture vessel and 1 ml of Accumax added for every 10 cm² of culture surface. The vessel is then placed in a 37°C incubator for exactly 5 minutes; the cells should not incubate in Accumax longer than this time. After the vessel is removed from the incubator, the cells are washed off the culture surface using a volume of HEScGRO (or HEScGRO Basal Medium™, which does not contain bFGF) that is equal to the volume of Accumax that was used; the cells are then removed to a conical tube. The flask is next washed with a fresh aliquot of the same amount of HEScGRO (or HEScGRO Basal medium), and this is added to the conical tube that has the cells. The cells are spun at 1,000 RPM (75 G) for 5 minutes, the supernatant removed, and the pelleted cells are resuspended in 5 ml HEScGRO (or HEScGRO Basal medium). The volume that will be plated (e.g., 1 ml from the tube would represent a 1:5 split) is transferred to a fresh conical tube, and an equal volume of HEScGRO (or HEScGRO Basal medium) is added. The cells are spun at 1,000 RPM for 5 minutes, the supernatant aspirated, and the pellet resuspended in the desired final volume of HEScGRO (HEScGRO Basal medium should not be used at this step). The suspension is transferred to a new culture vessel (with pre-plated Detroit 551 or WS1 fibroblasts), and placed in the incubator.

9.6   Future Directions for Human ES Cell Culture Optimization

While a number of potential improvements in human ES cell culture have been discussed, it is clear that much more needs to be done before human ES cells are either readily available for industrial applications or suitable for the derivation of therapeutically relevant cells. The most significant improvement in human ES cell culture since their original isolation has likely been the discovery of the ability of bFGF to maintain pluripotent human ES cells in culture. However, the fact that bFGF is required at very high levels to maintain human ES cells in the absence of feeders indicates that other critical factors for human ES cell pluripotency remain to be identified. Other improvements in human ES cell culture have been made toward the goals of industrial applications and therapeutics, including the ability to expand the cells as well as to grow them in xeno-free conditions, but continued work in these areas is critical to achieve the promise that human ES cells offer.

References

1. Amit M, Carpenter MK, Inokuma MS et al. (2000) Clonally derived human embryonic stem cell lines maintain pluripotency and proliferative potential for prolonged periods of culture. Dev Biol 227:271–278
2. Amit M, Margulets V, Segev H et al. (2003) Human feeder layers for human embryonic stem cells. Biol Reprod 68:2150–2156
3. Amit M, Sahriki C, Margulets V et al. (2004) Feeder-layer- and serum-free culture of human embryonic stem cells. Biol Reprod 70:837–845
4. Beattie GM, Lopez AD, Bucay N et al. (2005) Activin A maintains pluripotency of human embryonic stem cells in the absence of feeder layers. Stem Cells 23:489–495
5. Bendall SC, Stewart MH, Menendez P et al. (2007) IGF and FGF cooperatively establish the regulatory stem cell niche of pluripotent human cells in vitro. Nature 448:1015–1021
6. Bongso A, Fong CY, Ng SC et al. (1994) Isolation and culture of inner cell mass cells from human blastocysts. Hum Reprod 9:2110–2117
7. Evans MJ, Kaufman MH (1981) Establishment in culture of pluripotential cells from mouse embryos. Nature 292:154–156
8. Guhr A, Kurtz A, Friedgen K et al. (2006) Current state of human embryonic stem cell research: an overview of cell lines and their use in experimental work. Stem Cells 24:2187–2191
9. Hovatta O, Mikkola M, Gertow K et al. (2003) A culture system using human foreskin fibroblasts as feeder cells allows production of human embryonic stem cells. Hum Reprod 18: 1404–1409
10. Kahan BW, Ephrussi B (1970) Developmental potentialities of clonal in vitro cultures of mouse testicular teratoma. J Natl Cancer Inst 44:1015–1036
11. Kleinman HK, McGarvey ML, Liotta LA et al. (1982) Isolation and characterization of type IV procollagen, laminin, and heparan sulfate proteoglycan from the EHS sarcoma. Biochemistry 21:6188–6193
12. Kueh J, Richards M, Ng SW et al. (2006) The search for factors in human feeders that support the derivation and propagation of human embryonic stem cells: preliminary studies using transcriptome profiling by serial analysis of gene expression. Fertil Steril 85:1843–1846
13. Lee JB, Song JM, Lee JE (2004) Available human feeder cells for the maintenance of human embryonic stem cells. Reproduction 128:727–735
14. Levenstein ME, Ludwig TE, Xu RH et al. (2006) Basic fibroblast growth factor support of human embryonic stem cell self-renewal. Stem Cells 24:568–574
15. Li Y, Powell S, Brunette E et al. (2005) Expansion of human embryonic stem cells in defined serum-free medium devoid of animal derived products. Biotechnol Bioeng 91:688–698
16. Liu Y, Song Z, Zhao Y et al. (2006) A novel chemical-defined medium with bFGF and N2B27 supplements supports undifferentiated growth in human embryonic stem cells. Biochem Biophys Res Comm 346:131–139
17. Ludwig TE, Levenstein ME, Jones JM et al. (2006) Derivation of human embryonic stem cells in defined conditions. Nat Biotech 24:185–187
18. Martin GR (1981) Isolation of a pluripotent cell line from early mouse embryos cultured in medium conditioned by teratocarcinoma stem cells. Proc Natl Acad Sci USA 98:7634–7638
19. Martin MJ, Muotri A, Gage F et al. (2005) Human embryonic stem cells express an immunogenic nonhuman sialic acid. Nat Med 11:228–232
20. Ng ES, Davis RP, Azzola L et al. (2005) Forced aggregation of defined numbers of human embryonic stem cells into embryoid bodies fosters robust, reproducible hematopoietic differentiation. Blood 106:1601–1603
23. Pebay A, Raymond CB, Wong SM et al. (2005) Essential roles of sphingosine-1-phosphate and platelet-derived growth factor in the maintenance of human embryonic stem cells. Stem Cells 23:1541–1548
24. Pera MF, Reubinoff B, Trounson A (2000) Human embryonic stem cells. J Cell Sci 113:5–10

25. Price PJ, Goldsborough MD, Tilkins ML (1998) Embryonic stem cell serum replacement. International Patent W098/30679

26. Pyle AD, Lock LF, Donovan PJ (2006) Neurotrophins mediate human embryonic stem cell survival. Nat Biotech 24:344–350

27. Reubinoff BE, Pera MF, Fong CY et al. (2000) Embryonic stem cell lines from human blastocysts: somatic differentiation in vitro. Nature Biotech 18:399–404

28. Richards M, Fong CY, Chan WK et al. (2002) Human feeders support prolonged undifferentiated growth of human inner cell masses and embryonic stem cells. Nat Biotech 20:933–936

29. Schuldiner M, Yanuka O, Itskovitz-Eldor J et al. (2000) Effects of eight growth factors on the differentiation of cells derived from human embryonic stem cells. Proc Natl Acad Sci USA 97:11307–11312

30. Stojkovic P, Lako M, Stewart R et al. (2005) An autogeneic feeder cell system that efficiently supports growth of undifferentiated human embryonic stem cells. Stem Cells 23:306–314

31. Thomson JA, Kalishman J, Golos TG et al. (1995) Isolation of a primate embryonic stem cell line. Proc Natl Acad Sci USA 92:7844–7848

32. Thomson JA, Kalishman J, Golos TG et al. (1996) Pluripotent cell lines derived from common marmoset (*Callithrix jacchus*) blastocysts. Biol Reprod 55:254–259

33. Thomson JA, Itskovitz-Eldor J, Shapiro SS et al. (1998) Embryonic stem cell lines derived from human blastocysts. Science 282:1145–1147

34. Vallier L, Alexander M, Pedersen RA (2005) Activin/nodal and FGF pathways cooperate to maintain pluripotency of human embryonic stem cells. J Cell Sci 118:4495–4509

35. Watanabe K, Ueno M, Kamiya D et al. (2007) A ROCK inhibitor permits survival of dissociated human embryonic stem cells. Nat Biotech 25:681–686

36. Xiao L, Yuan X, Sharkis SJ (2006) Activin A maintains self-renewal and regulates FGF, Wnt and BMP pathways in human embryonic stem cells. Stem Cells 24:1476–1486

37. Xu C, Inokuma MS, Denham J et al. (2001) Feeder-free growth of undifferentiated human embryonic stem cells. Nat Biotech 19:971–974

38. Xu C, Rosler E, Jiang J et al. (2005) Basic fibroblast growth factor supports undifferentiated human embryonic stem cell growth without conditioned medium. Stem Cells 23:315–323

39. Xu RH, Peck RM, Li DS (2005) Basic FGF and suppression of BMP signaling sustain undifferentiated proliferation of human ES cells. Nat Meth 2:185–190

40. Yoo SJ, Yoon BS, Kim JM et al. (2005) Efficient culture system for human embryonic stem cells using autologous human embryonic stem cell-derived feeder cells. Exp Mol Med 37:399–407

41. Zwaka TP, Thomson JA (2005) A germ cell origin of embryonic stem cells? Development 132:227–233

Chapter 10
Potential of Stem Cells in Liver Regeneration

Madhava Pai, Nataša Levičar, and Nagy Habib*

Abstract Organ transplantation currently remains the definitive cure for several liver and pancreatic disorders. However, due to a major shortage of available organs many are turning to alternative sources for whole organ or cell-based transplantation. Stem cells have been proposed as an alternative to organ transplantation. The ethical and legal issues associated with embryonic stem cells have shifted the focus to adult stem cells and their regenerative potential has been under intense investigation. In this chapter we are reviewing the latest advances in stem cell therapy in liver diseases from bench to bedside.

Keywords Liver disease, stem cells, transplantation, regenerative medicine, immunosuppression

10.1   Introduction

Liver constitutes about 1.5% of our body mass and simultaneously performs a variety of different functions, such as the regulation of energy homeostasis, synthesis of plasma proteins, biotransformation and excretion of endogenous metabolic products and the production and secretion of bile [1]. It has the remarkable capacity to regenerate in response to injury. However, in severe cases of liver injury, its regenerative capacity may prove insufficient and the liver injury may progress to end stage liver disease (ESLD) and subsequent liver failure. Over 4,000 people died from cirrhosis in the last year of the 20th century, two thirds of them before their 65th birthday [2]. Cirrhosis of the liver is an important cause of illness and death. In 2000 it killed more men than Parkinson's disease and more women than cancer of the cervix [2]. Large rises in death rates from chronic liver disease and cirrhosis have occurred in most age groups. The rise in deaths from cirrhosis among younger

Department of Surgery, Hammersmith Campus, Imperial College London, UK

*Corresponding Author:
e-mail: nagy.habib@imperial.ac.uk

Y. Shi, D.O. Clegg (eds.) *Stem Cell Research and Therapeutics*,
© Springer Science+Business Media B.V. 2008

people is of particular concern where binge-drinking patterns appear to be common. In 2000 cirrhosis accounted for nearly 500 deaths in men aged 25–44 years and nearly 300 deaths in women of this age group [2].

Presently, orthotopic liver transplantation is the major therapeutic option for patients with acute and chronic ESLD. Because of the shortage of donated organs, up to 10–15% of these patients die while on the waiting list awaiting an organ [3]. Liver transplantation also has disadvantages such as the need for life-long immunosupression and follow-up, highlighting the need for research into alternative methods of treatment. Hepatocyte transplantation may be an alternative for liver transplantation, especially for hepatic disorders caused by inherited protein deficiency [4]. However, widespread application of hepatocyte transplantation is limited by organ availability, viability of isolated hepatocytes after cryopreservation and potential formation of hepatocyte aggregates during injection that can obstruct the liver sinusoids resulting in portal hypertension or lead to fatal emboli.

Recent advances in the understanding of stem cell biology and plasticity have raised expectations for using stem cells as new cellular therapeutics in regenerative medicine. Although stem cell therapy is not considered classically within the realm of clinical medicine, this technology will become increasingly important for clinicians in the future. Much of the excitement in stem cell research centers on embryonic stem (ES) cells because of their high plasticity, but this approach remains controversial for ethical reasons. Another major limiting factor for their usefulness in clinical therapy lies in their tumorigenicity when introduced *in vivo*. The injected ES cells formed teratomas when injected subcutaneously in NOD/SCID mice [5]. However, adult stem cells from bone marrow (BM) are well characterised and have long been used therapeutically [6].

The BM compartment is largely made up of haematopoietic stem cells (HSC) and committed progenitor cells, non-circulating stromal cells (called mesenchymal stem cells (MSC)) that have the ability to develop into mesenchymal lineages [7, 8]. HSC are adult stem cells and can be identified by their ability to differentiate into all blood cell types and reconstitute the haematopoietic system in a host that has been lethally myelo-ablated [9]. It was previously thought that adult stem cells were lineage restricted, but recent studies demonstrated that BM-derived progenitors in addition to haematopoiesis also participate in regeneration of ischemic myocardium [10], damaged skeletal muscle [11] and neurogenesis [12]. This chapter will focus on the potential of HSC in the management of liver disease. The discussion will concentrate on experimental models in animal and human tissues along with current status of clinical trials.

10.2 Indications for Stem Cell Therapy in Liver Disease

There are three broad groups of liver disease we can identify for the purpose of cell therapeutic options. First, fulminant hepatic failure is characterised by rapid failure of the liver and death of the patient if whole liver replacement does not occur urgently. Cell therapeutic trials for fulminant hepatic failure in the form of liver cell transplants have shown moderate success [13]. Bioartificial livers that could also theoretically employ stem cells (as opposed to the currently used hepatoma cell lines or porcine hepatocytes) are undergoing clinical trials to treat these patients as an alternative to cell transplantation while awaiting organ transplantation [14].

Second, chronic liver disease is characterised by simultaneous liver regeneration and development of fibrosis that results in end-stage cirrhosis if unchecked. Cirrhosis could be an inhibitor of cell engraftment through altered cytokine milieu for any form of cell therapy, whether using hepatocytes for transplantation or stem cells.

Third, metabolic liver diseases are characterised by an inherited defect of one hepatic enzyme resulting in the build up of toxic metabolites that are harmful to the individual but the rest of the function of the liver is normal. In some diseases, the pathology occurs extrahepatically and total replacement of the liver is not required. Metabolic liver diseases are ideal targets for development of cell therapeutic programs since only a small number of functional donor cells would effect disease correction through single enzyme replacement [15].

The liver in an adult healthy body maintains a balance between cell gain and cell loss. Though normally proliferatively quiescent, hepatocyte loss such as that caused by partial hepatectomy, uncomplicated by virus infection or inflammation, invokes a rapid regenerative response to restore liver mass. This restoration of moderate cell loss and 'wear and tear' renewal is largely achieved by hepatocyte self-replication. More severe liver injury can activate a potential stem cell compartment located within the intrahepatic biliary tree, giving rise to cords of bipotential, so-called, oval cells within the lobules that can differentiate into hepatocytes and biliary epithelial cells [16].

10.3 Role of BMSCs in Liver Repair

One of the first demonstrations of using bone marrow to reconstitute liver was reported by Petersen et al. [17]. Lethally irradiated female rats were rescued using bone marrow transplants from syngeneic males following induced hepatic injury and treatment with 2-aminoacetylfluorine to prevent hepatic proliferation. Markers for the Y-chromosome, dipeptidyl peptidase IV enzyme (DPPIV), and L21–6 antigen were used to identify liver cells of bone marrow origin. This cross-sex model allowed identification of male liver cells in the female rats' livers which indicated that bone marrow-derived HSC have the capacity to transdifferentiate into hepatocytes [17]. In similar sex-mismatched experiments in mice, Theise et al. [18] demonstrated the presence of Y-chromosome positive hepatocytes in lethally irradiated female mice following bone marrow transplants from males. In this case no liver injury was induced supporting the theory that marrow-derived HSC can differentiate into hepatocytes in the absence of acute liver injury [18].

Although evidence of transdifferentiation to hepatocytes is compelling from animal studies, few have examined this possibility in humans. Alison et al. [19] detected Y-chromosome positive cells in retrospective analysis of the livers of female recipients (n = 9) of bone marrow transplants from male donors. These cells were confirmed as being hepatocytes as they also expressed cytokeratin-8 [19]. The authors also looked for the presence of Y-chromosome-positive cells in female livers transplanted to male recipients (n = 11) that were later removed due to recurrent disease. They found some (0.5–2%) Y-chromosome-positive cells that expressed cytokeratin-8. This confirmed that circulating extra-hepatic stem cells may colonize the liver [19]. Theise et al. [20] reported their analysis of archival autopsy and biopsy specimens from female recipients of male donor bone marrow transplants and male recipients of female livers. The BM-derived cell engraftment in the liver ranged between 4% and 40%. The study showed that hepatocytes and cholangiocytes can be obtained from extrahepatic circulating stem cells, probably of marrow origin in humans [20]. Korbling et al. [21] reported that the frequency of hepatocytes generated from the bone marrow of recipients of sex-mismatched liver or bone marrow transplants varied from 4% to 7% and was unrelated to liver injury and to the time after transplantation.

10.4   Mechanism of Hepatocyte Regeneration

There is controversy about the mechanism by which BMSCs contribute to hepatocyte regeneration or to liver repair. Transdifferentiation into hepatocytes represents genomic plasticity in response to the microenvironment and has been shown in several experiments *in vivo* [22–24]. However, some authors have proposed that conversion to hepatocytes may occur via cell fusion [25, 26]. The bystander effect is postulated to be due to the factors secreted by BMSCs that are chemo-attracted to the site of injury, leading to the stimulation of mitosis of endogenous liver cells. This mechanism is thought to recruit endogenous BM for cardiac repair following myocardial infarction [27] following administration of granulocyte colony-stimulating factor (G-CSF).

Other possible explanations for target organ regeneration and improvement in function include facilitating the release of vascular endothelial growth factor (VEGF) by stem cells, thereby increasing the blood supply to the cells and thus helping to repair the damaged tissue [28]. Stem cells may act by up-regulating the Bcl-2 gene and suppressing apoptosis [29] and also by suppressing inflammation in the diseased organ via the interleukin-6 (IL-6) pathway [30]. Both these processes may help in the regeneration of normal cells in the damaged organ. Finally HSCs may stimulate the tissue specific stem cells, e.g., oval cells in liver, and facilitate regeneration of the target organ [16].

10.5 Animal Data Supporting BMSC Treatment of Liver Disease

Studies in animal models of liver diseases have demonstrated that BM cell transplantation decreases hepatic fibrosis and improves survival rate. Whether engraftment and organ restitution continues in the long term is unclear. Oyagi et al. transplanted MSCs (induced to adopt hepatocyte phenotype *in vitro*) intravenously into non-irradiated carbon tetrachloride (CCl_4) - damaged recipients and observed a rise in serum albumin and a histological decrease in hepatic fibrosis [31]. Similar results have been observed by Sakaida et al. [32] in mice with liver fibrosis induced by CCl_4 after infusion of BM sub-fraction.

Jang et al. transplanted 1×10^5 highly enriched HSC (CD45[+]) into lethally irradiated mice treated with a single dose of CCl_4 [24]. In this model 7.6% of liver cells were of donor origin within 7 days of transplantation. There was early amelioration of liver disease with some improvement in levels of alanine aminotransferase, prothrombin times and fibrinogen levels in transplanted mice compared to non-operative controls. Terai et al. [23] found that persistent injury induces efficient trans-differentiation of BM cells into functional hepatocytes. Mice with liver cirrhosis induced by CCl_4 were injected with 1×10^5 non-treated GFP-transfected BM cells via the tail vein. In these mice, transplanted GFP-positive BM cells efficiently migrated into the peri-portal area of liver lobules after 1 day, repopulating 25% of the recipient liver by 4 weeks. In contrast, no GFP-positive BM cells were detected following transplantation into control mice with undamaged livers. Serum albumin levels were significantly elevated to compensate for chronic liver failure in BM cell transplantation. These results reveal that recipient conditions and microenvironments represent key factors for successful cell therapy using BMCs.

The most promising study to date demonstrates liver disease correction following transplantation of enriched HSCs in FAH-deficient mice, an animal model of tyrosenimia type I [33]. In this study bone marrow from metabolically competent donor mice was transplanted into a lethally irradiated FAH-deficient mouse strain which resulted in the proliferation of large numbers of donor LacZ + hepatocytes, and animals had restored biochemical function of the liver. Wang et al. [34] used a similar mouse model to establish the kinetics of hepatocyte replacement after BM transplantation. Lethally irradiated FAH-deficient mice were transplanted with BM cells from wild type donors. Two months after transplantation, clusters of BM-derived hepatocytes were detected, while after 5 months significant liver repopulation was present. FAH-deficient mouse model has produced exciting results, while research using other models of liver injury such as administration of CCl_4 has not been as promising. It must be kept in mind that the CCl_4 model of liver disease differs from the FAH-deficient mouse in that there is no genetic survival advantage of the donor cells over the recipient liver. Not only is the type of liver injury likely to be important in deciding which stem cell repair mechanism is activated, but it is also likely to influence how rapidly liver repair or reconstitution occurs.

MSCs derived from adult marrow have demonstrated some promising results. Jiang et al. [35] isolated multipotent adult progenitor cells (MAPCs) from BM that were able to form hepatocytes *in vivo*. They transplanted ROSA26 mouse MAPCs into non-obese diabetic/severe combined immunodeficiency disease (NOD/SCID) mice and culled them 4–24 weeks later. The recipient liver contained 5–10% donor cells that co-localized with hepatocyte markers CK18 and albumin. Since there was no noxious liver injury creating a donor cell survival advantage, there was no increase in the number of donor cells in the 6-month post-transplant period.

10.6   Clinical Trials of BMSCs in Liver Disease

Pioneering clinical trials in cardiology have heightened the enthusiasm for stem cell therapies in other organs. The delivery of marrow-derived cells into the coronary circulation of human subjects was reported to improve blood flow and cardiac function in ischemic myocardium [36, 37]. In the published reports of human stem cell trials thus far, the use of mononuclear BM cells, delivered via the intracoronary route in patients with previous myocardial infarcts but a preserved ventricular ejection fraction, were shown to improve function and perfusion [38–41]. The application of BM cell treatment in hepatology is not as far advanced. G-CSF when given to increase the circulating CD34$^+$ cells in patients with cirrhosis of the liver has shown inconsistent improvement in liver function [42].

There are only a few of clinical trials conducted in hepatology (Table 10.1), all of which are safety and feasibility studies. Our group conducted a phase I clinical trial of the infusion of CD34$^+$ cells, into the portal vein or hepatic artery of five patients with chronic liver disease with no adverse effects [43]. Although these patients received relatively low numbers of cells (2×10^6), a moderate improvement in serum bilirubin was seen in three out of five patients which lasted for more than 18 months [44]. Our experience is in keeping with the observation by am Esch et al. [45], who demonstrated increased regeneration of liver following portal application of autologous bone marrow cells to the contra-lateral side during portal vein embolization. Accelerated hepatic regeneration was demonstrated in three of these patients after the infusion of autologous CD133$^+$ BM cells. By CT criteria, the left lateral segments hypertrophied by two and a half times more than in non-BM cell-treated controls. Terai et al. [46] have shown improvement in liver function following peripheral infusion of autologous BM cells in patients with liver cirrhosis. Nine patients with cirrhosis who received portal vein infusion of 5.2×10^9 autologous unsorted BM cells showed some improvement in Child–Pugh score and albumin. Liver biopsies were taken in some patients and showed increases in proliferating cell nuclear antigen staining, an indirect marker of hepatocyte turnover. Yannaki et al. [47] have reported two cases treated with boost infusions of autologous mobilized HSCs to regenerate cirrhotic liver. Each patient underwent three rounds

Table 10.1 Clinical trials of bone marrow stem cells in liver disease

Reference	Patient group	Number (n)	Site injection	BM cells	Outcome
Am Esch et al. [45]	Patients with liver cancer, no cirrhosis	Study =3 Control =3	Portal vein	Autologous, Iliac crest, CD133+	Procedure well tolerated 2.5 fold increase in left lobe in study group on CT volumetry
Gordon et al. [43]	Hepatitis B or C, alcoholic cirrhosis and primary sclerosing cholangitis	5	Portal vein-3 Hepatic artery-2	Autologous Peripheral blood, post G-CSF CD34+	Procedure well tolerated improvement in albumin or bilirubin in three/five patients
Terai et al. [46]	Hepatitis B or C cirrhosis	9	Peripheral vein	Autologous, Iliac crest, unsorted BM	Procedure well tolerated improvement in child's Pugh score and albumin
Yannaki et al. [47]	Alcoholic cirrhosis	2	Peripheral vein	Autologous Peripheral blood, post G-CSF CD34+	Procedure well tolerated improvement in child's Pugh and MELD score
Lyra et al. [48]	Alcoholic, hepatis C, cholestatic and cryptogenic cirrhosis	10	Hepatic artery	Autologous, Iliac crest, unsorted BM	Procedure well tolerated improvement in child's Pugh score, bilirubin and albumin
Gasbarrini et al. [49]	Drug induced acute liver failure	1	Portal vein	Autologous peripheral blood, post G-CSF CD34+	Procedure well tolerated improvement in clotting (PT), AST & ALT up to 30 days. Patient died of Sepsis at day 60

of G-CSF mobilization and infusion of CD34$^+$ cells into the peripheral vein. The procedure was well tolerated and both patients improved their baseline Child-Turcotte-Pugh (CTP) and model for end-stage liver disease (MELD) scores which remained for 30 months. The largest series published recently recruited ten patients with chronic liver disease [48]. BM aspirate from the iliac crest was infused into the hepatic artery of these patients. There was improvement in serum bilirubin, albumin and international normalized ratio (INR) in the study group. In an interesting case report the authors have described the use of autologous BMSCs as rescue treatment for a patient with drug induced acute liver failure, who was not suitable for liver transplantation [49]. Following G-CSF mobilization, 5×10^6 CD34$^+$ cells were infused into the portal vein of this patient. A liver biopsy performed at 20 days post infusion showed increased hepatocyte replication around necrotic foci. There was improvement in the synthetic liver function, coagulation in particular, in the first 30 days. However the patient died due to multi-organ failure related to bacterial infection.

10.7   Therapeutic Mass

The liver contains approximately 2.8×10^{11} hepatocytes and the required mass of cells to correct a single enzyme biochemical defect is likely to be significantly less than for treatment of either chronic or acute liver failure. There is evidence that provision of only 1–5% of liver mass by transplantation may be sufficient to restore adequate functional activity so that metabolic parameters are normalized [4, 50, 51]. The cells can be delivered into the patients using one of the following routes: through the peripheral vein, through the portal vein or the hepatic artery into the liver or through intra splenic injection as illustrated in Figs. 10.1–10.3. Since both fulminant and chronic liver failure may require replacement of more than 10% of functional liver, the cell mass required for transplantation into the liver will be significantly higher. The liver cell mass is restored primarily through division of the majority of mature hepatocytes. A stimulus to regeneration such as two-thirds partial hepatectomy promotes increases in carbamyl phosphate synthetase I activity [52] with subsequent liver hypertrophy. This early experience suggests that this therapeutic approach has the potential of enhancing and accelerating hepatic regeneration in a clinical setting.

BMSCs may be advantageous for liver regeneration compared to hepatocytes as availability of the hepatocytes depends on the procurement of cadaveric organs from deceased donors who are often immunologically disparate and also short in supply. Use of adult stem cells overcomes many of the moral and ethical barriers of ES cell manipulation. Moreover, BMSCs are multipotent and are an ideal source. The obvious advantage of BMSCs is that there is already considerable experience in their handling, they are relatively accessible and there is unlimited supply of these cells. The new findings in adult stem cell biology are transforming our understanding of tissue repair with promising hopes of regenerative hepatology.

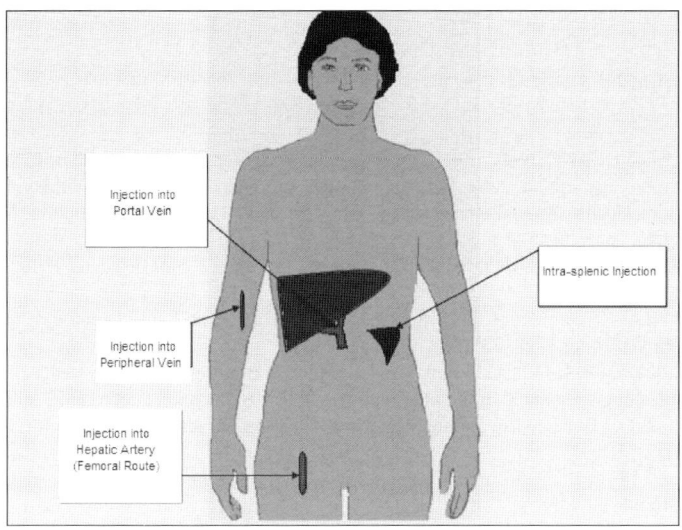

Fig. 10.1 Routes of administration of stem cells into the liver (*See Color Plates*)

Fig. 10.2 Infusion of stem cells into the portal vein

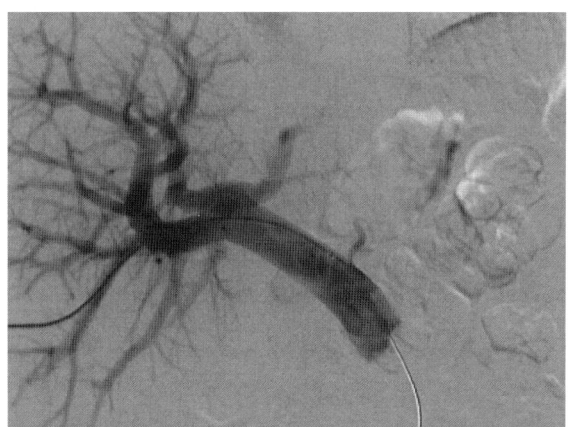

Fig. 10.3 Infusion of stem cells into the hepatic artery

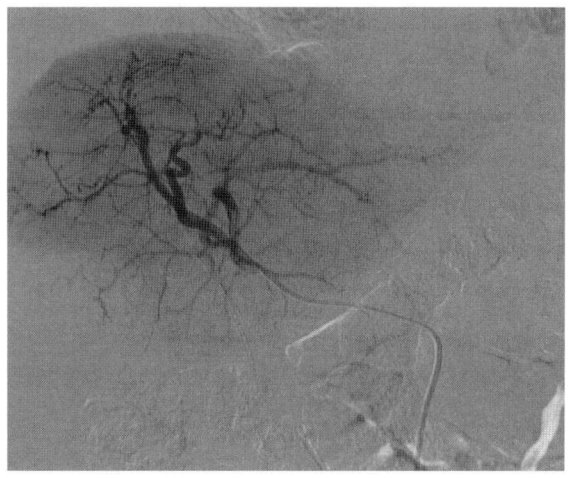

References

1. Arias, I.M., J.L. Boyer, N. Fausto, F.V. Chisari, D. Schachter, D.A. Shafritz, The Liver: Biology and Pathobiology. 4th ed. 2001, Philedelphia, PA: Lippincott Williams & Wilkins, 1088 pp.
2. Ministry of Health, Annual Report of the Chief Medical Officer. 2001, London: Ministry of Health, UK.
3. UNOS. United Network of Organ Sharing Online. http://www.unos.org/data. 2006 [cited 2006 February 21].
4. Fox, I.J. et al., Treatment of the Crigler-Najjar syndrome type I with hepatocyte transplantation. N Engl J Med, 1998. **338**(20): 1422–6.
5. Reubinoff, B.E., M.F. Pera, C.Y. Fong, A. Trounson, A. Bongso, Embryonic stem cell lines from human blastocysts: somatic differentiation in vitro. Nat Biotechnol, 2000. **18**(4): 399–404.
6. Thomas, E.D., Bone marrow transplantation from the personal viewpoint. Int J Hematol, 2005. **81**(2): 89–93.
7. Pittenger, M.F. et al., Multilineage potential of adult human mesenchymal stem cells. Science, 1999. **284**(5411): 143–7.
8. Bianco, P. et al., Bone marrow stromal stem cells: nature, biology, and potential applications. Stem Cells, 2001. **19**(3): 180–92.
9. Herzog, E.L., L. Chai, D.S. Krause, Plasticity of marrow-derived stem cells. Blood, 2003. **102**(10): 3483–93.
10. Orlic, D. et al., Mobilized bone marrow cells repair the infarcted heart, improving function and survival. Proc Natl Acad Sci U S A, 2001. **98**(18): 10344–9.
11. Gussoni, E. et al., Dystrophin expression in the mdx mouse restored by stem cell transplantation. Nature, 1999. **401**(6751): 390–4.
12. Mezey, E. et al., Turning blood into brain: cells bearing neuronal antigens generated in vivo from bone marrow. Science, 2000. **290**(5497): 1779–82.
13. Strom, S.C. et al., Hepatocyte transplantation as a bridge to orthotopic liver transplantation in terminal liver failure. Transplantation, 1997. **63**(4): 559–69.
14. Selden, C., H. Hodgson, Cellular therapies for liver replacement. Transpl Immunol, 2004. **12**(3–4): 273–88.
15. Neuberger, J. et al., Transplantation for alcoholic liver disease. Journal of Hepatology, 2002. **36**(1): 130–7.
16. Austin, T.W., E. Lagasse, Hepatic regeneration from hematopoietic stem cells. Mech Dev, 2003. **120**(1): 131–5.
17. Petersen, B.E. et al., Bone marrow as a potential source of hepatic oval cells. Science, 1999. **284**(5417): 1168–70.
18. Theise, N.D. et al., Derivation of hepatocytes from bone marrow cells in mice after radiation-induced myeloablation. Hepatology, 2000. **31**(1): 235–40.
19. Alison, M.R. et al., Hepatocytes from non-hepatic adult stem cells. Nature, 2000. **406**(6793): 257.
20. Theise, N.D. et al., Liver from bone marrow in humans. Hepatology, 2000. **32**(1): 11–6.
21. Korbling, M. et al., Hepatocytes and epithelial cells of donor origin in recipients of peripheral-blood stem cells. N Engl J Med, 2002. **346**(10): 738–46.
22. Krause, D.S. et al., Multi-organ, multi-lineage engraftment by a single bone marrow-derived stem cell. Cell, 2001. **105**(3): 369–77.
23. Terai, S. et al., An in vivo model for monitoring trans-differentiation of bone marrow cells into functional hepatocytes. J Biochem (Tokyo), 2003. **134**(4): 551–8.
24. Jang, Y.Y. et al., Hematopoietic stem cells convert into liver cells within days without fusion. Nat Cell Biol, 2004. **6**(6): 532–9.
25. Vassilopoulos, G., P.R. Wang, D.W. Russell, Transplanted bone marrow regenerates liver by cell fusion. Nature, 2003. **422**(6934): 901–4.
26. Wang, X. et al., Cell fusion is the principal source of bone-marrow-derived hepatocytes. Nature, 2003. **422**(6934): 897–901.

27. Takano, H. et al., Pleiotropic effects of cytokines on acute myocardial infarction: G-CSF as a novel therapy for acute myocardial infarction. Curr Pharm Des, 2003. **9**(14): 1121–7.

28. Tang, J. et al., Mesenchymal stem cells participate in angiogenesis and improve heart function in rat model of myocardial ischemia with reperfusion. Eur J Cardiothorac Surg, 2006. **30**(2): 353–61.

29. Chen, Z. et al., Overexpression of Bcl-2 attenuates apoptosis and protects against myocardial I/R injury in transgenic mice. Am J Physiol Heart Circ Physiol, 2001. **280**(5): H2313–20.

30. Wang, M. et al., Pretreatment with adult progenitor cells improves recovery and decreases native myocardial proinflammatory signaling after ischemia. Shock, 2006. **25**(5): 454–9.

31. Oyagi, S. et al., Therapeutic effect of transplanting HGF-treated bone marrow mesenchymal cells into CCl4-injured rats. J Hepatol, 2006. **44**(4): 742–8.

32. Sakaida, I. et al., Transplantation of bone marrow cells reduces CCl4-induced liver fibrosis in mice. Hepatology, 2004. **40**(6): 1304–11.

33. Lagasse, E. et al., Purified hematopoietic stem cells can differentiate into hepatocytes in vivo. Nat Med, 2000. **6**(11): 1229–34.

34. Wang, X. et al., Liver repopulation and correction of metabolic liver disease by transplanted adult mouse pancreatic cells. Am J Pathol, 2001. **158**(2): 571–9.

35. Jiang, Y. et al., Pluripotency of mesenchymal stem cells derived from adult marrow. Nature, 2002. **418**(6893): 41–9.

36. Tse, H.F. et al., Angiogenesis in ischaemic myocardium by intramyocardial autologous bone marrow mononuclear cell implantation. Lancet, 2003. **361**(9351): 47–9.

37. Assmus, B. et al., Transplantation of progenitor cells and regeneration enhancement in acute myocardial infarction (TOPCARE-AMI). Circulation, 2002. **106**(24): 3009–17.

38. Perin, E.C. et al., Transendocardial, autologous bone marrow cell transplantation for severe, chronic ischemic heart failure. Circulation, 2003. **107**(18): 2294–302.

39. Bartunek, J. et al., Intracoronary injection of CD133-positive enriched bone marrow progenitor cells promotes cardiac recovery after recent myocardial infarction: feasibility and safety. Circulation, 2005. **112**(9 Suppl): I178–83.

40. Ge, J. et al., Efficacy of emergent transcatheter transplantation of stem cells for treatment of acute myocardial infarction (TCT-STAMI). Heart, 2006. **92**(12): 1764–7.

41. Janssens, S. et al., Autologous bone marrow-derived stem-cell transfer in patients with ST-segment elevation myocardial infarction: double-blind, randomised controlled trial. Lancet, 2006. **367**(9505): 113–21.

42. Gaia, S. et al., Feasibility and safety of G-CSF administration to induce bone marrow-derived cells mobilization in patients with end stage liver disease. J Hepatol, 2006. **45**(1): 13–9.

43. Gordon, M.Y. et al., Characterization and clinical application of human CD34 + stem/progenitor cell populations mobilized into the blood by granulocyte colony-stimulating factor. Stem Cells, 2006. **24**(7): 1822–30.

44. Levicar, N. et al., Long-term clinical results of autologous infusion of mobilised adult bone marrow derived CD34 + cells in patients with chronic liver disease. Cell Prolif, 2008. 41: 115–25.

45. am Esch, J.S., 2nd et al., Portal application of autologous CD133 + bone marrow cells to the liver: a novel concept to support hepatic regeneration. Stem Cells, 2005. **23**(4): 463–70.

46. Terai, S. et al., Improved liver function in patients with liver cirrhosis after autologous bone marrow cell infusion therapy. Stem Cells, 2006. **24**(10): 2292–8.

47. Yannaki, E. et al., Lasting amelioration in the clinical course of decompensated alcoholic cirrhosis with boost infusions of mobilized peripheral blood stem cells. Exp Hematol, 2006. **34**(11): 1583–7.

48. Lyra, A.C. et al., Feasibility and safety of autologous bone marrow mononuclear cell transplantation in patients with advanced chronic liver disease. World J Gastroenterol, 2007. **13**(7): 1067–73.

49. Gasbarrini, A. et al., Rescue therapy by portal infusion of autologous stem cells in a case of drug-induced hepatitis. Dig Liver Dis., 2007. **39**(9): 878–82.

50. Selden, C. et al., Histidinemia in mice: a metabolic defect treated using a novel approach to hepatocellular transplantation. Hepatology, 1995. **21**(5): 1405–12.
51. Muraca, M. et al., Hepatocyte transplantation as a treatment for glycogen storage disease type 1a. Lancet, 2002. **359**(9303): 317–8.
52. Selden, A.C., H.J. Hodgson, Growth factors and the liver. Gut, 1991. **32**(6): 601–3.

Chapter 11
Cell Transplantation Therapy for Myocardial Repair: Current Status and Future Challenges

Wangde Dai and Robert A. Kloner*

Abstract Recent experimental studies and clinical trials have demonstrated that cell transplantation therapy has the potential to improve cardiac function after myocardial infarction. However, the mechanisms responsible for the observed therapeutic effects remain unknown. Different mechanisms have been proposed to explain the beneficial effects, including regeneration of contractile myocardial tissue, therapeutic neovascularization, prevention of left ventricular remodeling, release of paracrine growth factors, induction of nerve fiber regeneration, and potential influences on the cardiac stem cell niche. Furthermore, the clinical application of stem cell transplantation therapy still faces many challenges, such as tumor formation and unexpected differentiation, immunogenicity, arrhythmogenesis of engrafted stem cells, as well as how to prevent cell loss after transplantation. In this chapter, we review the current status of cell transplantation therapy, and discuss future challenges for its application in treating ischemic heart disease.

Keywords Cell transplantation therapy, myocardial infarction, stem cell

Abbreviations ESC Embryonic stem cell; MSC Mesenchymal stem cell; SCID Severe combined immunodeficient; MMP Matrix metalloproteinase; TIMP Tissue inhibitor of matrix metalloproteinase; TK Herpes Simplex Virus; GCV Ganciclovir; FGF Fibroblast growth factor; TGF Transforming growth factor; IGF Insulin-like growth factor; G-CSF Granulocyte-colony-stimulating factor

The Heart Institute, Good Samaritan Hospital, Division of Cardiovascular Medicine of the Keck School of Medicine at University of Southern California, Los Angeles, CA 90017-2395, USA

*Corresponding Author:
1225 Wilshire Boulevard, Los Angeles, CA 90017, USA
e-mail: Rkloner@goodsam.org

Y. Shi, D.O. Clegg (eds.) *Stem Cell Research and Therapeutics*,
© Springer Science+Business Media B.V. 2008

11.1   Introduction

Myocardial infarction results in the irreversible loss of cardiac muscle, thinning and stretching of the necrotic area referred to as infarct expansion, eccentric hypertrophy of the nonischemic myocardium with global dilation of the left ventricle – phenomena which in toto make up the concept of ventricular remodeling. The progressive cardiac remodeling ultimately leads to heart failure, and left ventricular dilation correlates with death. Currently, pharmacological and interventional procedures are not able to regenerate functional cardiomyocytes. Therefore, there is a need to seek new approaches to address this pathophysiologic condition resulting from the loss of cardiomyocytes and viable blood vessels caused by the ischemic insult.

Over the past 15 years, cell transplantation therapy for cardiac regeneration has been extensively investigated in both experimental studies and clinical trials. In this chapter, we focus on the underlying mechanism of benefits of cell transplantation, and related side effects and problems.

11.2   Underlying Mechanism and Potential Strategies of Cell Transplantation Therapy in Heart Disease

A wide range of cells, including immature cardiomyocytes (such as fetal or neonatal cardiomyocytes), stem cells from various sources (embryonic or adult somatic tissue) and other non-myogenic cell types, have been transplanted into infarcted myocardium in animal laboratory studies and early clinical trials. Experimental and clinical data have demonstrated that cell transplantation therapy results in an improvement in ventricular function. However, the underlying mechanism remains unclear. The major controversy in interpretation is whether cell transplantation therapy truly replaces the damaged myocardium with newly formed cardiac cells.

11.2.1   Regeneration of Contractile Myocardial Tissue

The aim of cell transplantation is to restore the cardiac function after myocardial infarction by regeneration of healthy myocardial tissue. Transplanted fetal [1] and neonatal rat cardiomyocytes [2] exhibited long-term survival in a rat myocardial infarct model, developed sarcomeric structures and other morphological features of mature cardiomyocytes, thickened the infarcted left ventricular wall, and enhanced left ventricular ejection fraction. Engrafted rat neonatal cardiomyocytes formed cell junctions with the host cardiomyocytes at the border zone of rat myocardial infarction demonstrated by immunohistochemistry and confocal microscopy using antibodies against connexin43, desmoplakin, and cadherin at 4–7 days after transplantation [3]. Grafted cardiomyocytes might have electrical pathways with host counterparts through the gap junction. However, within the infarct scar, the engrafted cells appeared to be hindered by scar tissue and formed discrete lumps, separating them from the host cardiomyocytes [4]. The limitation of human fetal or neonatal donor cells for clinical application is the lack of availability of sufficient numbers and ethical restrictions.

Embryonic stem cells (ESC) have also been used to repair damaged myocardium due to their pluripotent nature. ESCs have the potential to differentiate into cell types of all three germ layers (ectoderm, mesoderm and endoderm). Cardiomyocytes derived from ESCs have the structural and functional properties of early-stage cardiomyocytes [5]. Transplanted undifferentiated mouse ESCs differentiated into cardiomyocytes, vascular smooth muscle, and endothelial cells within the infarcted mouse heart, and reduced post-myocardial infarction remodeling of the heart and improved cardiac function [6]. ESCs have also been induced to differentiate into cardiomyocytes *ex vivo*, then transplanted into infarcted myocardium. Engrafted mouse cardiac-committed ESCs survived and differentiated into mature cardiomyocytes that expressed connexin within infarcted myocardium, and improved left ventricular ejection fraction in a clinically relevant large-animal model of heart failure [7]. Recently, our research group [8] observed that transplanted human ESC-derived cardiomyocytes survived, expressed cardiac muscle markers, exhibited sarcomeric structure, and were well interspersed with the endogenous myocardium at 4 weeks after transplantation in hearts of nude rats subjected to ischemia/reperfusion. The advantage is that human ESCs can potentially provide an unlimited supply of cardiomyocytes for cell therapy procedures. Tumorigenesis is the major hurdle for their application in clinical medicine. In our study we did not observe teratomas at 4 weeks.

Recently, investigators have focused on cardiac resident stem cells as a potential therapeutic approach. Messina et al [9] isolated undifferentiated cells from subcultures of postnatal atrial or ventricular human biopsy specimens and from murine hearts. These cells appeared to have the properties of adult cardiac stem cells, and were capable of long-term self-renewal in vitro. After transplantation into the hearts of severe combined immunodeficient (SCID) beige mice, these cells differentiated into cells with cardiomyocyte markers and cells with endothelial or smooth muscle markers. Smith et al. [10] demonstrated that resident cardiac stem cells isolated from human and porcine biopsy specimens exhibited biophysical signatures characteristic of myocytes when cocultured with neonatal rat ventricular myocytes, including calcium transients synchronous with those of neighboring myocytes. After injection into the border zone of acute myocardial infarcts in immunodeficient mice, these cells promoted cardiac regeneration and improved heart function at 20 days after treatment. However, the isolation and *ex vivo* expansion of autologous cardiac stem cells is time consuming. It would be difficult to transplant cardiac stem cells in a timely fashion following an acute myocardial infarction in clinical practice.

Other types of cells, such as skeletal myoblasts and bone marrow-derived stem cells, have also been extensively investigated in myocardial regeneration [11]. However, skeletal myoblasts cannot differentiate into true cardiomyocytes and do not express connexin. Transplanted skeletal myoblasts do not electrically couple with viable host myocardium in vivo [12, 13]. Although Orlic et al. [14] demonstrated that transplanted bone marrow cells transdifferentiated into myocytes and regenerated functional myocardium within infarcted regions at 9 days after transplantation in mice hearts, the plasticity of bone marrow-derived stem cells remains controversial [15]. Therefore, compared with other sources of stem cells, human ESC-derived cardiomyocytes may be the most promising cells for true cardiac regeneration [16].

11.2.2   Therapeutic Neovascularization

The network of blood vessels within the infarcted tissue and border zone is not enough to supply oxygen and nutrients to the greater demands of the hypertrophied myocardium within the infarct or border zone, resulting in progressive loss of viable tissue, infarct extension and fibrous replacement. Transplanted cells can induce new blood vessel formation in the infarct and peri-infarct region (vasculogenesis) and proliferation of preexisting vasculature (angiogenesis) after the experimental myocardial infarction. The neovascularization induced by cell therapy can decrease apoptosis of hypertrophied myocytes, induce cardiomyocyte proliferation and regeneration, improve long-term salvage and survival of viable myocardium, reduce collagen deposition, prevent left ventricular remodeling, and sustain improvement in cardiac function [17]. Tang et al. [18] injected autologous mesenchymal stem cells (MSC) or culture medium directly into the periinfarct zone in a rat myocardial infarction model. Compared with medium-treated hearts, the expression of angiogenic factors, basic fibroblast growth factor, vascular endothelial growth factor, and stem cell homing factor significantly increased, and capillary density increased about 40% in cell-treated hearts. Cardiac function was also improved in the cell-treated hearts at 8 weeks after implantation. The results suggested engrafted cells improved cardiac performance through enhanced angiogenesis induced by paracrine action. Our research group demonstrated that transplanted allogeneic MSCs expressed von Willebrand factor and significantly increased blood vessel density within the scar tissue at 6 months after cell transplantation in a rat myocardial infarction model [19]. We also observed that transplanted rat immature cardiomyocytes induced neo-angiogenesis in zones of successful cell engraftment within the scar and effectively enhanced regional myocardial blood flow at 4 weeks after transplantation in a rat myocardial infarction model [20].

11.2.3 Prevention of Left Ventricular Remodeling

Myocardial infarction induces deleterious remodeling of the myocardium, resulting in ventricular dilation and pump dysfunction. The benefit of cell transplantation therapy for myocardial infarction may result from mechanisms of prevention of left ventricular remodeling, not from true myocardial regeneration. Cell transplantation can increase the elastin content [21] and decrease the mRNA and protein expressions of collagen type I, collagen type III, matrix metalloproteinase (MMP)-1, tissue inhibitor of matrix metalloproteinase (TIMP)-1 [22, 23] within the infarcted myocardium. Fazel et al. [24] injected bone marrow-derived MSCs from beta-galactosidase transgenic mice into the anterior wall of the left ventricle after coronary artery ligation. Compared with the medium control group, cell transplantation significantly increased myocardial angiogenesis, reduced infarct scar area, resulted in smaller ventricular volumes and greater cardiac function without observation of mitogenesis in host cardiomyocytes or beta-galactosidase-expressing cardiomyocytes. Berry et al. [25] injected human MSCs into the acutely ischemic myocardium of Lewis rats. Two weeks later, myocardial elasticity was assessed by atomic force microscopy. The infarct region in hearts that had received MSCs was more compliant than myocardium from vehicle-treated hearts, although it was twofold stiffer than myocardium from noninfarcted animals. At 8 weeks after treatment, MSCs transplantation significantly reduced myocardial fibrosis, left ventricular dilation and apoptosis of cardiac cells; increased myocardial thickness, and preserved systolic and diastolic cardiac function compared with vehicle treatment. The engrafted human cells expressed a cardiomyocyte protein but stopped short of full differentiation and did not stimulate significant angiogenesis. These results demonstrated that MSC transplantation preserved cardiac function after myocardial infarction through the mechanisms of reduction of the stiffness of the subsequent scar and attenuation of postinfarction remodeling, but not through regeneration of contracting cardiomyocytes.

11.2.4 Release of Paracrine Mediators

Transplanted cells may promote cardiac function by release of paracrine mediators instead of or besides the replacement of lost cells after myocardial infarction. Our research group [19] injected allogeneic MSCs or saline into the scar of a 1-week-old myocardial infarction in Fischer rats, and observed that transplanted MSCs significantly improved left ventricular function compared with saline at 4 weeks after treatment, but the benefits of MSC treatment were lost at 6 months. Although the transplanted cells expressed muscle-specific markers alpha-actinin, myosin heavy chain, phospholamban, and tropomyosin, they did not fully evolve into an adult cardiac phenotype at 6 months. Cell treatment had no effects on cardiac remodeling. The results suggested that the early transient benefit at 4 weeks might be due to a possible paracrine effect. Recent published data provide evidence of a paracrine effect of cell transplantation therapy [18, 26, 27]. Gnecchi et al. [27] demonstrated conditioned culture medium of bone marrow-derived MSCs overexpressing Akt markedly inhibited hypoxia-induced apoptosis, triggered vigorous spontaneous contraction of adult rat cardiomyocytes in vitro, and significantly limited infarct size and improved ventricular function when injected into infarcted hearts in rats. These data support the hypothesis that paracrine mechanisms play an important role in myocardial protection and functional improvement of cell therapy in the injured heart. Recently, our research group [28] injected saline, fresh medium, conditioned medium (collected at 4 days of culture of MSCs), or two million MSCs in fresh medium directly into 1-week-old myocardial infarction in Fischer rats. Four weeks later, left ventricular angiograms showed that left ventricular ejection fraction was better preserved in the fresh medium, conditioned medium and MSC groups than in the saline group. Since the culture medium contains nutrients and bovine serum, which contain various cytokines, the soluble factors might play a crucial role in the improvement of cardiac function.

11.2.5 Induction of Nerve Fiber Regeneration

Ischemia leads to denervation of infarcted myocardium. Nerve fiber regeneration within the damaged myocardium may have occurred either via the growth of pre-existing fibers and/or the mobilization of neural stem cells. Stem cell transplantation may improve the nerve fiber regeneration after myocardial infarction. Pak et al. [29] injected MSCs into 1-month-old myocardial infarctions in a swine model. Two months later, MSC transplantation increased the magnitude of cardiac nerve sprouting in both atria and ventricles, and increased the magnitude of atrial sympathetic hyperinnervation within the infarct. Lin et al. [30] transplanted autologous bone marrow mononuclear cells into the border zone of myocardial infarcts at 2 weeks after injury in a rabbit model, and observed that cell transplantation induced angiogenesis and nerve sprouting and improved left ventricular diastolic function at 2 months after treatment. However, the correlation between enhanced nerve fiber regeneration and cardiac function remains to be determined.

11.2.6 Potential Influences on the Cardiac Stem Cell Niche

Endogenous adult stem cells, such as bone marrow stem cells and cardiac resident stem cells, may be involved in the healing process after myocardial infarction. In order to form new myocardium, stem cells either from the cardiac tissue or migrating from other tissue must successfully settle in an empty niche of the damaged cardiac tissue. Stem cell niche is a specialized physical location which constitutes a three-dimensional microenvironment in the host tissue [31]. The self-renewing capacity and differentiation of stem cells in myocardium are protected and controlled by the environmental tissue niche. Transplanted cells may stimulate endogenous repair by the regeneration of stem cell niches in damaged myocardium. Mazhari et al. [32] demonstrated that direct injection of allogeneic MSCs into infarcted myocardium improved the ejection fraction, reduced infarct size, and regenerated a rim of new cardiac tissue in a porcine myocardial infarction model. The authors observed that the host porcine cardiac myocytes entered the cell cycle, new blood vessels formed, and levels of apoptosis were reduced in the recipient hearts, but the engrafted MSCs did not exhibit transdifferentiation into adult cardiomyocytes. Therefore the authors suggested that the heart could contain stem cell niches, and transplanted cells could lead to restoration of these niches through multifaceted cell-cell interactions.

11.2.7   Cell-Based Gene Therapy

Adult stem cells could be used as a vehicle for delivery of specific therapeutic genes. The advantages of cell-based gene therapy are their reliable efficiency of transfection and controllable expression. Therapeutic genes can be stably transfected into cells *ex vivo*, and their efficiency of transfection can be assessed before transplantation. Mizuno et al. [33] transfected syngeneic rat endothelial cells with the rat elastin gene, and transplanted these cells into the infarct scar in rats. At 3 months after transplantation, recombinant elastin was detected in the scar tissue, and the elastic fibers were organized. Compared with the control group, expression of recombinant elastin reduced scar expansion, prevented left ventricular enlargement, and improved the cardiac function. The results suggested that altering matrix remodeling by cell-based gene therapy may preserve the cardiac function after myocardial infarction. Yau et al. [34] transplanted (1) bone marrow cells; (2) bone marrow cells transfected with either vascular endothelial growth factor gene or basic fibroblast growth factor gene, or both genes simultaneously; or (3) medium into myocardial infarction in Lewis rats. Four weeks later, the combined transfection with vascular endothelial growth factor and basic fibroblast growth factor genes resulted in the greatest vascular densities and regional perfusion in the scar, as well as the greatest improvement in left ventricular ejection fraction. Therefore cell-based gene therapy may be used for multimodal gene delivery to enhance angiogenesis and cardiac function.

The expression of cell-based delivered therapeutic genes is controllable. Miyagawa et al. [35] demonstrated that the thymidine kinase gene of Herpes Simplex Virus (TK) and the Ganciclovir (GCV) system can be used to regulate cell-based gene therapy. Cells transfected with TK can be killed when exposed to GCV. Combined transfection of TK can control the expression of therapeutic genes through the control of cell growth in cell-based gene therapy.

11.3 Side Effects, Controversial Issues and Problems to Be Solved

11.3.1 Tumorigenesis and Unexpected Differentiation

Transplanted undifferentiated stem cells might form teratomas. Swijnenburg et al. [36] transplanted mouse ESCs into murine hearts of both allogeneic and syngeneic recipients after left anterior descending coronary artery ligation by direct myocardial injection. The ESC grafts remained stable and there was no evidence of differentiation at 2 weeks after transplantation; however, the grafts showed the presence of teratomas in the hearts of both allogeneic and syngeneic recipients at 4 weeks. Cao et al. [37] injected murine ESCs into the myocardium of adult nude rats, and demonstrated that transplanted murine ESCs formed intracardiac teratomas at 5 weeks after transplantation.

Besides teratoma formation, engrafted stem cells might differentiate into other unexpected tissues. Grinnemo et al. [38] demonstrated that transplanted human MSCs differentiated into fibroblasts, not cardiomyocytes in a rat myocardial infarction model. Ribeiro et al. [39] observed that unselected bone marrow cell transplantation resulted in bone-like formations (including bone, cartilage, and marrow-like structures) in the left ventricular wall of infarcted rats. Yoon et al. [40] injected unselected bone marrow cells into acute myocardial infarction in rats. At 2 weeks after cell transplantation, echocardiography indicated intramyocardial calcification which was confirmed by histological examination with hematoxylin and eosin staining and von Kossa staining. The acellular calcific areas were surrounded by transplanted cells, suggesting the direct involvement of transplanted cells in myocardial calcification. Recently, Chiavegato et al. [41] reported the chondro-osteogenic differentiation of transplanted human amniotic fluid-derived stem cells in a rat model of myocardial infarction. Therefore, the possibility of teratoma formation and unexpected differentiation after transplantation poses a daunting challenge for clinical application of stem cell therapy.

In order to prevent spontaneous differentiation of stem cells into undesired lineages and reduce the risk of teratoma formation, it is necessary to find a way to guide cardiomyogenic differentiation of stem cells in vitro prior to transplantation or in vivo after transplantation. Various techniques that could possibly be used to direct and control the cardiomyogenic differentiation of stem cells have been developed (for review, see [42]). For example, Bartunek et al. [43] reported that pretreatment of adult bone marrow MSCs with cardiomyogenic growth factors (including basic FGF, IGF-1, and bone morphogenetic protein-2) resulted in enhanced cardiomyogenic differentiation and in superior effects on cardiac function in chronically infarcted canine myocardium. Kofidis et al. [44] added recombinant mouse vascular endothelial growth factor, fibroblast growth factor (FGF), and transforming growth factor (TGF) to a mouse ESC suspension, and injected the cell suspension into the ischemic area after left anterior descending artery ligation in allogeneic (BALB/c) mice. These growth factors promoted in vivo cardiac-specific differentiation of early ESCs and improved myocardial function. However, additional successful strategies to guide cardiac differentiation of stem cells need to be established and will depend upon the understanding of the basic mechanisms of cardiac differentiation of stem cells [45, 46].

11.3.2 Immunogenicity

Transplanted allogeneic stem cells may be rejected by immune responses following the engraftment. Whether stem cells (ESCs and adult stem cells) are "immune privledged" remains controversial. For example, Menard et al. [7] demonstrated that engrafted cardiac-committed mouse ESCs survived for 1 month without immunosuppresion, and differentiated into mature cardiomyocytes with connexin expression within the infarcted myocardium in sheep. In contrast, our research group observed that transplanted human ESC-derived cardiomyocytes induced a brisk lymphocytic infiltrate typical of rejection in the hearts of immune competent Sprague-Dawley rats at 4 weeks after transplantation [8]. Grinnemo et al. [47] reported that transplanted adult human MSCs caused significant infiltration of round cells, mostly macrophages when injected into the myocardium of host Sprague-Dawley rats, suggesting that MSCs caused an immune reaction in this xenogenic model. In our study [19], engrafted rat-derived allogeneic MSCs survived and expressed cardiac muscle markers at 6 months after transplantation into the scar of a 1-week-old myocardial infarction in Fischer rats, and no immune responses were observed.

Nuclear transfer techniques may provide an unlimited supply of histocompatible ES cells (therapeutic cloning) [48]. Stem cell banks may be another alternative approach.

11.3.3 Arrhythmogenesis of Cell Therapy

A clinical trial demonstrated that skeletal myoblast transplantation in a post-myocardial infarction population increased the risk of left ventricular arrhythmias [49]. Thus the potential arrhythmogenic risk of various transplanted cells should be investigated before clinical application. Some cells show intrinsic arrhythmic potential. Zhang et al. [50] demonstrated that cultured mouse ESC-derived cardiomyocytes had arrhythmogenic properties in the whole-cell patch-clamp mode, including spontaneous activity, low dV/dt, prolonged AP duration, and easily inducible triggered arrhythmias. Chang et al. [51] showed that human bone marrow-derived MSCs decreased conduction velocity and induced reentrant arrhythmias in co-cultured neonatal rat ventricular myocytes, and suggested that MSCs could produce an arrhythmogenic substrate and had proarrhythmic potential. Skeletal myoblasts lack gap junctions and are not able to couple to each other and to surrounding host ventricular cardiomyocytes [52, 53], and in such a manner may induce arrhythmias once implanted into conducting tissue. Furthermore, the transplanted cells may increase the risk of arrhythmias by inducing nerve sprouting [54] or promoting myocyte hypertrophy [55] of the host heart.

Although the underlying mechanisms of arrhythmogenesis after cell transplantation remain unknown [55], some strategies have been proposed to prevent the arrhythmogenesis of cell therapy. Genetic manipulation of the expression of the different cardiac ion channels, modulators of ion channel function, or proteins involved in cell-to-cell interactions may modify electrophysiological properties of the ESC (for review, see reference [56]). Abraham et al. [57] demonstrated that the reentrant arrhythmias observed in co-cultures of human skeletal myoblasts and rat cardiomyocytes were decreased when the skeletal myoblasts were genetically modified to express the gap junction protein connexin43. Implantation of automatic cardiac defibrillators may be useful for controlling the arrhythmic risk in patients receiving skeletal myoblast transplantation [49].

11.3.4 Plasticity of Adult Stem Cells Within Myocardium

Adult stem cells have been suggested to possess a much broader differentiation potential than previously appreciated. Transplanted adult stem cells have been reported to extensively regenerate cardiomyocytes through transdifferentiation. However, recent studies raised the issue that the observed transdifferentiation may be through the cell fusion of donor stem cells with the host cardiomyocytes. Yeh et al. [58] injected human peripheral blood CD34 +-enriched cells into myocardial infarction in SCID mice, and observed that transplanted cells transdifferentiated into cardiomyocytes, mature endothelial cells, and smooth muscle cells in vivo at 2 months after injection. Nygren et al. [59] delivered transgenically marked unfractionated bone marrow cells and a purified population of hematopoietic stem cells to the injured myocardium, and observed bone marrow-derived cardiomyocytes outside the infarcted myocardium at a low frequency. The identified bone marrow-derived cardiomyocytes were derived exclusively through cell fusion. Zhang et al. [60] transplanted human peripheral blood CD34-positive cells into the injured hearts of SCID mice. The human CD34 + cell-derived cardiomyocytes were isolated from the hearts of mice. Interphase fluorescence in situ hybridization showed that 73.3% of human CD34 + cell-derived cardiomyocytes contained both human and mouse X chromosomes and 23.7% contain only human X chromosomes. The data suggested that the transformation of peripheral blood CD34 + cells into cardiomyocytes resulted from both cell fusion and transdifferentiation. Murry et al. [15] tracked the fate of haematopoietic stem cells by expression of reporter transgenes after 145 transplants into normal and injured adult mouse hearts, and demonstrated that no transdifferentiation into cardiomyocytes was detectable. These results indicate that plasticity of adult stem cells within myocardium remains uncertain, and raise a cautionary note for their clinical studies of cardiac repair.

11.3.5 Cell Loss After Transplantation

Therapeutic impact of cell transplantation may be limited by the low survival of grafted cells within the recipient heart. Muller-Ehmsen et al. [61] injected mononuclear or mesenchymal bone marrow cells of male Fischer rats into the border zone of myocardial infarction in syngeneic female Fischer rats immediately or 7 days after left coronary artery occlusion. Quantitative real-time PCR with Y-chromosome specific primers showed that there were 34–80% of injected donor-cells in the recipient heart at 0 hour after transplantation. This percentage decreased rapidly to 0.3–3.5% 6 weeks later. The decrease was independent of cell type and application time. The early cell loss after transplantation may be due to the washout through the vascular system of the heart. Dow et al. [62] demonstrated that transplanted neonatal rat cardiac cells were acutely washed out of the infarcted myocardium to other organs (lungs, liver, kidneys and spleen) through the vascular system of the heart in both reperfusion and non-reperfusion myocardial ischemia models in rats. At the present time, no efficient way is available to prevent the washout.

Another cause of cell loss is death induced by poor supply of oxygen and nutrients within the ischemic area. Genetic modification may be a useful approach to increase the survival of transplanted cells in ischemic tissue. Liu et al. [63] transfected male smooth muscle cells with insulin-like growth factor 1 (IGF-1) gene, and transplanted these IGF-1-transfected cells into myocardial scar tissue in female rats. IGF-1-transfected smooth muscle cells increased IGF-1, VEGF and Bcl2 expression in the myocardium, enhanced vessel formation, and limited cell apoptosis in the myocardial scar compared with the two control groups (received smooth muscle cells transfected with a plasmid vector and nontransfected with gene). IGF-1 transfection significantly improved donor cell proliferation, survival, and engraftment after cell transplantation in the implanted region. The mechanism may be due to enhanced angiogenesis and reduced apoptosis. Nakamura et al. [64] pretreated male Lewis rat aortic smooth muscle cells with antiapoptotic Bcl-2 gene transfection, and then implanted them into the infarcted myocardium in syngenic female rats. At days 7 and 28 after transplantation, apoptosis was significantly reduced in Bcl-2-treated cells, whereas survival was increased. Transfection of other genes, such as heme oxygenase-1 [65], Akt [66, 67], fibroblast growth factor-2 [68], vascular endothelial growth factor [69], have also been reported to increase the survival of grafted cells in myocardial ischemia.

Besides genetic modification, there are other approaches to increase grafted cell survival. Bonaros et al. [70] demonstrated that co-transplantation of skeletal myoblasts with angiopoietic progenitor cells increased vascular density and reduced apoptotic index in a nude rat myocardial infarction model. Therefore, co-transplantation of angioblasts might be used to generate a network of blood vessels to provide vascular structures for supply of oxygen and nutrients for the implanted cells. Wang et al. [71] pretreated myocardial infarct areas with angiogenic therapy induced by transmyocardial revascularization, and then transplanted ESCs into the injured heart in a rat myocardial infarction model. Pretreatment of transmyocardial revascularization significantly increased capillary density and enhanced the efficacy of cell grafts at 4 weeks after cell transplantation. Niagara et al. [72] pharmacologically preconditioned skeletal myoblasts from male Fischer rats for 30 minutes with 200 micromol/L diazoxide, and injected these cells into the myocardial infarctions of female Fischer rats. Pharmacologic preconditioning significantly promoted cell survival at 4 days after transplantation assessed by Real-time PCR for sry gene. Davis et al. [73] mixed IGF-1 with biotinylated peptide nanofibers, and delivered this mixture combined with transplanted cardiomyocytes into rat myocardial infarction. IGF-1 delivery by biotinylated nanofibers significantly improved the efficiency of cell therapy. Kutschka et al. [74] demonstrated that collagen matrices as cell delivery vehicles could enhance early survival of transplanted cardiomyoblasts after transplantation into ischemic hearts in rats.

11.3.6   Other Adverse Effects

There are some other unexpected adverse effects that have been reported in the cell transplantation literature. Vulliet et al. [75] injected early passage autologous MSCs derived from bone marrow into the left circumflex coronary artery in dogs, and observed ST segment elevation and T wave changes characteristic of acute myocardial ischaemia during administration. Histological examination showed evidence of myocardial infarction at 7 days later, including scattered regions of dense fibroplasia accompanied by macrophage infiltrates in areas where the MSCs were observed. The results suggested that intracoronary arterial injection of MSCs caused acute myocardial ischaemia and subacute myocardial microinfarction in healthy dogs. Kang et al. [76] and Steinwender et al. [77] reported that granulocyte-colony stimulating factor application combined with transcoronary peripheral blood stem cell transplantation in patients with myocardial infarction who underwent coronary stenting led to significantly higher rates of in-stent restenosis during the 6 months of follow-up. Thus, unexpected effects should be carefully monitored in future studies.

11.4   Clinical Trials

Skeletal myoblasts and bone marrow-derived cells were used for cell transplantation therapy of acute myocardial infarction and ischemic cardiomyopathy in early clinical trials. These autologous stem cells were delivered to infarcted myocardium by direct injection, intravascular injection, or by bone marrow stimulation with granulocyte-colony-stimulating factor (G-CSF). The available clinical trial data suggested that stem cell transplantation therapy is technically feasible and some studies showed that stem cell therapy resulted in beneficial effects on cardiac function.

Skeletal myoblasts are easily isolated from autologous skeletal muscle biopsies and can be expanded *ex vivo*. Siminiak et al. [78] selected ten patients who survived an acute myocardial infarction for skeletal myoblast transplantation therapy. Autologous myoblasts were isolated from the skeletal muscle biopsy and cultured for 3 weeks in vitro. Myoblasts were injected into the akinetic/dyskinetic area when coronary artery bypass grafting was performed. The left ventricular ejection fraction significantly increased during the 12 months of follow-up. However, sustained ventricular tachycardia was observed in four patients during 2 weeks of follow-up. Prophylactic amiodarone infusion was used to prevent sustained ventricular tachycardia episodes in this study. Recently, Hagege et al. [49] reported data of a long-term follow-up of the first phase I cohort of patients (n = 9). These patients with ischemic heart failure received autologous skeletal myoblast transplantation in a post-myocardial infarction scar during bypass surgery. NYHA class and left ventricular ejection fraction significantly improved during 52 (18–58) months follow-up after myoblast transplantation. Five patients were implanted with an automatic cardiac defibrillator for nonsustained (n = 1) or sustained (n = 4) ventricular tachycardia. Another two patients received a resynchronization pacemaker. These early clinical trials with autologous skeletal myoblast transplantation for the treatment of postinfarction heart failure are small sample sizes and lack a control group. The available data demonstrated that myoblast transplantation is feasible, but have a potential risk of increased ventricular arrhythmias.

Bone marrow stem cells are isolated from bone marrow which is easily obtained from an iliac crest biopsy as routinely done in clinical haematology. Recently, several groups have reported the results of randomized, controlled clinical trials which investigated the effect of bone marrow cells on ventricular function after a myocardial infarction. In a multicenter randomized, double-blind trial, Schächinger et al. [79] assigned 204 patients with acute myocardial infarction to receive an intracoronary infusion of progenitor cells derived from bone marrow (n = 101) or placebo medium (n = 98) into the infarct artery 3–7 days after successful reperfusion therapy. The absolute improvement in the global left ventricular ejection fraction was significantly greater in the cell group (5.5 ± 7.3%) than in the control group (3.0 ± 6.5%; p = 0.01) at 4 months. Adverse clinical events, including death, recurrence of myocardial infarction, and any revascularization procedure were significantly reduced in the cell group at 1 year after treatment. In another randomized, crossover trial, Assmus et al. [80] assigned 75 post-myocardial infarction patients with stable ischemic heart disease to receive bone marrow-derived progenitor cells (n = 28), circulating blood-derived progenitor cells (n = 24), or no cells (n = 23) by intracoronary infusion. At 3 months, there were moderate but significant improvements in the left ventricular ejection fraction in the bone marrow-derived progenitor cells compared with the other two groups. However, Lunde et al. [81] reported a negative result in their randomized trial. In this trial, patients with acute ST-elevation myocardial infarction of the anterior wall received intracoronary injection of autologous mononuclear bone marrow cells (n = 47) or no cell infusion (n = 50). At 6 months follow up, there was no significant difference in left ventricular end-diastolic volume, infarct size, or adverse events rates between the two groups. Meyer et al. [82]

demonstrated that intracoronary autologous bone marrow cell infusion significantly increased left ventricular ejection fraction after 6 months but not after 18 months in patients with percutaneous coronary intervention with stent implantation (n = 30) compared with the control group (no infusion, n = 30). Currently, the clinical trial results of bone marrow cell transplantation therapy are mixed. It may be due to the differences in patient selection and time point, or some other unknown reasons.

Mobilization of bone marrow stem cells by G-CSF has been suggested to be able to prevent left ventricular remodeling and improve cardiac function after acute myocardial infarction in early-phase clinical trials [83]. However, Zohlnhofer et al. [84] randomly assigned 114 patients with acute myocardial infarction to receive subcutaneously either a daily dose of 10 μg/kg of G-CSF (n = 56) or placebo (n = 58) for 5 days. Although G-CSF significantly induced mobilization of bone marrow stem cells, the treatment of G-CSF had no influence on infarct size and left ventricular function at 6 months of follow-up in this randomized, double-blind, placebo-controlled trial. Although this study yielded negative results, it is one of the first, controlled, larger, and more carefully designed studies to assess the effect of mobilization of bone marrow stem cells by G-CSF to an acute myocardial infarction [85]. Ripa et al. [86] also reported that G-CSF treatment after myocardial infarction did not lead to further improvement in ventricular function compared with the placebo group at 6 months of follow-up in the double-blind, randomized, placebo-controlled stem cells in myocardial infarction (STEMMI) trial.

The adult stem cells used in current clinical trials have their disadvantages. The plasticity of skeletal myoblasts and bone marrow cells remains controversial. Most of the clinical trials have thus far included relatively small sample sizes, lacked randomization and lacked double-blind assessment of outcomes. Therefore, the available clinical trial results have not yet clearly answered the question of whether stem cell therapy should be utilized in routine clinical practice.

11.5 Summary

Currently, experimental studies and early-phase clinical trials suggest that cell transplantation therapy for myocardial infarction is feasible and safe. Accumulated evidence indicates that cell therapy may induce a modest preservation of cardiac function through true cardiac regeneration, new blood vessel formation, prevention of ventricular remodeling, paracrine effect, or possibly other unknown mechanisms. However, most of the fundamental knowledge needed to develop guidelines for the application of stem cell therapy in cardiac disease, such as the optimal type of donor cells, dosage regimen, and timing of administration, is still lacking. Numbers of questions and problems, including the risk of teratoma formation, immune rejection, poor cell viability associated with transplantation, etc., remain to be resolved. Therefore in our opinion the routine clinical application of cell transplantation in the prevention and treatment of post-myocardial infarction congestive heart failure should be delayed until these fundamental questions are answered.

References

1. Yao M, Dieterle T, Hale SL, Dow JS, Kedes LH, Peterson KL, Kloner RA. Long-term outcome of fetal cell transplantation on postinfarction ventricular remodeling and function. *J Mol Cell Cardiol* 2003;35(6):661–70.
2. Muller-Ehmsen J, Peterson KL, Kedes L, Whittaker P, Dow JS, Long TI, Laird PW, Kloner RA. Rebuilding a damaged heart: long-term survival of transplanted neonatal rat cardiomyocytes after myocardial infarction and effect on cardiac function. *Circulation* 2002;105(14):1720–6.
3. Matsushita T, Oyamada M, Kurata H, Masuda S, Takahashi A, Emmoto T, Shiraishi I, Wada Y, Oka T, Takamatsu T. Formation of cell junctions between grafted and host cardiomyocytes at the border zone of rat myocardial infarction. *Circulation* 1999;100(19 Suppl):II262–8.
4. Reffelmann T, Leor J, Muller-Ehmsen J, Kedes L, Kloner RA. Cardiomyocyte transplantation into the failing heart-new therapeutic approach for heart failure? *Heart Fail Rev* 2003;8 (3):201–11.
5. Kehat I, Kenyagin-Karsenti D, Snir M, Segev H, Amit M, Gepstein A, Livne E, Binah O, Itskovitz-Eldor J, Gepstein L. Human embryonic stem cells can differentiate into myocytes with structural and functional properties of cardiomyocytes. *J Clin Invest* 2001;108(3):407–14.
6. Singla DK, Hacker TA, Ma L, Douglas PS, Sullivan R, Lyons GE, Kamp TJ. Transplantation of embryonic stem cells into the infarcted mouse heart: formation of multiple cell types. *J Mol Cell Cardiol* 2006;40(1):195–200.
7. Menard C, Hagege AA, Agbulut O, Barro M, Morichetti MC, Brasselet C, Bel A, Messas E, Bissery A, Bruneval P, Desnos M, Puceat M, Menasche P. Transplantation of cardiac-committed mouse embryonic stem cells to infarcted sheep myocardium: a preclinical study. *Lancet* 2005;366(9490):1005–12.
8. Dai W, Field LJ, Hale SL, Zweigerdt R, Graichen RE, Kay GL, Jyrala AJ, Davidson B, Pera M, Kloner RA. Survival and maturation of human embryonic stem cell-derived cardiomyocytes implanted into rat hearts exposed to ischemia (abstract) *J Am Coll Cardiol* 2007;49(9)(Suppl A):233 A.
9. Messina E, De Angelis L, Frati G, Morrone S, Chimenti S, Fiordaliso F, Salio M, Battaglia M, Latronico MV, Coletta M, Vivarelli E, Frati L, Cossu G, Giacomello A. Isolation and expansion of adult cardiac stem cells from human and murine heart. *Circ Res* 2004;95(9):911–21.
10. Smith RR, Barile L, Cho HC, Leppo MK, Hare JM, Messina E, Giacomello A, Abraham MR, Marban E. Regenerative potential of cardiosphere-derived cells expanded from percutaneous endomyocardial biopsy specimens. *Circulation* 2007;115(7):896–908.
11. Dai W, Hale SL, Kloner RA. Stem cell transplantation for the treatment of myocardial infarction. *Transpl Immunol* 2005;15(2):91–97.
12. Fouts K, Fernandes B, Mal N, Liu J, Laurita KR. Electrophysiological consequence of skeletal myoblast transplantation in normal and infarcted canine myocardium. *Heart Rhythm* 2006;3(4):452–61.
13. Mills WR, Mal N, Kiedrowski MJ, Unger R, Forudi F, Popovic ZB, Penn MS, Laurita KR. Stem cell therapy enhances electrical viability in myocardial infarction. *J Mol Cell Cardiol* 2007;42(2):304–14.
14. Orlic D, Kajstura J, Chimenti S, Jakoniuk I, Anderson SM, Li B, Pickel J, McKay R, Nadal-Ginard B, Bodine DM, Leri A, Anversa P. Bone marrow cells regenerate infarcted myocardium. *Nature* 2001;410(6829):701–5.
15. Murry CE, Soonpaa MH, Reinecke H, Nakajima H, Nakajima HO, Rubart M, Pasumarthi KB, Virag JI, Bartelmez SH, Poppa V, Bradford G, Dowell JD, Williams DA, Field LJ. Haematopoietic stem cells do not transdifferentiate into cardiac myocytes in myocardial infarcts. *Nature* 2004;428(6983):664–8.
16. Dai W, Kloner RA. Myocardial regeneration by embryonic stem cell transplantation: present and future trends. *Expert Rev Cardiovasc Ther* 2006;4(3):375–83.
17. Kocher AA, Schuster MD, Szabolcs MJ, Takuma S, Burkhoff D, Wang J, Homma S, Edwards NM, Itescu S. Neovascularization of ischemic myocardium by human bone-marrow-derived

angioblasts prevents cardiomyocyte apoptosis, reduces remodeling and improves cardiac function. *Nat Med* 2001;7(4):430–6.

18. Tang YL, Zhao Q, Qin X, Shen L, Cheng L, Ge J, Phillips MI. Paracrine action enhances the effects of autologous MSC transplantation on vascular regeneration in rat model of myocardial infarction. *Ann Thorac Surg* 2005;80(1):229–36.

19. Dai W, Hale SL, Martin BJ, Kuang JQ, Dow JS, Wold LE, Kloner RA. Allogeneic mesenchymal stem cell transplantation in postinfarcted rat myocardium: short- and long-term effects. *Circulation* 2005;112(2):214–23.

20. Reffelmann T, Dow JS, Dai W, Hale SL, Simkhovich BZ, Kloner RA. Transplantation of neonatal cardiomyocytes after permanent coronary artery occlusion increases regional blood flow of infarcted myocardium. *J Mol Cell Cardiol* 2003;35(6):607–13.

21. Fujii T, Yau TM, Weisel RD, Ohno N, Mickle DA, Shiono N, Ozawa T, Matsubayashi K, Li RK. Cell transplantation to prevent heart failure: a comparison of cell types. *Ann Thorac Surg* 2003;76(6):2062–70.

22. Xu X, Xu Z, Xu Y, Cui G. Effects of mesenchymal stem cell transplantation on extracellular matrix after myocardial infarction in rats. *Coron Artery Dis* 2005;16(4):245–55.

23. Xu X, Xu Z, Xu Y, Cui G. Selective down-regulation of extracellular matrix gene expression by bone marrow derived stem cell transplantation into infarcted myocardium. *Circ J* 2005;69(10):1275–83.

24. Fazel S, Chen L, Weisel RD, Angoulvant D, Seneviratne C, Fazel A, Cheung P, Lam J, Fedak PW, Yau TM, Li RK. Cell transplantation preserves cardiac function after infarction by infarct stabilization: augmentation by stem cell factor. *J Thorac Cardiovasc Surg* 2005;130(5):1310.

25. Berry MF, Engler AJ, Woo YJ, Pirolli TJ, Bish LT, Jayasankar V, Morine KJ, Gardner TJ, Discher DE, Sweeney HL. Mesenchymal stem cell injection after myocardial infarction improves myocardial compliance. *Am J Physiol Heart Circ Physiol* 2006;290(6):H2196–203.

26. Noiseux N, Gnecchi M, Lopez-Ilasaca M, Zhang L, Solomon SD, Deb A, Dzau VJ, Pratt RE. Mesenchymal stem cells overexpressing Akt dramatically repair infarcted myocardium and improve cardiac function despite infrequent cellular fusion or differentiation. *Mol Ther* 2006;14(6):840–50.

27. Gnecchi M, He H, Noiseux N, Liang OD, Zhang L, Morello F, Mu H, Melo LG, Pratt RE, Ingwall JS, Dzau VJ. Evidence supporting paracrine hypothesis for Akt-modified mesenchymal stem cell-mediated cardiac protection and functional improvement. *FASEB J* 2006;20(6):661–9.

28. Dai W, Hale SL, Kloner RA. Role of a paracrine action of mesenchymal stem cells in the improvement of left ventricular function after coronary artery occlusion in rats. *Regen Med* 2007;2(1):63–8.

29. Pak HN, Qayyum M, Kim DT, Hamabe A, Miyauchi Y, Lill MC, Frantzen M, Takizawa K, Chen LS, Fishbein MC, Sharifi BG, Chen PS, Makkar R. Mesenchymal stem cell injection induces cardiac nerve sprouting and increased tenascin expression in a Swine model of myocardial infarction. *J Cardiovasc Electrophysiol* 2003;14(8):841–8.

30. Lin GS, Lu JJ, Jiang XJ, Li XY, Li GS. Autologous transplantation of bone marrow mononuclear cells improved heart function after myocardial infarction. *Acta Pharmacol Sin* 2004;25(7):876–86.

31. Diaz-Flores L Jr, Madrid JF, Gutierrez R, Varela H, Valladares F, Alvarez-Arguelles H, Diaz-Flores L. Adult stem and transit-amplifying cell location. *Histol Histopathol* 2006;21 (9):995–1027.

32. Mazhari R, Hare JM. Mechanisms of action of mesenchymal stem cells in cardiac repair: potential influences on the cardiac stem cell niche. *Nat Clin Pract Cardiovasc Med* 2007;4(1 Suppl):S21–6.

33. Mizuno T, Yau TM, Weisel RD, Kiani CG, Li RK. Elastin stabilizes an infarct and preserves ventricular function. *Circulation* 2005;112(9 Suppl):I81–8.

34. Yau TM, Kim C, Li G, Zhang Y, Fazel S, Spiegelstein D, Weisel RD, Li RK. Enhanced angiogenesis with multimodal cell-based gene therapy. *Ann Thorac Surg* 2007;83(3):1110–9.

35. Miyagawa S, Sawa Y, Fukuda K, Hisaka Y, Taketani S, Memon IA, Matsuda H. Angiogenic gene cell therapy using suicide gene system regulates the effect of angiogenesis in infarcted rat heart. *Transplantation* 2006;81(6):902–7.

36. Swijnenburg RJ, Tanaka M, Vogel H, Baker J, Kofidis T, Gunawan F, Lebl DR, Caffarelli AD, de Bruin JL, Fedoseyeva EV, Robbins RC. Embryonic stem cell immunogenicity increases upon differentiation after transplantation into ischemic myocardium. *Circulation* 2005;112(9 Suppl):I166–72.

37. Cao F, Lin S, Xie X, Ray P, Patel M, Zhang X, Drukker M, Dylla SJ, Connolly AJ, Chen X, Weissman IL, Gambhir SS, Wu JC. In vivo visualization of embryonic stem cell survival, proliferation, and migration after cardiac delivery. *Circulation* 2006;113(7):1005–14.

38. Grinnemo KH, Mansson-Broberg A, Leblanc K, Corbascio M, Wardell E, Siddiqui AJ, Hao X, Sylven C, Dellgren G. Human mesenchymal stem cells do not differentiate into cardiomyocytes in a cardiac ischemic xenomodel. *Ann Med* 2006;38(2):144–53.

39. Ribeiro KC, Mattos EC, Werneck-de-castro JP, Ribeiro VP, Costa-e-Sousa RH, Miranda A, Olivares EL, Farina M, Mill JG, Goldenberg JR, Masuda MO, de Carvalho AC. Ectopic ossification in the scar tissue of rats with myocardial infarction. *Cell Transplant* 2006;15(5):389–97.

40. Yoon YS, Park JS, Tkebuchava T, Luedeman C, Losordo DW. Unexpected severe calcification after transplantation of bone marrow cells in acute myocardial infarction. *Circulation* 2004;109(25):3154–7.

41. Chiavegato A, Bollini S, Pozzobon M, Callegari A, Gasparotto L, Taiani J, Piccoli M, Lenzini E, Gerosa G, Vendramin I, Cozzi E, Angelini A, Iop L, Zanon GF, Atala A, De Coppi P, Sartore S. Human amniotic fluid-derived stem cells are rejected after transplantation in the myocardium of normal, ischemic, immuno-suppressed or immuno-deficient rat. *J Mol Cell Cardiol* 2007;42(4):746–59.

42. Heng BC, Haider HKh, Sim EK, Cao T, Ng SC. Strategies for directing the differentiation of stem cells into the cardiomyogenic lineage in vitro. *Cardiovasc Res* 2004;62(1):34–42.

43. Bartunek J, Croissant JD, Wijns W, Gofflot S, de Lavareille A, Vanderheyden M, Kaluzhny Y, Mazouz N, Willemsen P, Penicka M, Mathieu M, Homsy C, De Bruyne B, McEntee K, Lee IW, Heyndrickx GR. Pretreatment of adult bone marrow mesenchymal stem cells with cardiomyogenic growth factors and repair of the chronically infarcted myocardium. *Am J Physiol Heart Circ Physiol* 2007;292(2):H1095–104.

44. Kofidis T, de Bruin JL, Yamane T, Tanaka M, Lebl DR, Swijnenburg RJ, Weissman IL, Robbins RC. Stimulation of paracrine pathways with growth factors enhances embryonic stem cell engraftment and host-specific differentiation in the heart after ischemic myocardial injury. *Circulation* 2005;111(19):2486–93.

45. Sachinidis A, Fleischmann BK, Kolossov E, Wartenberg M, Sauer H, Hescheler J. Cardiac specific differentiation of mouse embryonic stem cells. *Cardiovasc Res* 2003;58(2):278–91.

46. Lev S, Kehat I, Gepstein L. Differentiation pathways in human embryonic stem cell-derived cardiomyocytes. *Ann N Y Acad Sci* 2005;1047:50–65.

47. Grinnemo KH, Mansson A, Dellgren G, Klingberg D, Wardell E, Drvota V, Tammik C, Holgersson J, Ringden O, Sylven C, Le Blanc K. Xenoreactivity and engraftment of human mesenchymal stem cells transplanted into infarcted rat myocardium. *J Thorac Cardiovasc Surg* 2004;127(5):1293–300.

48. Lanza R, Moore MA, Wakayama T, Perry AC, Shieh JH, Hendrikx J, Leri A, Chimenti S, Monsen A, Nurzynska D, West MD, Kajstura J, Anversa P. Regeneration of the infarcted heart with stem cells derived by nuclear transplantation. *Circ Res* 2004;94(6):820–7.

49. Hagege AA, Marolleau JP, Vilquin JT, Alheritiere A, Peyrard S, Duboc D, Abergel E, Messas E, Mousseaux E, Schwartz K, Desnos M, Menasche P. Skeletal myoblast transplantation in ischemic heart failure: long-term follow-up of the first phase I cohort of patients. *Circulation* 2006;114(1 Suppl):I108–13.

50. Zhang YM, Hartzell C, Narlow M, Dudley SC Jr. Stem cell-derived cardiomyocytes demonstrate arrhythmic potential. *Circulation* 2002;106(10):1294–9.

51. Chang MG, Tung L, Sekar RB, Chang CY, Cysyk J, Dong P, Marban E, Abraham MR. Proarrhythmic potential of mesenchymal stem cell transplantation revealed in an in vitro coculture model. *Circulation* 2006;113(15):1832–41.

52. Al Attar N, Carrion C, Ghostine S, Garcin I, Vilquin JT, Hagege AA, Menasche P. Long-term (1 year) functional and histological results of autologous skeletal muscle cells transplantation in rat. *Cardiovasc Res* 2003;58(1):142–8.

53. Fernandes S, Amirault JC, Lande G, Nguyen JM, Forest V, Bignolais O, Lamirault G, Heudes D, Orsonneau JL, Heymann MF, Charpentier F, Lemarchand P. Autologous myoblast transplantation after myocardial infarction increases the inducibility of ventricular arrhythmias. *Cardiovasc Res* 2006;69(2):348–58.

54. Makkar RR, Lill M, Chen PS. Stem cell therapy for myocardial repair: is it arrhythmogenic? *J Am Coll Cardiol* 2003;42(12):2070–2.

55. Kolettis TM. Arrhythmogenesis after cell transplantation post-myocardial infarction. Four burning questions–and some answers. *Cardiovasc Res* 2006;69(2):299–301.

56. Gepstein L, Feld Y, Yankelson L. Somatic gene and cell therapy strategies for the treatment of cardiac arrhythmias. *Am J Physiol Heart Circ Physiol 2004*;286:H815–22.

57. Abraham MR, Henrikson CA, Tung L, Chang MG, Aon M, Xue T, Li RA, O' Rourke B, Marban E. Antiarrhythmic engineering of skeletal myoblasts for cardiac transplantation. *Circ Res* 2005;97(2):159–67.

58. Yeh ET, Zhang S, Wu HD, Korbling M, Willerson JT, Estrov Z. Transdifferentiation of human peripheral blood CD34 + -enriched cell population into cardiomyocytes, endothelial cells, and smooth muscle cells in vivo. *Circulation* 2003;108(17):2070–3.

59. Nygren JM, Jovinge S, Breitbach M, Sawen P, Roll W, Hescheler J, Taneera J, Fleischmann BK, Jacobsen SE. Bone marrow-derived hematopoietic cells generate cardiomyocytes at a low frequency through cell fusion, but not transdifferentiation. *Nat Med* 2004;10(5):494–501.

60. Zhang S, Wang D, Estrov Z, Raj S, Willerson JT, Yeh ET. Both cell fusion and transdifferentiation account for the transformation of human peripheral blood CD34-positive cells into cardiomyocytes in vivo. *Circulation* 2004;110(25):3803–7.

61. Muller-Ehmsen J, Krausgrill B, Burst V, Schenk K, Neisen UC, Fries JW, Fleischmann BK, Hescheler J, Schwinger RH. Effective engraftment but poor mid-term persistence of mononuclear and mesenchymal bone marrow cells in acute and chronic rat myocardial infarction. *J Mol Cell Cardiol* 2006;41(5):876–84.

62. Dow J, Simkhovich BZ, Kedes L, Kloner RA. Washout of transplanted cells from the heart: a potential new hurdle for cell transplantation therapy. *Cardiovasc Res* 2005;67(2):301–7.

63. Liu TB, Fedak PW, Weisel RD, Yasuda T, Kiani G, Mickle DA, Jia ZQ, Li RK. Enhanced IGF-1 expression improves smooth muscle cell engraftment after cell transplantation. *Am J Physiol Heart Circ Physiol* 2004;287(6):H2840–9.

64. Nakamura Y, Yasuda T, Weisel RD, Li RK. Enhanced cell transplantation: preventing apoptosis increases cell survival and ventricular function. *Am J Physiol Heart Circ Physiol* 2006;291(2):H939–47.

65. Tang YL, Tang Y, Zhang YC, Qian K, Shen L, Phillips MI. Improved graft mesenchymal stem cell survival in ischemic heart with a hypoxia-regulated heme oxygenase-1 vector. *J Am Coll Cardiol* 2005;46(7):1339–50.

66. Lim SY, Kim YS, Ahn Y, Jeong MH, Hong MH, Joo SY, Nam KI, Cho JG, Kang PM, Park JC. The effects of mesenchymal stem cells transduced with Akt in a porcine myocardial infarction model. *Cardiovasc Res* 2006;70(3):530–42.

67. Jiang S, Haider HKh, Idris NM, Salim A, Ashraf M. Supportive interaction between cell survival signaling and angiocompetent factors enhances donor cell survival and promotes angiomyogenesis for cardiac repair. *Circ Res* 2006;99(7):776–84.

68. Song H, Kwon K, Lim S, Kang SM, Ko YG, Xu Z, Chung JH, Kim BS, Lee H, Joung B, Park S, Choi D, Jang Y, Chung NS, Yoo KJ, Hwang KC. Transfection of mesenchymal stem cells with the FGF-2 gene improves their survival under hypoxic conditions. *Mol Cells* 2005;19(3):402–7.

69. Yau TM, Kim C, Li G, Zhang Y, Weisel RD, Li RK. Maximizing ventricular function with multimodal cell-based gene therapy. *Circulation* 2005;112(9 Suppl):I123–8.

70. Bonaros N, Rauf R, Wolf D, Margreiter E, Tzankov A, Schlechta B, Kocher A, Ott H, Schachner T, Hering S, Bonatti J, Laufer G. Combined transplantation of skeletal myoblasts and angiopoietic progenitor cells reduces infarct size and apoptosis and improves cardiac function in chronic ischemic heart failure. *J Thorac Cardiovasc Surg* 2006;132(6):1321–8.

71. Wang Y, Tang H, Wang D, Li R, Dong Y, Liu W, Zhang X. Pretreatment with transmyocardial revascularization might improve ischemic myocardial function performed with cell transplantation. *Circ J* 2006;70(5):625–30.
72. Niagara MI, Haider HKh, Jiang S, Ashraf M. Pharmacologically preconditioned skeletal myoblasts are resistant to oxidative stress and promote angiomyogenesis via release of paracrine factors in the infarcted heart. *Circ Res* 2007;100(4):545–55.
73. Davis ME, Hsieh PC, Takahashi T, Song Q, Zhang S, Kamm RD, Grodzinsky AJ, Anversa P, Lee RT. Local myocardial insulin-like growth factor 1 (IGF-1) delivery with biotinylated peptide nanofibers improves cell therapy for myocardial infarction. *Proc Natl Acad Sci U S A* 2006;103(21):8155–60.
74. Kutschka I, Chen IY, Kofidis T, Arai T, von Degenfeld G, Sheikh AY, Hendry SL, Pearl J, Hoyt G, Sista R, Yang PC, Blau HM, Gambhir SS, Robbins RC. Collagen matrices enhance survival of transplanted cardiomyoblasts and contribute to functional improvement of ischemic rat hearts. *Circulation* 2006;114(1 Suppl):I167–73.
75. Vulliet PR, Greeley M, Halloran SM, MacDonald KA, Kittleson MD. Intra-coronary arterial injection of mesenchymal stromal cells and microinfarction in dogs. *Lancet* 2004;363(9411):783–4.
76. Kang HJ, Kim HS, Zhang SY, Park KW, Cho HJ, Koo BK, Kim YJ, Soo Lee D, Sohn DW, Han KS, Oh BH, Lee MM, Park YB. Effects of intracoronary infusion of peripheral blood stem-cells mobilised with granulocyte-colony stimulating factor on left ventricular systolic function and restenosis after coronary stenting in myocardial infarction: the MAGIC cell randomised clinical trial. *Lancet* 2004;363(9411):751–6.
77. Steinwender C, Hofmann R, Kammler J, Kypta A, Pichler R, Maschek W, Schuster G, Gabriel C, Leisch F. Effects of peripheral blood stem cell mobilization with granulocyte-colony stimulating factor and their transcoronary transplantation after primary stent implantation for acute myocardial infarction. *Am Heart J* 2006;151(6):1296.e7–13.
78. Siminiak T, Kalawski R, Fiszer D, Jerzykowska O, Rzezniczak J, Rozwadowska N, Kurpisz M. Autologous skeletal myoblast transplantation for the treatment of postinfarction myocardial injury: phase I clinical study with 12 months of follow-up. *Am Heart J* 2004;148(3):531–7.
79. Schachinger V, Erbs S, Elsasser A, Haberbosch W, Hambrecht R, Holschermann H, Yu J, Corti R, Mathey DG, Hamm CW, Suselbeck T, Assmus B, Tonn T, Dimmeler S, Zeiher AM. Intracoronary bone marrow-derived progenitor cells in acute myocardial infarction. *N Engl J Med* 2006;355(12):1210–21.
80. Assmus B, Honold J, Schachinger V, Britten MB, Fischer-Rasokat U, Lehmann R, Teupe C, Pistorius K, Martin H, Abolmaali ND, Tonn T, Dimmeler S, Zeiher AM. Transcoronary transplantation of progenitor cells after myocardial infarction. *N Engl J Med* 2006;355(12):1222–32.
81. Lunde K, Solheim S, Aakhus S, Arnesen H, Abdelnoor M, Egeland T, Endresen K, Ilebekk A, Mangschau A, Fjeld JG, Smith HJ, Taraldsrud E, Grogaard HK, Bjornerheim R, Brekke M, Muller C, Hopp E, Ragnarsson A, Brinchmann JE, Forfang K. Intracoronary injection of mononuclear bone marrow cells in acute myocardial infarction. *N Engl J Med* 2006;355(12):1199–209.
82. Meyer GP, Wollert KC, Lotz J, Steffens J, Lippolt P, Fichtner S, Hecker H, Schaefer A, Arseniev L, Hertenstein B, Ganser A, Drexler H. Intracoronary bone marrow cell transfer after myocardial infarction: eighteen months' follow-up data from the randomized, controlled BOOST (BOne marrOw transfer to enhance ST-elevation infarct regeneration) trial. *Circulation* 2006;113(10):1287–94.
83. Ince H, Petzsch M, Kleine HD, Eckard H, Rehders T, Burska D, Kische S, Freund M, Nienaber CA. Prevention of left ventricular remodeling with granulocyte colony-stimulating factor after acute myocardial infarction: final 1-year results of the Front-Integrated Revascularization and Stem Cell Liberation in Evolving Acute Myocardial Infarction by Granulocyte Colony-Stimulating Factor (FIRSTLINE-AMI) Trial. *Circulation* 2005;112(9 Suppl):I73–80.
84. Zohlnhofer D, Ott I, Mehilli J, Schomig K, Michalk F, Ibrahim T, Meisetschlager G, von Wedel J, Bollwein H, Seyfarth M, Dirschinger J, Schmitt C, Schwaiger M, Kastrati A, Schomig A; REVIVAL-2 Investigators. Stem cell mobilization by granulocyte colony-stimulating factor in

patients with acute myocardial infarction: a randomized controlled trial. *JAMA* 2006;295(9):1003–10.

85. Kloner RA. Attempts to recruit stem cells for repair of acute myocardial infarction: a dose of reality. *JAMA* 2006;295(9):1058–60.

86. Ripa RS, Jorgensen E, Wang Y, Thune JJ, Nilsson JC, Sondergaard L, Johnsen HE, Kober L, Grande P, Kastrup J. Stem cell mobilization induced by subcutaneous granulocyte-colony stimulating factor to improve cardiac regeneration after acute ST-elevation myocardial infarction: result of the double-blind, randomized, placebo-controlled stem cells in myocardial infarction (STEMMI) trial. *Circulation* 2006;113(16):1983–92.

Chapter 12
Surgical Stem Cell Therapy for the Treatment of Heart Failure

Federico Benetti[1]*, Luis Geffner[2], Daniel Brusich[3], Agustin Fronzutti[3], Roberto Paganini[3], Juan Paganini[3], and Amit Patel[4]

Abstract Congestive heart failure (CHF) is a complex clinical syndrome resulting from myocardial dysfunction that impairs the cardiovascular system's function. Both medical and surgical therapy still results in a large number of patients with very few options and persistent ventricular dysfunction. The major process to reverse ventricular remodeling would be the enhancement of regeneration of cardiac myocytes, as well as the stimulation of neovascularization within the affected area of the myocardium. This can be achieved by introducing progenitor cells that are capable of differentiating into cardiac myocytes or that promote neovascularization and restore the normal characteristics of myocardium environment. However a number of issues remain as to the type of cells, delivery, timing, and mechanisms involved. There have been a number of clinical trials based on very early small and large animal experiments that investigate stem cell therapy for heart failure, most of which have employed bone marrow stem cells or myoblasts. The majority of studies demonstrate an improvement in ventricular function, reduction in scar, or improvement in symptoms. There are a few trials that show no improvement at all. Here we present our surgical experience over the past 4 years with autologous and fetal liver stem cells in patients with heart failure.

Keywords Stem cell, heart failure, regeneration

---

[1] President, Benetti Foundation, Rosario, Argentina

[2] Director, Stem cell Program, Junta de Beneficencia, Guayaquil, Ecuador

[3] Cardiac Surgical and Heart Failure Department, Asociacion Espanola, Montevideo, Uruguay

[4] University of Pittsburgh, McGowan Institute for Regenerative Medicine; Consultant, Benetti Foundation, Rosario, Argentina

* Corresponding Author:
e-mail: federicobenetti@hotmail.com

Y. Shi, D.O. Clegg (eds.) *Stem Cell Research and Therapeutics*,
© Springer Science+Business Media B.V. 2008

12.1   Introduction

Congestive heart failure (CHF) is a complex clinical syndrome that results from myocardial dysfunction that impairs the heart's ability to circulate blood at a rate sufficient to maintain the metabolic needs of peripheral tissues and various organs. Heart failure is a relatively common clinical disorder, estimated to affect more than 5 million patients in the United States, and it remains the predominant cause of mortality in the western world. About 400,000 new patients are diagnosed with CHF each year. Morbidity and mortality rates are high; annually, approximately 900,000 patients require hospitalization for CHF, and up to 200,000 patients die from this condition. The average annual mortality rate is 40–50% in patients with severe (New York Heart Association [NYHA] class IV) heart failure. In the United States CHF treatment is estimated to cost more than 25 billion dollars for 2004 [1]. CHF has multiple etiologies including ischemic myocardial disease, the main cause of heart failure, and infective agents such as bacteria, viruses and protozoa. The protozoa Trypanosome cruzi is the causative agent of Chagas disease. Chagas disease may also be transmitted through blood transfusion and to the newborn from infected mothers. Trypanosome cruzi infects 10–18 million people in the Americas [2] and infection leads to a myocarditis with immunological pathogenesis that results in CHF. CHF is the natural evolution of a good part of Chagas patients. A progressive destruction of the myocardium occurs in approximately 30% of infected persons [3].

   CHF is a systemic disease that affects many different organs including activation of the immune system with release of proinflammatory cytokines, activation of the complement system, and production of antibodies [4]. Animals with CHF after a prior myocardial infarction show a reduced immune response to an inflammatory challenge [5]. Inflammatory mediators are important in the pathogenesis and maintenance of CHF, contributing to cardiac remodeling and peripheral vascular disturbances. An imbalance in favor of inflammatory cytokines, such as tumor necrosis factor alpha (TNF-alpha), interleukin (IL)-1beta and IL-6 is present in both plasma and circulating leukocytes and the myocardium itself [6]. Considering the natural release of proinflammatory cytokines in infectious myocarditis that progress to CHF, it is very important in that the potential direct or indirect immunomudolatory effects of transplanted cells may have on progression of the disease [3].

   The initial stages of heart failure are managed with medical therapy, and end-stage heart failure is managed with surgical procedures in addition to medical therapy. Some of the proven surgical procedures include myocardial revascularization, ventricular assist devices, and heart transplantation [7]. Although surgical and catheter-based revascularization of ischemic myocardium can treat angina, reduce the risk of myocardial infarction, and improve function of viable myocardium, the viability of severely ischemic myocardium, necrotic myocardium, or both cannot be restored. The major process to reverse the left ventricular remodeling would be the enhancement of regeneration of cardiac myocytes, as well as the stimulation of neovascularization within the affected area of the myocardium [8]. Thus the aim of cardiac cellular transplantation is to repopulate the ailing myocardium with cells that could restore contractility and blood supply. This can be achieved by introducing progenitor cells that are capable of differentiating into cardiac myocytes or that promote neovascularization or generate a favorable atmosphere for native stem cell proliferation and differentiation via release of pro-homeostatic cytokines.

12.2 Stem Cells and Chronic Heart Failure

Recently the concept has been accepted that the heart is no longer considered a post-mitotic organ, and this condition is particularly important in relation to new therapeutic possibilities. Like other organs, the heart contains resident stem cells [9–12], some of them with recognized proliferative activity, similar to blood [13] and other, more static tissues such as the central nervous system [14]. Cardiac stem cells have been isolated from human and murine hearts and well characterized [15]. Cytokines that control of cardiac stem cells through positive autocrine loops have also been described [16]. However, the progression of CHF in patients demonstrates that, even in presence of native stem cells, self-renewal of the myocardium is, at least, an insufficient mechanism to resolve the damage incurred in the heart. The changes in regional environment, including vascularization, extracellular matrix and cytokine profiles, could act synergistically to stimulate the heart's regenerative capacity, but often resident stem cells are also lost. CHF maybe suitable for treatment by stem cell transplantation, especially in elderly patients, where the population of resident stem cells is reduced. In humans, regeneration is reduced in favor of reparation and efficient wound healing with scar formation. This resolution is a complex and multifactor process. A defective resolution will result in temporary compensatory mechanisms that at some moment start a cascade that will progress to decreased cardiac function and eventually CHF.

At the beginning of the process and especially after acute damage, it is highly possible that the recruitment of other stem cells, circulating and mostly originating in the bone marrow, help to generate structures other than cardiac muscle to restore the regional architecture and to generate the adequate niche for native and migrating stem cells. An adequate level of inflammation, with reparative characteristics should be critical not only to limit the local necrosis but also to support regulatory cytokines and generate a facilitating environment. For reasons that are unclear, this process is unstable and the generation of neo-tissues and the reparative character of the inflammatory process are insufficient to achieve the *restituto ad-integrum*. The lesion size in which these mechanisms are efficient is unclear and may not have clinical relevance. The formation of connective tissue is prevalent. Immune activation by direct antigenic stimulation secondary to cardiac injury, due in part to generation of neo-antigens, together with a cytokine imbalance [4] may increase heart damage. The imbalance of this inflammatory process could be very important in infectious myocarditis.

The use of stem cells for the treatment of CHF may provide exogenous stem cells to improve the ineffective reparative activity and reduce or avoid the associated processes mentioned above that increase cardiac damage. These cells not only should have a replacement effect but also will modify the myocardial environment that influences the physiology of resident cells. This action will be mainly mediated by cytokine secretion, including angiogenic, antiapoptotic and mitogenic factors. These cytokines could be secreted by the injected or recruited cells in a paracrine action, as has been demonstrated after bone marrow-mesenchymal derived stem cells injection [17], with a direct effect on resident cells and their autocrine circuits.

Many different types of cells have been studied in a large body of animal research and many others have been applied in patients, most of them in the immediate period after an acute infarct. Although there are a number of cells that have been used in a variety of cardiac disorders, the experience in CHF is more limited and mostly restricted to bone-marrow cells and myoblasts. It has been well established that adult bone marrow is a rich reservoir of tissue-specific stem and progenitor cells. Several studies have shown that bone marrow–derived cells functionally contribute to neoangiogenesis during wound healing and limb ischemia [18–23], postmyocardial infarction [24–29], endothelialization of vascular grafts [30–33], atherosclerosis [34], retinal and lymphoid organ neovascularization [35–37], and vascularization during neonatal growth [38]. It is well known that adult bone marrow cells can differentiate into different cell lineages, including cardiac cell lineages [39], although it is still a question if these cells are homogeneous population or heterogeneous sub-population s of tissue-committed stem cells [40]. In human subjects, whole autologous bone marrow mononuclear cells have been delivered by means of arterial and venous catheters into the coronary vessels feeding the infarcted and ischemic tissue [41–44], by transendocardial injections [45], by guided electrochemical mapping directly into infarcted myocardium [46, 47], by stem cells mobilization or by direct epicardial injections [48]. The use of cytokines to mimic the natural stem cells mobilization after a cardiac injury should be considered carefully by evaluating the risk of adverse events and the theoretical tumorogenesis induced by agents closely associated with natural oncogenesis [49]. In another study the efficacy of the *ex vivo* expanded peripheral blood mononuclear cells was compared with bone marrow–derived endothelial progenitor cells in restoring revascularization after acute myocardial infarction [50]. In all of these studies, there was improved blood flow and left ventricular function, suggesting that infusion of autologous progenitor cells appears to be feasible and safe and might confer a short-term therapeutic benefit [51]. Bone-marrow mononuclear cell fraction increased collateral neovascularization in infarcted hearts and significantly improved cardiac function in acute (6 hours) and chronic (4 weeks) myocardium infarction with a significant increases of vascular endothelial growth factor (VEGF) and basic fibroblast growth factor (FGF2) after cell implantation. The presence of proliferative and activated myocardial cells in infarcted hearts has also been reported [29]. Bone-marrow derived cell injection has positive effects on the affected myocardium and the extra cellular matrix. In a rat model the injection of bone-marrow mesenchymal stem cells significantly increased capillary density and decreased the collagen volume fraction in the myocardium, resulting in decreased left ventricular end-diastolic pressure and increased left ventricular maximum dP/dt [52]. It is pertinent to note that cell therapy in cardiac disease is not only oriented to restore an efficient systole but also diastole, resulting in improved ventricular compliance.

Unlike myoblasts, bone-marrow stem cells have not been associated with arrhythmia episodes [53]. This safety issue associated with the relatively easy access to cell source and the lack of tissue culture make bone-marrow cells a first option in cardiac cell therapy. The cells may be delivered by means of direct surgical injection, intracoronary infusion, retrograde venous infusion, and transendocardial injection. Stem cells may directly increase cardiac contractility or passively limit infarct expansion and remodeling. Cell therapy is generally well tolerated, but the potential for accelerated atherogenesis remains a concern. Postmortem findings, 11 months after treatment, in the injection site of autologous bone-marrow cells suggested similar results in humans and in animal models: an active process of angiogenesis in the cicatricial tissue and adjacent myocardium [54]. Negative findings in the myocardium or local vessels have not been reported. Bone-marrow derived mesenchymal stem-cells have been used preferentially in the acute ischemia model. However, data from animal studies suggest an equivalent beneficial effect in chronic disease [55]. Additionally, bone marrow cells injected intravenously into chronic chagasic mice migrated to the heart and caused a significant reduction in the inflammatory infiltrates and in the interstitial fibrosis. After intravenous injection, a massive apoptosis of myocardial inflammatory cells was observed [3]. Another potential alternative is the use of combined cell therapies. Considering the most angiogenic effects of bone-marrow cells in relation to contractile enhancing of myoblasts injections, a mixed cell treatment has been proposed. A recent report showed that a combined autologous cell therapy induced both myogenesis and angiogenesis with enhancement of cardiac performance and reduction of cardiac remodeling which has a potential direct effect in resolution of CHF [56].

In spite of the therapeutic efficacy of bone-marrow stem cells in humans and the huge amount of data available in different animal models, some studies have presented negative results [57–59]. A pilot trial that included 5 patients with chronic ischemic cardiomyopathy that were treated with intracoronary transplantation of autologous, mononuclear bone-marrow cells did not show that any significant improvement in myocardial function and physical performance occurred after 1 year after treatment [60]. It should be mentioned that there are a number of well-documented technical issues and variables, in both basic research and clinical studies that need to be considered when evaluating outcomes of cell therapy [61]. The technical modality used to implant the cells appears to have influence on the efficacy of bone-marrow cell transplants. In an animal model it has been reported that bone-marrow cells injected intramyocardially are more effective than those delivered intravenously for inducing angiogenesis and repair of injured myocardium [62]. Intracoronary and endoventricular catheter-based cell delivery procedures have been clinically performed [46, 63, 64]. These studies reinforce the necessity to develop efficient injection devices for intramyocardial injection in patients with non-immediate indication of thoracotomy. The type of cell chosen and the addition of cytokines are other unresolved issues. Cardiac cell therapy with granulocyte-colony stimulating factor (G-CSF) mobilized bone-marrow stem-cells (CD 34+) has been shown to improve ventricular function in patients with more than 1 year old myocardial infraction [65]. In a similar manner, subepicardial autologous stem cells (CD 34+) led to significant improvement in cardiac function in patients with ischemic cardiomyopathy with an ejection fraction of less than 35% undergoing off-pump coronary artery bypass grafting. The use of G-SCF as a mobilizer of bone-marrow derived stem cells into the circulation has been used in patients with chronic heart failure due to dilated or ischemic cardiomyopathy as an alternative to avoid injection of cells. This strategy has shown to have therapeutic effects in 9 to 12 patients with increased risk of angina and arrhythmias in the group of patients with ischemic cardiomyopathy [66]. The use of genetically modified cells in combination with an artificial myocardial patch developed by tissue-engineering technologies may be the next generation of cardiac cell therapy.

12.3 Surgical Implantation of Autologous Bone Marrow Stem Cells and Fetal Liver Stem Cells

From March 2003–2007, we surgically treated 29 heart failure patients with stem cells injections; 19 of them received autologous bone marrow stem cells and 10 received fetal liver stem cells. The origin and characterization of these cells is described below.

To obtain autologous bone marrow stem cells, the bone marrow was placed in a blood collection bag with 5,000 units of sodium heparin and kept on ice. We also added 400 micromoles of lysine acetvlsalicvlate, to avoid platelet clumping. Once the harvest was completed, an aliquot of the sample was sent for hematocrit, leukocyte, mononuclear cell, CD34+ and CD34+, CD45-counts. The bone marrow was processed and FACS analysis performed to obtain CD 34+ /CD 45- cells. If cells were used more than 4 hours after harvest, they were processed in a refrigerated laminar flow hood at 4°C to increase longevity and decrease contamination risks. The cells were washed twice by adding 500 ml normal saline with an identical centrifugal procedure. After the last washing, cells were resuspended in 50 ml of saline, and final CD 34+ and CD34+ /CD45- counts were performed.

Fetal liver cells were harvested from 5 to 12 weeks of gestation fetuses obtained from non compensated donors with ectopic pregnancy or spontaneous abortion, provided by the Institute of Regenerative Medicine Barbados. The tissue was obtained under full Ethical Committee approval at the Institute for Problems in Cryobiology in Kharkov, Ukraine. Fetal liver was disrupted using a fine gauge sterile stainless steel mesh, followed by repeated aspiration via syringe. The single cell suspension thus formed was centrifuged cells were resuspended in freezing medium. A serum-free sucrose-based medium was used in the study containing 5% DMSO as a penetrating cryoprotectant. The cells were cooled down to −40°C with a low (−1°C/min) rate, with equilibration at −27°C, then down to −80°C with high (−10°C/min) rate, after which they were plunged into liquid nitrogen. The thawing was performed in a 37°C water bath. The viability of the cell preparations was determined using trypan blue exclusion.

The specific cell phenotype contained with each cell preparation was determined using CD34 (marker for hematopoietic progenitor cells), CD 133 (considered to be a marker of more primitive hematopoietic stem cells), CD45 (expressed by all myeloid and lymphoid committed cells as well as by some erythroid progenitor cells) and glycophorin-A (Gly-A: expressed by committed erythroid cell precursors and mature red blood cells). The proportion of cell types analyzed in an human fetal liver preparation: CD34⁻ cells 0.89 ± 0.09%, CD45⁻ cells 2.33 ± 0.25%. The CD34+CD45+cell fraction comprised 0.82 ± 0.09%. Gly-A⁺ cells comprised 90.0 ± 2.54% and CD133⁺ cell content was 0.39 ± 0.07%. The majority (>70%) of the CD133⁺ cells co-expressed CD34.

Patients were divided into 3 groups. The first group (15 patients) included patients with ischemic heart disease that were treated with an off-pump coronary artery bypass (OPCAB) or minimally invasive direct coronary artery bypass (MIDCAB) operation plus implantation of autologous bone marrow stem cells. The second group consisted of 4 patients with non-ischemic idiopathic myocadiopathy that were treated by surgical injection of autologous bone marrow stem cells using a minimally invasive thoracoscopic procedure. The third group consisted of 10 patients with idiopathic myocardiopathy that were treated by surgical injection of fetal liver cells (9 through sternotomy, 1 via minithoracotomy).

In the first group of ischemic patients, 1 patient passed away immediately post operation due to heart failure. In the idiopathic myocardiopathy group, all survived the operation with both types of cells. In the long term follow up at 4 years, 4 patients in the ischemic group had died; 3 from heart failure and 1 from a pulmonary infection. All of the idiopathic myocardiopathy patients treated with autologous bone marrow stem cells were alive after 3 years. In the group of idiopathic myocardiopathy patients treated with fetal liver stem cells, 4 patients died after 2 years and 7 months; 3 from cardiac causes and 1 from complications of diabetes.

Figures 12.1–12.3 show that the postoperative ejection fraction (EF) is clearly greater than the preoperative level after 1, 2 and 3 years. The probability of survival is presented in Fig. 12.4 (autologous bone marrow stem cells) and Fig. 12.5 (fetal liver stem cells).

12.4   Conclusion

In summary, surgical cell therapy is a new alternative or adjunct for CHF treatment with incredible possibilities. Some evidence gives hope for the possibility to change the natural course of heart failure from different etiologies. However, cardiac cell therapies, and especially CHF cell therapy, are in the early frontier of knowledge and many questions remain to be answered until an ideal cell treatment for each

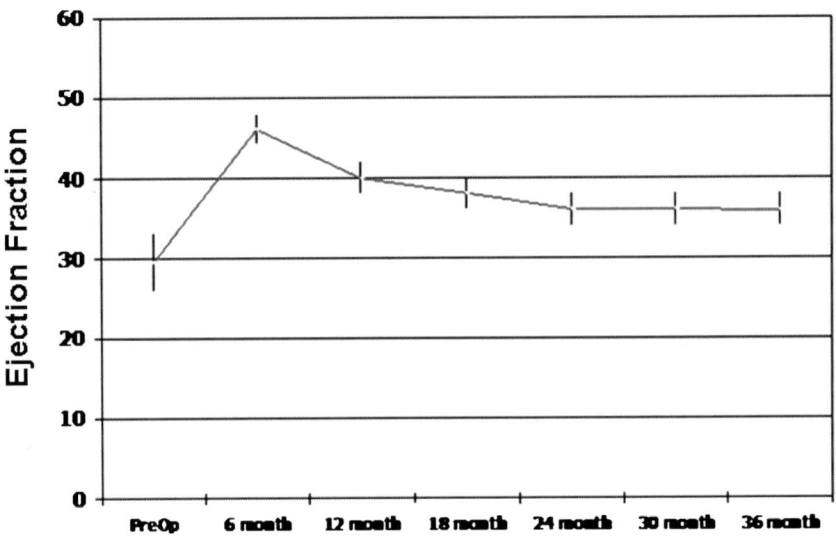

Fig. 12.1 Cardiac function in group 1 patients. These patients received a transplantation of autologous bone marrow stem cells plus coronary surgery off pump (OPCAB and MIDCAB). Ejection fraction is plotted versus time after surgery (*See Color Plates*)

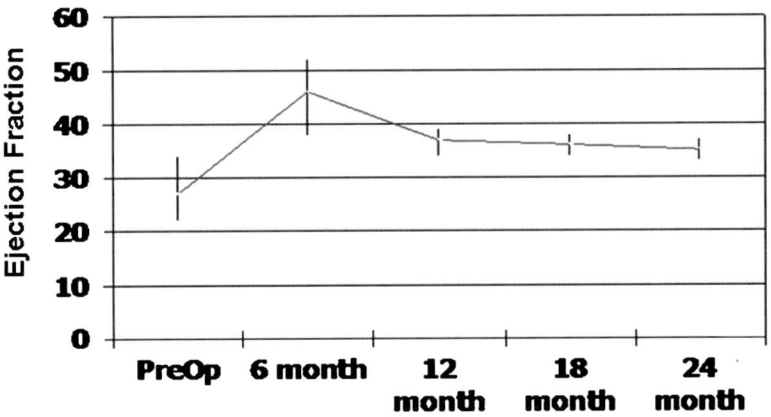

Fig. 12.2 Cardiac function in group 2 patients. Idiopathic non-ischemic cardiomyopathy patients were treated with autologous bone marrow stem cells. Ejection fraction is plotted versus time after surgery (*See Color Plates*)

patient is found. The choices of cell type, or cell combination, mode of cell delivery, cytokines, scaffold material or genetic modification of cells are just some of the questions to answer. The definition of target patient population for treatment that would be universal is not a minor problem. Only the application of rigorous scientific methodology, from observation to experimentation, a careful evaluation of

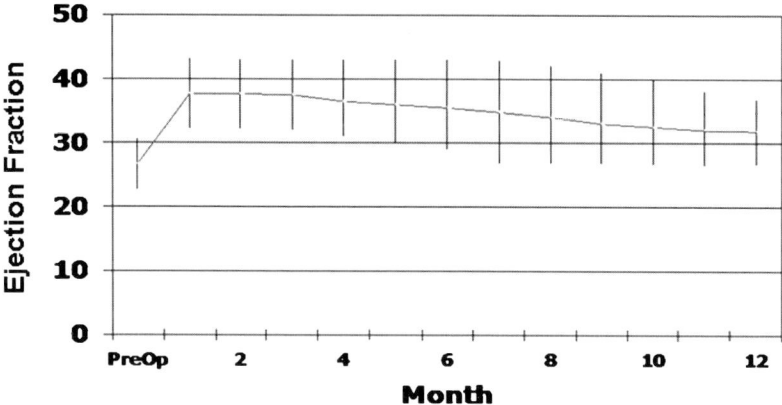

Fig. 12.3 Cardiac function in group 3 patients. Idiopathic non-ischemic cardiomyopathy patients were treated with fetal liver stem cells. Ejection fraction is plotted versus time after surgery (*See Color Plates*)

Fig. 12.4 Survival of patients treated with autologous bone marrow stem cells. The fraction surviving is plotted versus post operative time (*See Color Plates*)

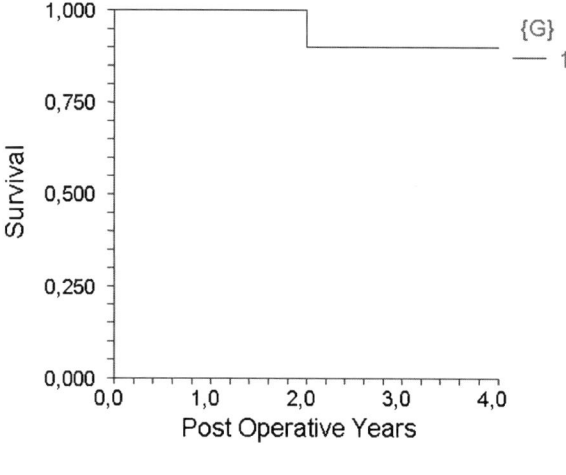

Survival Plot

Fig. 12.5 Survival of patients treated with fetal liver stem cells. The fraction surviving is plotted versus post operative time (*See Color Plates*)

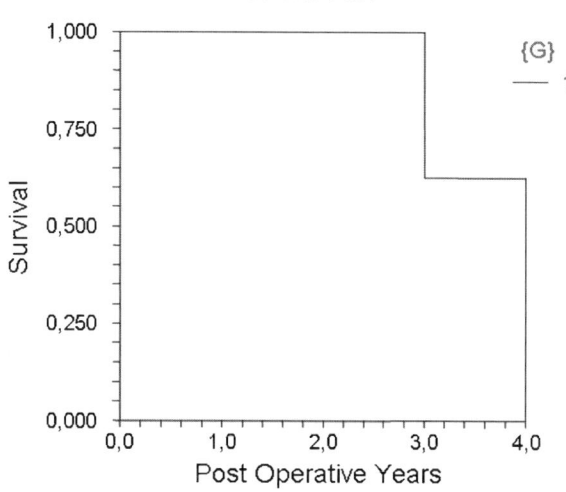

preliminary clinical results, and a careful design of controlled randomized double blind trials will address these problems. Along the way, a parallel analysis of many fundamental aspects of stem cell biology should be resolved through basic research. Few technologies have generated such great expectations is such a short time. A coordinated effort, "from bench to the bedside", will be required to deliver on this promise while providing for the safety of patients.

Bibliography

1. Carbajal EV, Deedwania PC. Congestive heart failure. In Crawford MH, editor. Current diagnosis and treatment in cardiology, 2nd ed. New York: McGraw-Hill, 2003.
2. Gürtler RE, Segura EL, Cohen JE. Congenital transmission of *Trypanosoma cruzi* infection in Argentina. Emerg Infect Dis. 2003 Jan;9(1):29–32.
3. Soares MB, Lima RS, Rocha LL, et al. Transplanted bone marrow cells repair heart tissue and reduce myocarditis in chronic chagasic mice. Am J Pathol. 2004 Feb;164(2):441–7.
4. Torre-Amone G. Immune activation in chronic heart failure. Am J Cardiol. 2005 June 6;95(11A):3C–8C
5. Iversen PO, Woldbaek PR, Christensen G. Reduced immune responses to an aseptic inflammation in mice with congestive heart failure. Eur J Haematol. 2005 Aug;75(2):156–63.
6. Gullestad L, Aukrust P. Review of trials in chronic heart failure showing broad-spectrum anti-inflammatory approaches. Am J Cardiol. 2005 June 6;95(11A):17C–23C
7. Schachinger V, Assmus B, Britten MB, et al. Transplantation of progenitor cells and regeneration enhancement in acute myocardial infarction (TOPCARE-AMI). Circulation. 2002; 106:3009–17.
8. American Heart Association. Heart disease and stroke statistics 2004 update. Available at: www.americanheart.org. Accessed March 2005.
9. Linke A, Muller P, Nurzynska D, et al. Stem cells in the dog heart are self-renewing, clonogenic, and multipotent and regenerate infracted myocardium, improving cardiac function. Proc Natl Acad Sci U S A. 2005;102:8966–71
10. Matsuura K, Nagai T, Nishigaki N, et al. Adult cardiac sca-1-positive cells differentiate into beating cardiomyocytes. J Biol Chem. 2004;279:11384–91.
11. Oh H, Bradfute SB, Gallardo TD, et al. Cardiac progenitor cells from adult myocardium: homing, differentiation, and fusion after infarction. Proc Natl Acad Sci U S A. 2003;100:12313–8.
12. Urbanek K, Quaini F, Tasca G, et al. Intense myocyte formation from cardiac stem cells in human cardiac hypertrophy. Proc Natl Acad Sci U S A. 2003;100:10440–5.
13. Jaffredo T, Nottingham W, Liddiard K, et al. From hemangioblast to hematopoietic stem cell: an endothelial connection? Exp Hematol. 2005;33:1029–40.
14. Sanai N, Alvarez-Buylla A, Berger MS. Neural stem cells and the origin of gliomas. N Engl J Med. 2005;353:811–22.
15. Messina E, De Angelis L, Frati G, et al. Isolation and expansion of adult cardiac stem cells from human and murine heart. Circ Res. 2004;95:911–21.
16. Urbanek K, Rota M, Cascapera S, et al. Cardiac stem cells possess growth factor-receptor systems that after activation regenerate the infarcted myocardium, improving ventricular function and long-term survival. Circ Res. 2005 Sep 30;97(7):663–73.
17. Tang YL, Zhao Q, Qin X, et al. Paracrine action enhances the effects of autologous mesenchymal stem cell transplantation on vascular regeneration in rat model of myocardial infarction. Ann Thorac Surg. 2005;80:229–36.
18. Majka SM, Jackson KA, Kienstra KA, et al. Distinct progenitor populations in skeletal muscle are bone marrow derived and exhibit different cell fates during vascular regeneration. J Clin Invest. 2003;111:71–9.

19. Asahara T, Murohara T, Sullivan A, et al. Isolation of putative progenitor endothelial cells for angiogenesis. Science. 1997;275:964–7.
20. Schatteman GC, Hanlon HD, Jiao C, et al. Blood derived angioblasts accelerate blood-flow restoration in diabetic mice. J Clin Invest. 2000;106:571–8.
21. Crosby JR, Kaminski WE, Schatteman G, et al. Endothelial cells of hematopoietic origin makes a significant contribution to adult blood vessel formation. Circ Res. 2000;87:728–30.
22. Takahashi T, Kalka C, Masuda H, et al. Ischemia and cytokineinduced mobilization of bone marrow-derived endothelial progenitor cells for neovascularization. Nat Med. 1999;5: 434–8.
23. Luttun A, Carmeliet G, Carmeliet P. Vascular progenitors: from biology to treatment. Trends Cardiovasc Med. 2002;12:88–96.
24. Orlic D, Kajstura J, Chimenti S, et al. Bone marrow cells regenerate infarcted myocardium. Nature. 2001;410:701–5.
25. Orlic D, Kajstura J, Chimenti S, et al. Mobilized bone marrow cells repair the infarcted heart, improving function and survival. Proc Natl Acad Sci U S A. 2001;98:10344–9.
26. Kocher AA, Schuster MD, Szabolcs MJ, et al. Neovascularization of ischemic myocardium by human bone-marrow-derived angioblasts prevents cardiomyocyte apoptosis, reduces remodeling and improves cardiac function. Nat Med. 2001;7:430–6.
27. Jackson KA, Majka SM, Wang H, et al. Regeneration of ischemic cardiac muscle and vascular endothelium by adult stem cells. J Clin Invest. 2001;107:1395–402.
28. Edelberg JM, Tang L, Hattori K, et al. Young adult bone marrowderived endothelial precursor cells restore aging-impaired cardiac angiogenic function. Circ Res. 2002;90:E89–E93.
29. Yokoyama S, Fukuda N, Li Y, et al. A strategy of retrograde injection of bone marrow ononuclear cells into the myocardium for the treatment of ischemic heart disease. J Mol Cell Cardiol. 2006 Jan;40(1):24–34.
30. Shi Q, Rafii S, Wu MH, et al. Evidence for circulating bone marrowderived endothelial cells. Blood. 1998;92:362–7.
31. Bhattacharya V, McSweeney PA, Shi Q, et al. Enhanced endothelialization and microvessel formation in polyester grafts seeded with CD34_ bone marrow cells. Blood. 2000;95: 581–5.
32. Kaushal S, Amiel GE, Guleserian KJ, et al. Functional small-diameter neovessels created using endothelial progenitor cells expanded ex vivo. Nat Med. 2001;7:1035–40.
33. Noishiki Y, Tomizawa Y, Yamane Y, et al. Autocrine angiogenic vascular prosthesis with bone marrow transplantation. Nat Med. 1996;2:90–3.
34. Sata M, Saiura A, Kunisato A, et al. Hematopoietic stem cells differentiate into vascular cells that participate in the pathogenesis of atherosclerosis. Nat Med. 2002;8:403–9.
35. Otani A, Kinder K, Ewalt K, et al. Bone marrow derived stem cells target retinal astrocytes and can promote or inhibit retinal angiogenesis. Nat Med. 2002;8:1004–10.
36. Grant MB, May WS, Caballero S, et al. Adult hematopoietic stem cells provide functional hemangioblast activity during retinal neovascularization. Nat Med. 2002;8:607–12.
37. Crisa L, Cirulli V, Smith KA, et al. Human cord blood progenitors sustain thymic T-cell development and a novel form of angiogenesis. Blood. 1999;94:3928–40.
38. Young PP, Hofling AA, Sands MS. VEGF increases engraftment of bone marrow-derived endothelial progenitor cells (EPCs) into vasculalture of newborn murine recipients. Proc Natl Acad Sci U S A. 2002;99:11951–6.
39. Kajstura J, Rota M, Whang B, et al. Bone marrow cells differentiate in cardiac cell lineages after infarction independently of cell fusion. Circ Res. 2005 Jan 7;96(1):127–37.
40. Kucia M, Ratajczak J, Ratajczak MZ. Are bone marrow stem cells plastic or heterogenous – that is the question. Exp Hematol. 2005 June;33(6):613–23.
41. Strauer BE, Brehm M, Zeus T, et al. Repair of infarcted myocardium by autologous intra-coronary mononuclear bone marrow cell transplantation in humans. Circulation. 2002; 106:1913–8.
42. Viña RF, Saslavsky J, Vrsalovick F, et al. Repair of infarcted myocardium by autologous intracoronary stems cells implant. Available at: www.TCTMD.com. Accessed January 2004.

43. Viña RF, Saslavsky J, Vrsalovick F, et al. Trans (coronary) LIMA implantation of stems cells in chronic coronary disease. Available at: www.TCTMD.com. Accessed September 2003.
44. Viña RF, Saslavsky J, Vrsalovick F, et al. Angiogenesis: trans (coronary) venous implantation of stems cells in chronic coronary disease. Available at: www.TCTMD.com. Accessed May 2003.
45. Perin EC, Dohmann HF, Borojevic R, et al. Transendocardial, autologous bone marrow cell transplantation for severe, chronic ischemic heart failure. Circulation. 2003;107:2294–302.
46. Tse HF, Kwong YL, Chan JK, et al. Angiogenesis in ischaemic myocardium by intramyocardial autologous bone marrow mononuclear cell implantation. Lancet. 2003;361:47–9.
47. Patel AN, Geffner L, Vina R, et al. Surgical treatment for congestive heart failure with autologous adult stem cell transplantation: a prospective randomized study. J Thorac Cardiovasc Surg. 2005 Dec;130(6):1631–8.
48. Benetti F, Viña RF, Patel AN, et al. OPCABG plus simultaneous autologous stem cells implants. Available at: www.TCTMD.com.
49. Perin EC, Lopez J. Methods of stem cell delivery in cardiac diseases. Nat Clin Pract Cardiovasc Med. 2006 Mar;3(Suppl 1):S110–3.
50. Rabbany SY, Heissig B, Hattori K, Rafii S. Molecular pathways regulating mobilization of marrow-derived stem cells for tissue revascularization. Trends Mol Med. 2003;9:109–17.
51. Perin EC, Dohmann HF, Borojevic R, et al. Transendocardial, autologous bone marrow cell transplantation for severe, chronic ischemic heart failure Circulation. 2003;107:2294–302.
52. Nagaya N, Kangawa K, Itoh T, et al. Transplantation of mesenchymal stem cells improves cardiac function in a rat model of dilated cardiomyopathy. Circulation. 2005 Aug 23;112(8):1128–35.
53. Fernandes S, Amirault JC, Lande G, et al. Autologous myoblast transplantation after myocardial infarction increases the inducibility of ventricular arrhythmias. Cardiovasc Res. 2006 Feb 1;69(2):348–58.
54. Dohmann HF, Perin EC, Takiya CM, et al. Transendocardial autologous bone marrow mononuclear cell injection in ischemic heart failure: postmortem anatomicopathologic and immunohistochemical findings. Circulation. 2005 July 26;112(4):521–6.
55. Silva GV, Litovsky S, Assad JA, et al. Mesenchymal stem cells differentiate into an endothelial phenotype, enhance vascular density, and improve heart function in a canine chronic ischemia model. Circulation. 2005;111:150–6.
56. Memon IA, Sawa Y, Miyagawa S, et al. Combined autologous cellular cardiomyoplasty with skeletal myoblasts and bone marrow cells in canine hearts for ischemic cardiomyopathy. J Thorac Cardiovasc Surg. 2005 Sep;130(3):646–53.
57. Murry CE, Soonpaa MH, Reinecke H, et al. Haematopoietic stem cells do not transdifferentiate into cardiac myocytes in myocardial infarcts. Nature. 2004;428:664–8.
58. Balsam LB, Wagers AJ, Christensen JL, et al. Haematopoietic stem cells adopt mature haematopoietic fates in ischaemic myocardium. Nature. 2004;428:668–73.
59. Deten A, Volz HC, Clamors S, et al. Hematopoietic stem cells do not repair the infarcted mouse heart. Cardiovasc Res. 2005 Jan 1;65(1):52–63.
60. Kuethea FT, Richartza BM, Kasper C, et al. Autologous intracoronary mononuclear bone marrow cell transplantation in chronic ischemic cardiomyopathy in humans. Int J Cardiol. 2005;100:485–91.
61. Leri A, Kajstura J, Anversa P. Cardiac stem cells and mechanisms of myocardial regeneration. Physiol Rev. 2005 Oct;85(4):1373–416.
62. Hayashi M, Li TS, Ito H, Mikamo A, et al. Comparison of intramyocardial and intravenous routes of delivering bone marrow cells for the treatment of ischemic heart disease: an experimental study. Cell Transplant. 2004;13(6):639–47.
63. Willerson JT, Yeh ET, Geng YJ, et al. Blood-derived progenitor cells after recanalization of chronic coronary artery occlusions in humans. Circ Res. 2005 Oct 14;97(8):735–6.
64. Silva GV, Perin EC, Dohmann HF, et al. Catheter-based transendocardial delivery of autologous bone-marrow-derived mononuclear cells in patients listed for heart transplantation. Tex Heart Inst J. 2004;31(3):214–9.

65. Archundia A, Aceves JL, Lopez Hernandez M, et al. Direct cardiac injection of G-CSF mobilized bone-marrow stem-cells improves ventricular function in old myocardial infarction. Life Sci. 2005 Dec 5;78(3):279–83.
66. Hüttmann A, Dührsen U, Stypmann J, et al. Granulocyte colony-stimulating factor induced blood stem cell mobilization in patients with chronic heart failure. Feasibility, safety and effects on exercise tolerance and cardiac function. Basic Res Cardiol. 2005;100:1–9.

Chapter 13
Use of Combinatorial Screening to Discover Protocols That Effectively Direct the Differentiation of Stem Cells

Yen Choo

Abstract Embryonic stem cells (ESCs) have the rare ability to differentiate into all cell types that comprise the human adult, offering an unprecedented opportunity to perform developmental studies *in vitro* and promising unlimited supplies of somatic cells for numerous biomedical applications including transplantation medicine. Reliably controlling the differentiation of ESCs *in vitro* by conventional methods requires an understanding of complex developmental pathways, the availability of a series of phenotypic markers and involves technically demanding and time-consuming empirical determination of cell culture conditions. Directed differentiation of ESCs has thus proved a robust challenge and is likely to become the first major bottleneck in the stem cell field, particularly when the time comes to substitute costly recombinant growth factors by small molecule functional mimetics. This chapter briefly examines the benefits and shortcomings of various approaches currently used to differentiate stem cells, from mechanism-based rational approaches to the emerging systematic and higher throughput methods, and ultimately describes a novel 'directed evolution' method called 'Combinatorial Cell Culture' which has the potential to increase the throughput of directed differentiation experiments by orders of magnitude.

Keywords Stem Cell; Differentiation; Combinatorial; Screening

13.1 Introduction

A major driver of biomedical industry growth this century is predicted to be the availability of high quality stem cell-derived human tissue for which there is currently an increasing and unmet need.

Plasticell Ltd., Imperial Bioincubator, Bessemer Building (RSM), Prince Consort Road, South Kensington, London SW7 2BP, UK

First, increased demand for organ transplantation from an aging population combined with a severe shortage of healthy organ donors, means that amongst those patients currently on hospital waiting lists only one in five will eventually receive treatment [1]. It is thought that stem-cell derived tissue could functionally substitute the whole organs currently used in transplantation and thus form the basis of numerous cell-replacement therapies to treat a remarkable variety of serious degenerative conditions.

Secondly, the pharmaceutical industry is clearly suffering from a lack of simple *in vitro* pharmacological models that can accurately predict the body's response to drug candidates. Over-dependence on unreliable animal models and costly human clinical trials, both of which often fail to detect ineffective or toxic compounds at a sufficiently early stage, has driven the average cost of developing a single drug almost to the billion dollar mark. The availability of quality controlled stem-cell derived human tissue for use in drug development would go a long way towards increasing efficiency and reducing the cost of medicines [2, 3].

13.2   Stem Cells

An increasing number of embryonic-, foetal- and adult- derived stem cell preparations and lines are readily available today through various cell banks and commercial suppliers. Stem cells constitute a virtually inexhaustible supply of raw material from which to derive the specific differentiated cell types required for current biomedical research and future cell replacement therapy. Pluripotent stem cells are of the widest applicability and by their nature the most challenging stem cell types to differentiate reliably. This chapter is thus focused on these cells and makes repeated reference to ESCs; but the reader should note that much of what is described is not limited to ESCs but also applies to induced pluripotent stem cells (iPS) [4], as well as foetal and adult stem cells.

13.2.1   Embryonic Stem Cells

ESC lines are indefinitely self-renewing and pluripotent [5–7]. Over 400 human ESC (hESC) lines from laboratories in more than 20 countries are available [8]. The International Stem Cell Initiative has characterised 59 of these lines [9], a subset of which are available from centralised cell banks (e.g. UK Stem Cell Bank; www.ukstemcellbank.org.uk) that ensure the lines are ethically derived and properly characterised using accredited quality control systems.

It is generally agreed that the immediate challenges in the stem cell field are to develop: (i) industrial scale culture of research and clinical grade undifferentiated stem cell lines [10] and (ii) effective, reproducible and economical differentiation protocols that generate the particular, specialised cell types required for a given application [11].

13.2.2 Scale Up of hESC Culture

While scale up of hESC culture currently presents a variety of technical challenges, these are expected to yield to near term advances in cell handling, laboratory automation and substrate and/or media formulation [12–16]. It is beyond the scope of this chapter to examine this topic in any detail, however it is worthwhile citing certain recent developments in passing. For example, original growth conditions for hESC required coculture with a feeder layer of mitotically inactivated mouse embryonic fibroblasts to maintain cell pluripotency and self-renewal [7]. Since use of feeders is cumbersome, there has been much progress in providing functional substitutes such as cell-free lysates or combinations of defined growth substrate and media formulations, and also in humanising the sources of these reagents for future clinical use [17–19]. Furthermore, hESC lines which previously required laborious manual mechanical dissection for efficient propagation can be passaged with automated protocols [20] or have been adapted for passage as enzymatically-dissociated single cell cultures [21], and compounds are emerging which are capable of increasing the survival of dissociated hESCs [22].

The handling of stem cells has been automated, increasing the ease of culture and also reproducibility. Robotic liquid handling systems adapted from machines originally designed to carry out cell-based drug screens on microtitre plates now support fully automated culture at least of mouse ESCs (mESCs). A typical reconfigured system such as Hamilton's CellHost consists of a liquid handling robot in a sterile housing flanked by tissue culture incubators which provide plates and media to the robot using transfer units [23].

Historically, many different cell lines besides hESC have been 'domesticated' through technical advances or via adaptation/selection while maintaining the essential characteristics that underpin their utility. Assuming researchers maintain the impressive rate of progress in improving culture conditions for hESC, it is reasonable to expect large-scale production of these cells to be available in the foreseeable future. Production of clinical grade hESC, which is more cumbersome owing to regulatory (and not merely practical) concerns, may take a little longer but is also anticipated [24, 25].

13.3 Stem Cell Differentiation

While large quantities of undifferentiated hESCs may soon be at hand, reliably directing their differentiation towards the mature cellular phenotypes found in adult tissues continues to be an extremely thorny problem, essentially because we know relatively little about the precise pathways involved in early human development and organogenesis (despite the power of comparative developmental biology) and even less about how to replicate the process *in vitro* using the hESC model.

13.3.1   Multilineage Differentiation of ESCs

hESCs spontaneously differentiate in the absence of a feeder layer (which provides surrogate pluripotency signals), when dissociated in the absence of optimised conditions or when overgrown in culture. Indeed a common and heretofore useful method of precipitating spontaneous differentiation is to culture ESCs as three-dimensional multicellular aggregates referred to as embryoid bodies [26]. In this system, spontaneous differentiation occurs mainly through a process of intercellular signalling akin to that in the early embryo: thus it cannot be placed under full experimental control. It generally gives rise to a large number of differentiated cell types (i.e. a large degree of cell heterogeneity) but yields relatively few if any cells of a given lineage of interest. This multilineage differentiation is of little practical use, other than as an indication that ESCs are indeed pluripotent: i.e. capable of differentiating into the various cell types found in the three major embryonic lineages (ectoderm, mesoderm and endoderm).

13.3.2   Directed Stem Cell Differentiation

Directing cell differentiation towards any one phenotype can be achieved through one of two generally complementary means: (i) by expression of transcription factor or other transgenes (genetic modification) and more importantly (ii) by manipulating the culture conditions (sometimes called epigenetic methods).

13.3.2.1   Directing ESC Differentiation by Expression of Transgenes

Examples of the genetic modification approach include the use of Hoxb4 in hematopoietic differentiation [27]; constitutive expression of Pax4 [28] or inducible expression of Pdx1 [29] in the differentiation of mESC to pancreatic islet-like cells; and the transient expression of Nurr1 [30] or a combination of Nurr1 and Pitx3 [31] in mESC differentiation to dopaminergic neurons. In these instances the transfected genes are transcription factors that provide instructive differentiation signals by either up- or down- regulating expression of developmental genes. Alternatively, this genetic modification approach can be used to increase the purity (but not necessarily the yield) of a differentiated cell type, for instance by enabling lineage-specific positive or negative selection – a strategy which is discussed further below.

Obvious drawbacks of genetic modification include the low efficiency of transfection (and therefore differentiation) of hESCs or partly differentiated developmental intermediates and the difficulty of obtaining or maintaining transgene expression at the correct level. Over and above these practical issues, genetic modification of stem cells for therapeutic applications introduces complicating regulatory and safety considerations which are well known in gene therapy; most obviously the risk that transfected cells may have (or may acquire in future) some altered characteristics as a result of hosting the transgene [32].

Genetic modification is likely to be a valuable tool in directing differentiation of ESCs, though its full potential awaits better understanding of the gene networks which regulate various aspects of development [33] and improved methods of gene delivery, stable transfection and inducible expression in hESCs.

13.3.2.2 Directing ESC Differentiation by Culturing Under Specific Conditions

By far the most common and important method of directing the differentiation of ESCs is to manipulate the conditions under which they are cultured. Development involves a series of cell fate decisions that are largely controlled by a cascade of extrinsic signals and this process can be recapitulated *in vitro* through the use of appropriate instructive or selective cell culture conditions applied in the correct sequence, at the right time and for a suitable duration.

Many examples of ESC differentiation by this method are reviewed by Keller [11, 34] and Trounson [35] and include differentiation into lineages such as definitive endoderm [36], haematopoietic cells [37], cartilage [38], mesenchymal precursors [39], photoreceptors [40], cardiomyocytes [41–44] and skeletal muscle [45] to name but a few.

The most commonly manipulated extrinsic variables are the basal cell culture media and their supplements, in particular soluble signals such as morphogens, growth factors, hormones, organic compounds (e.g. nutrients, lipids, vitamins), synthetic small molecules (e.g. DMSO) and even ions (e.g. Li^+). Distinct cell types respond differently to these variations in the media, so while some cells in a culture interpret a given signal as instruction to differentiate, other cells may be induced to proliferate, become quiescent or die, leading to a selective enrichment of certain cell types in a population. With some imagination one might picture how consecutive waves of differentiation, phenotypic selection and proliferation of particular cell populations lead to the appearance of progressively specified cell lineages.

Another common variable in the control of stem cell behaviour is the extracellular microenvironment, in particular insoluble factors present in/on the growth substrate or on adjacent cells. The extracellular matrix (ECM), which is comprised of proteins such as the collagens, fibronectins and laminins, can directly affect cell signalling, attachment and activity. It is well known that stem cell differentiation can be affected by the composition of the culture substrate and the ECM, examples of which are the longstanding use of polylysine or laminin to support neural differentiation or conversely the use of matrigel in maintenance of hESC pluripotency [17]. Of particular interest in this field is the testing of combinatorial mixtures of ECM components [46] and the development of synthetic biomaterials [47, 48] that can be used to affect the differentiation of stem cells either alone or more likely in conjunction with soluble factors.

13.3.2.3 Examples of Directed Differentiation Through Cell Culture Under Specific Conditions

Unlike conventional cell culture, in which cells are usually grown in a single medium, directed differentiation of ESCs requires culture in a number of media, each of which has a different composition and must be applied in the correct series over a period of time.

Embryonic neural progenitors exhibit considerable developmental plasticity and neuronal fate depends on the timing and dose of different morphogens to which cells are exposed during development. This principle was applied by Jessell and colleagues to produce motor neurons from mESCs by differentiation through a pathway which recapitulated the physiological process, giving rise to the term 'directed-differentiation' [49]. mESCs were first neuralised by culturing embryoid bodies with stromal cell conditioned medium, after which these cells were caudalised by retinoic acid treatment and finally ventralised by Sonic hedgehog agonist treatment to produce the required motor neurons. Selective neuronal differentiation of hESCs was first shown by Thomson and by Reubinoff and colleagues [50, 51], and it was subsequently shown that the protocols devised by Jessell and coworkers to direct motor neuron differentiation could be adapted for use with human cultures [52].

The principles of directed differentiation have been extended to a number of other neuronal subtypes. In further examples of stepwise cell culture, a number of groups have adapted serial culture protocols for the derivation of midbrain dopaminergic neurons from mESCs [30] to achieve the same using hESCs [53–55]. Once again, regional specification is achieved by the sequential application of defined patterning molecules (such as FGF8 and Sonic hedgehog) that direct midbrain development *in vivo*. Dopamine neurons are heterogeneous in character and elicit different functions with distinct physiologies; in further studies it was shown that manipulation of *in vitro* neural patterning cues could selectively generate hypothalamic as opposed to midbrain DA neurons [56].

Examples of differentiation to other neuronal lineages include cerebellar neurons [57], neural crest cells with the potential for subsequent differentiation to sensory neurons, autonomic neurons, smooth muscle cells and glial cells [58–60]. Both mouse and human oligodendrocytes can also be derived from ESCs and in both cases have been shown to exhibit major restorative function by remyelinating damaged neurons in models of disease [61, 62].

Outside of the neural lineage a particularly clear example of serial cell culture to direct differentiation is the conversion of hESCs into hormone secreting cells similar to those found in the pancreas. D'Amour et al. devised a relatively effective protocol based on thorough knowledge of pancreatic organogenesis and the presence of a substantial body of literature describing the importance of such factors as activins, Wnt3a, BMPs, TGFs, FGFs, HGF, IGFs and others. These were assayed in various concentrations and combinations, in a background of different basal media with and without serum supplementation and at variable time intervals. Optimisation of the protocol was performed in a stepwise fashion and at each stage known markers of differentiation were assayed by RT-PCR and immunocytochemistry, to validate progression of the cells through predetermined stages of lineage commitment. Eventually, a five-step method was devised in which hESCs undergo six media changes over a 2–3 week period! The protocol yielded a mixed population of cells, around 7% of which contained insulin and could release it in response to treatment with various secretagogues, but not in response to glucose challenge.

The above works are important milestones in stem cell research, not only as definitive validation of the serial cell culture approach to directed differentiation, but as clear illustration of how a rationale based on detailed understanding of lineage development is normally required in this process. However, these papers also demonstrate that despite profound knowledge of natural developmental processes there is no *a priori* method of deducing the conditions that will lead to the differentiation of one cell type into another *in vitro*. These must be discovered empirically, entailing lengthy and costly experimentation – research that unfortunately is all too often rewarded only by low efficiency differentiation into phenotypes which approximate but do not fully resemble the desired cell type.

13.4 General Strategies for Achieving Stem Cell Differentiation

Directed differentiation of ESCs is technically challenging and threatens to form a robust bottleneck in an otherwise rapidly advancing field. The key to this problem is to adopt novel, generally applicable methods that can accelerate progress by increasing experimental throughput whilst reducing cost and the well-known day-to-day variability and tedium that are burdensome hallmarks of cell culture.

13.4.1 Genetic Lineage Selection of Differentiated Cells

One of the earliest, generally applicable techniques for 'directing' stem cell differentiation was the use of selectable genetic markers to purify differentiated lineages. This approach requires genetic modification of ESCs to place an antibiotic resistance gene (or other marker, e.g. green fluorescent protein (GFP) [63]) under the control of a tissue-specific promoter. Following differentiation, whether spontaneous or directed, selective pressure is applied to yield cultures of differentiated cells that express the selectable marker. Field and colleagues described a mESC line stably transformed with a construct in which aminoglycoside phosphotransferase was driven by the α–cardiac myosin heavy chain promoter, enabling G418 selection of essentially pure cardiomyocytes [64]. An alternative strategy demonstrated by Smith and colleagues using the Sox2 gene [65], was to integrate antibiotic resistance directly into the gene locus by homologous recombination, thus bringing it under specific control of the endogenous promoter.

Genetic lineage selection is a widely applicable technique. Though it is dependent on knowing tissue specific markers (and their specific promoter elements which can be elusive or complex), these are not limited to cell-surface antigens as is the case for selection by e.g. immunopurification or fluorescence activated cell sorting (FACS), and moreover the selection step is facile and effective. An important point to note is that genetic selection does not solve the problem of directed differentiation *per se*, but rather is a purification technique that is applied post differentiation to ablate non- or wrongly-differentiated cells. If differentiation of ESCs into the desired lineage is highly efficient then it is possible to isolate relatively large numbers of target cells, however if this is not the case then the yield will be minimal. Thus, even for relatively 'easy-to-obtain' lineages such as cardiomyocytes [66] and neuronal precursors [67–70], lineage selection must be used in conjunction with serial cell culture methods that direct large numbers of ESCs towards defined cell types.

13.4.2   Guided Walks Along Differentiation Pathways

The great difficulty with directing ESC differentiation in general is that (unlike some of the better studied neural lineages) most of the 200 or so basic cell types in the human body arise through cellular intermediates bearing phenotypic markers which are largely unknown at present, or which are common and therefore shared between different lineages. Indeed, progress towards devising instructive culture conditions towards endodermal lineages such as pancreas was held up considerably while there were no unique markers capable of distinguishing visceral and definitive endoderm, only the latter of which ultimately gives rise to the pancreas, liver and other organs [71, 72]. Without such a cell type-specific marker, it was in turn impossible to devise assays for cell culture media capable of directing differentiation.

The lack of specific lineage markers for stem cell differentiation is a serious obstacle in the field, however if a series of highly specific markers does exist, such that a fairly informative developmental roadmap can be assembled, the biotechnologist can attempt a guided walk from marker to marker towards a defined endpoint (i.e. A → →B → C → → → Z). Nevertheless, guessing the composition of the appropriate tissue culture medium for each step is still a complicated process that normally involves testing a multitude of factors in various combinations in order to arrive at an optimised formula. In principle, this process might be simplified (though not necessarily hastened) by screening the cells for the presence of cell surface growth factor receptors which signify the ability to respond to cognate soluble factors. An example of this approach was the RT-PCR screen of 5-day-old embryoid bodies comprising hESCs for expression of eight different growth factor receptors [73] and subsequent screening of the corresponding ligands to determine their effect on differentiation. The approach of screening for cellular receptors to home in on putative differentiating agents is potentially advantageous but the benefits may be outweighed by the fact that it is laborious and time consuming, and technically dependent on having a sufficiently pure population of cells at hand. Since in practice cell culture homogeneity is greatly reduced as ESC culture is progressed towards a terminally differentiated fate, it may be necessary to purify marked cells in order to carry out receptor analysis [63]. Finally, in the example above, all eight receptor types screened were found to be present in embryoid bodies, thus the screen was not particularly instructive and the experiment might have been quicker and just as instructive if the factors had been tested blindly.

13.4.3 Systematic Screening of Differentiation Conditions

Systematic screens of differentiation conditions are possible using current methods but are extremely complex owing to the large number of interacting variables (e.g. timing of addition, concentration and combination of multiple factors).

The pharmaceutical industry has recently embraced cell-based screens, together with related automation such as the high content screening systems of Cellomics, Evotech, GE Healthcare, Becton Dickinson et al., that allow highly parallel differentiation assays and quantitative analysis of results. A few groups to date have exploited the pharmaceutical screening approach to search libraries of synthetic small molecules and natural products for their effect on the self-renewal and differentiation of ESCs [74]. Takahashi et al. [75] and Wu et al. [76] performed chemical screens using mESCs bearing reporters for cardiomyocytes and identified known and novel compounds (including some from chemical libraries produced by combinatorial synthesis) that increased the efficiency of differentiation to spontaneously beating cardiomyocytes. Conversely, high throughput chemical screening has been used to identify a compound that promotes mESC self renewal in serum- and feeder- free culture [77].

Systematic tests of interacting variables can be performed using 'factorial' experimental designs in which two or more factors, each with discrete levels (e.g. concentrations), are tested in all possible combinations and the outputs subjected to statistical analysis. An example of this approach is Chang and Zandstra's quantitative screen of mESC differentiation to endoderm in which an initial experiment involving five factors tested at two levels revealed the interactions between the various media supplements, and a further experiment in which two factors tested at three levels allowed limited testing of concentration effects [78].

The number of experiments required for complete factorial designs rapidly gets out of hand as the complexity of a process increases. The vast majority of these experiments are carried out in two levels (i.e. factor present or absent) and the number of variables that can be tested is limited even when using automated cell culture and screening systems. In practice, factorial experiments to determine conditions for stem cell differentiation are possible for individual steps in guided walks along differentiation pathways, but probably not for substantial leaps (i.e. A $\rightarrow \rightarrow$ F) nor the entire journey (i.e. A $\rightarrow \rightarrow \rightarrow$ Z) both of which would require massive screens over a prolonged period. Large screens are expensive (the cost of growth factors alone is prohibitive) and the behaviour of biological cultures in the long-term often becomes unstable, making it difficult to correlate results from well to well. Thus factorial experiments are likely limited to testing individual steps in a differentiation pathway, for each of which a separate assay must be devised and validated (this is very frequently the most challenging part of the workflow). The screen itself must be repeated (typically three times on separate days) to obtain statistically relevant data and well content should be replicated and randomised on each plate to eliminate position-specific effects. Statistical analysis of results can also be prolonged depending on the complexity of the screen.

An important additional consideration is that each screen requires large numbers of quality-controlled input cells, which is a relatively simple matter during early stages of differentiation (i.e. A $\rightarrow$ B $\rightarrow$ C) but later becomes progressively harder. It is therefore no coincidence that differentiation factor screens have been performed predominantly on mESCs (which are easier to amplify than hESCs) and that the endpoints of these screens have been either ESC self-renewal or differentiation into readily obtained lineages.

In conclusion, conventional cell-based screening approaches, even if facilitated by robotic systems, are not easily adapted to the study of the directed differentiation of ESCs which is dependent on unusually large numbers of variables. The state of the art enables testing of a modest number of interacting variables per run, and is confounded by the stepwise aspect of the differentiation process that brings to play temporal variables such as the timing of addition of and duration of exposure to each medium.

13.5 'Directed Evolution' and Directed Differentiation

The remainder of this chapter is essentially concerned with the practical application of protein engineering principles to stem cell differentiation: these are seemingly disparate fields but in fact have interesting parallels. In ESC differentiation, cellular phenotypes with desirable functions (e.g. β-islet cell, dopaminergic neuron etc.) are created from a common building block (i.e. stem cell) that is changed through a combination of signals. In principle this process is highly analogous to protein engineering, in which protein phenotypes with desirable functions (e.g. antigen binding, DNA recognition or catalytic activity) are created from a common building block (e.g. antibody, zinc finger or enzyme motif) that is changed through a combination of mutations. Since the two disciplines are faced with precisely the same problem – namely finding effective combinations of variables that impinge on a biological process – they may also have solutions in common. This is a valuable insight because protein engineering is a mature field in which a number of practical approaches, ranging from rational design to random mutagenesis, have been tested. Interestingly, for all but the simplest cases of protein engineering it has emerged that the strategy of selecting or screening functional clones from a randomised combinatorial library of variants is the method of choice both in terms of ease and efficacy. Examples include panning large phage display libraries for novel antibodies and zinc fingers, or screening libraries created by DNA shuffling for improved enzyme activities. These methods are commonly referred to as combinatorial biology or 'directed evolution' [79] approaches because like the natural evolutionary process they sample random permutations of variables (typically amino acids or polypeptides) followed by phenotypic screening in order to identify combinations that result in improved or novel function.

13.5.1 Features of Directed Evolution Techniques: Example of Phage Display

A number of directed evolution techniques have been developed for protein engineering, notably phage display [80] and more recently *in vitro* compartmentalisation [81]. These techniques have a certain rationale in common: (i) a naïve protein scaffold is randomly mutated to create a large library of variants; (ii) selection or screening is used to isolate those variants which have improved function; and (iii) there is a coding mechanism allowing sequence information to be extracted from the system (typically the protein is somehow linked to its coding gene).

Phage display is the best-known directed evolution technique and is commonly used to engineer highly specific binding proteins such as antibodies or zinc finger proteins. Protein variants are cloned as fusions to the coat protein of a bacteriophage and therefore exposed (or 'displayed') on the outer surface of phage. Combinatorial libraries encoding millions of random variants are created in which key amino acids or peptides are present in many, if not all, possible permutations. Phage displaying variants with high binding affinities for a ligand of interest are affinity purified on a column of immobilised ligand, and non binding phage washed off. The binding phage are subsequently eluted, amplified by infection of bacteria and used in further rounds of selection to enrich for the tightest binders. Finally the genomes of the phage that have survived this 'natural selection' are sequenced to deduce the amino acid sequence of the tightest binding protein.

One can only imagine what a protein engineer of the old school must have thought when originally presented with such nonsense! At first it seems counterintuitive that such a haphazard approach could be more effective than an orthodox rational design strategy. But in fact combinatorial biology is a highly effective protein engineering tool and by far the method of choice when large numbers of trial and error experiments need to be performed. Notably, the approach of engineering proteins using a purely rational or knowledge-guided strategy has consistently performed unfavourably relative to the comparatively random evolutionary approach described above.

Highly complex biological problems such as protein folding, intermolecular interactions and very probably embryonic development can be tackled using high throughput empirical experimentation and combinatorial selection techniques are designed to test large numbers of interacting variables. Given the above, it is worthwhile exploring whether a 'directed evolution' or 'combinatorial selection' technique can be applied to a complex cellular engineering problem such as the directed differentiation of ESCs.

13.5.2 A Combinatorial Screen for ESC Differentiation Conditions: Combinatorial Cell Culture

Combinatorial Cell Culture is a technology which allows screening of multitude combinations of cell culture conditions to identify complex protocols that result in rare cell biological events [82].

A schematic overview of a simple Combinatorial Cell Culture experiment is provided in Fig. 13.1 (an animated version of which is available at http://www.plasticell. co.uk/technology_animated.php). In the first step of this process stem cells are seeded on specialized microscopic beads (microcarriers) to yield groups of 'cell units'. Using a 'split-pool' process, cell units are shuffled systematically through all pre-determined combinations of various differentiation conditions (e.g. media that contain growth factors, drugs etc.) and labeled with unique tags that attach to the

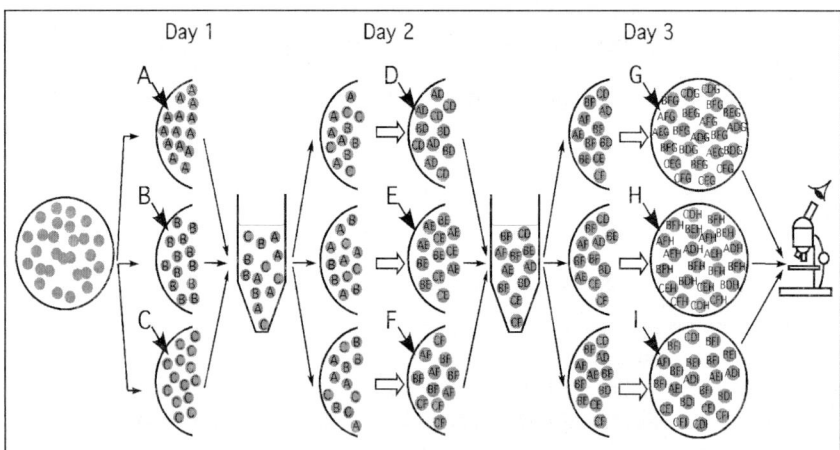

Fig. 13.1 Example of combinatorial cell culture. Cells are seeded on microcarrier beads (green). On day 1 these are split equally into three sets that are cultured under different conditions and the beads labeled using corresponding tags (A, B and C). On day 2 beads are mixed and re-partitioned into three sets that are cultured under different conditions and the beads again labeled using corresponding tags (D, E and F). On day 3 the procedure is repeated and further unique tags are added (G, H and I). At the end of the experiment, beads are screened for the desired cell type (shown as magenta) using an appropriate assay. The tags present on these 'positive' beads provide a record of the cell culture history (in this case tags C, D and H indicate cell culture in condition C on Day 1, D on Day 2 and H on Day 3) (Figure courtesy of J Green) (*See Color Plates*)

microcarrier substrate. Cell units that undergo directed differentiation as a result of fortuitous passage through appropriate conditions are later identified using a suitable cell-based screen. Finally, these are isolated and the associated tags are analysed to infer the cell culture history.

This method has been used to discover novel protocols for the directed differentiation of ESCs and very likely will find numerous other applications throughout cell biology. The various aspects of the Combinatorial Cell Culture workflow are discussed in more detail below.

13.5.2.1 Formation of Cell Units Through Microcarrier Cell Culture

Microcarriers are commonly used in basic research and industry for the scale up of adherent cell culture and in particular for commercial production of biological molecules and viruses in fermenters of up to 4,000 l [83]. Many systems have been developed in which carriers range in shape, size and porosity, and are manufactured using different processes and using a variety of materials including polystyrene, collagen and dextrans (see Table 13.1). In addition to solid carriers a number of porous systems featuring a network of open, interconnecting pores are available with greatly increased surface area for cell growth. These carriers are well characterised in terms of physical properties such as the specific gravity of the beads, the diameter and the surface area available for cell growth. Some of the carriers described and many besides are available as dried products that can be weighed accurately, and subsequently prepared by swelling in liquid medium.

Table 13.1 Examples of commercially available microcarriers for the formation of cell units

Microcarrier	Supplier	Size (μM)	Material
Cytodex 1	GE healthcare	180	Dextran
Cytodex 3	GE healthcare	175	Dextran and collagen
Cytopore1	GE healthcare	250	Cellulose
Cytopore2	GE healthcare	250	Cellulose
Cellagen	MP biomedicals	100–400	Bovine corium collagen
Fact102	Hyclone(SoloHill)	125–212	Polystyrene and porcine collagen
Cgen 102	Hyclone	125–212	Polystyrene and porcine collagen
ProF102L	Hyclone	125–212	Polystyrene and recombinant fibronectin
P102L	Hyclone	125–212	Polystyrene
Pplus 102	Hyclone	125–212	Polystyrene
Hlx 112	Hyclone	90–212 μM	Polysteryne and trymethyl ammonium
Polybeads	Polysciences	100–600	Polystyrene
Spherobeads	Spherotech	90–249	Polystyrene
Cultispher G	Percell Biolytica	50–400	Porcine gelatin
Cultispher S	Percell Biolytica	50–400	Porcine gelatin

Fig. 13.2 Example of a cell unit. Macroporous, crosslinked cellulose microcarriers with a diameter of about 250 microns (Cytopore 2; GE Healthcare) seeded with mouse ESCs. Cells are stained for alkaline phosphatase activity indicating pluripotency (*See Color Plates*)

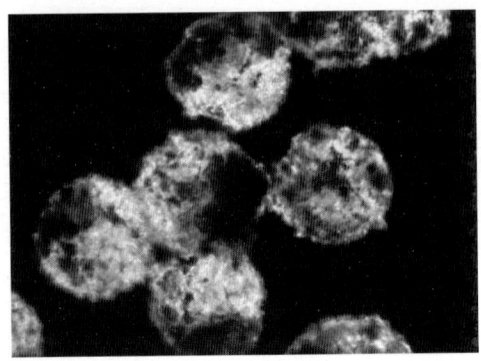

Mouse or human ESCs seeded onto most of these microcarriers will readily form cell colonies on the surface of the carrier (Fig. 13.2). In general, healthy adherent cells are not readily dissociated from their growth substrate, and so the integrity of each cell unit largely persists despite mechanical manipulation of the microcarrier, agitation of the culture medium, or transfer of the carriers from one vessel to another.

Growing cells in integral units that are suspended in the liquid phase allows individual units to be removed at will and conveniently transferred to a different culture vessel. By successively transferring cell units through a set of different tissue culture media, all cells in the unit are exposed to the same series of culture conditions, in the same order and for the same period of time. Importantly, passaging of cells in different media can be achieved without perturbing any niche that has formed on the carrier and which may be important in the process of differentiation.

Since not all cells are adherent, it is worthwhile noting that cells may also be grouped into units by immurement, i.e. confined within a medium permeable barrier or by cell encapsulation in semi-solid polymer matrices comprised of e.g. gelatin, polylysine, alginate or agarose.

13.5.2.2 Split-Pool Microculture of Cells

Forming cell units is useful for sampling multiple tissue culture conditions as each cell unit constitutes an easily handled element that can be exposed to a variety of cell culture conditions. 'Split-pool microculture' is an efficient, systematic method for testing multiple combinations of cell culture conditions. In this process, large numbers of cell units are divided randomly (but equally) into a number of sets and grown separately for a given time under different culture conditions and in the presence of unique tags which label the cell units (see section 13.5.2.3). The segregated cell units are subsequently washed to remove excess media and tags, then pooled and mixed thoroughly, and once again split randomly into equal sets that are cultured under further conditions. This split-pool procedure can be repeated for any number of cycles. In many respects the principle of this procedure resembles that of split synthesis of large combinatorial chemical libraries (known as combinatorial chemistry), which samples all possible combinations of chemical building block groups [84, 85].

Cell units subjected to this iterative split-pool process systematically sample all possible combinations of conditions in a predetermined experimental matrix (see Fig. 13.1). The number of different cell culture protocols sampled in an experiment where beads are split T times into N number of sets is equal to N^T (the 'complexity' of the experiment). However, this experiment can be carried out conveniently and cost effectively using only (N.T) number of different culture vessels and tag types. It is thus feasible to sample many thousands of combinations of conditions in a single run.

In theory, the split-pool procedure can be repeated over any number of rounds, and any number of conditions can be sampled at each round, so long as the number of cell units is greater than or equal to the number of different conditions sampled. In practice, the number of cell units used in the experiment should be approximately tenfold greater than the complexity of the experiment to compensate for losses of cell units in transit and to provide statistical confidence that each putative differentiation pathway has been sampled by at least one cell unit.

The practical complexity of a Combinatorial Cell Culture experiment is limited by the number of available tags, by the bead numbers (or culture volume) that can be conveniently handled and by the availability of starting cell material and/or the cost of reagents such as recombinant growth factors. In this latter respect the experimental schema is highly efficient because multiple cell units share a common vessel (i.e. are multiplexed) resulting in huge savings in reagents. The complexity of experiments that can be performed today is easily in reach of the hundred thousand range and with technical improvements will probably be in the millions.

The variables which can be sampled using this technique are not limited to the growth factors and morphogens present in different culture media but may include growth substrate (e.g. fibronectin on microcarrier), cell type, cell grouping (e.g. microcarrier culture, cell encapsulation, organotypic culture), duration of cell culture round, temperature, infection with viruses, addition of transgenes or antisense molecules, etc.

13.5.2.3 Use of Tags to Track Cell Culture History

Combinatorial Cell Culture necessarily involves mixing cell units, so to avoid confusing the chronology and the exact nature of the culture conditions to which any one cell unit has been exposed the process is performed in conjunction with labelling of the cell units using tags (Fig. 13.1).

A variety of tagging systems comprising distinctive chemical or non-chemical labels have been developed for use in combinatorial chemistry, but the vast majority of these are better suited to tagging chemical reactions rather than biological assays [86]. The ideal tag for Combinatorial Cell Culture should (i) exist in a large number of unique varieties ('flavours') which are easily distinguishable, preferably using an automated method; (ii) attach easily and permanently to cell units (and not transfer

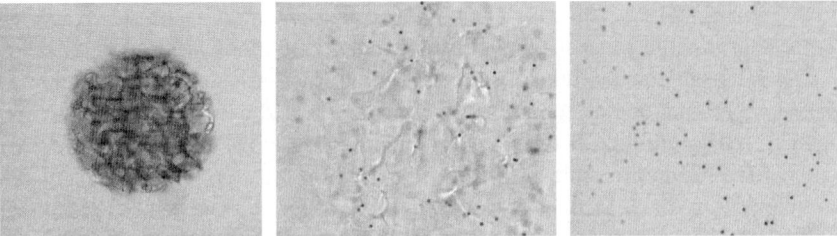

Fig. 13.3 Tagging of cell units and isolation of tags for analysis. Left panel: a Cytopore 2 micro-carrier (Ø 250 microns) bearing cells and black coloured polystyrene microsphere tags (Ø 5 microns) is placed in a drop of acid on a glass slide. Middle panel: after 20 minutes the microcarrier shows signs of hydrolysis, revealing the tags. Right panel: after 40 minutes the microcarrier sub-strate has disappeared, arraying the tags on the slide and allowing tag analysis by microscopy

or 'hop' between them); (iii) be physically stable, non-toxic and otherwise biologically inert; and (iv) be easily detected in a background of cells and biomolecules.

Cell unit substrates such as microcarriers can be derivatised or coated with sub-stances that facilitate tagging and do not interfere with cell growth, and it may be possible to selectively elute tags from colonised beads or to strip off the cells from tagged beads using selective conditions to facilitate detection (Fig. 13.3).

There are two general strategies for tagging cell units. If a different tag is stably associated with (the growth substrate) of each cell unit at the beginning of the experiment and the tags are read following each split, this would provide for a log of the series of cell culture conditions to which every cell unit was exposed. Alternatively, if tags are sequentially associated with the cell units as they are exposed to each different culture condition, one could infer the movement of any cell unit at the end of the experiment by analyzing the associated tags. Both strate-gies have advantages and disadvantages. For example, the first allows the tags to be very stably associated with the growth substrate under harsh chemical conditions but obviously requires an enormous number of tag 'flavours' (one for each cell unit) and repeated reading of the tags after each split; the second method requires repeated tagging of cell units but uses a relatively smaller number of tag 'flavours' (one for each cell culture condition sampled).

In practice, the tagging strategy used in Combinatorial Cell Culture will likely depend on the state of the art of various alternative tagging technologies. For instance, an attractive tagging strategy would be to use radio-frequency identification (RFID), where electronic memory is used to record the history of a sample and where information is read remotely via radiofrequency transmission [87, 88]. RFID for Combinatorial Cell Culture ideally would comprise a very large number of tags each with a unique binary code, and cell unit tracking would be carried out remotely during the cell culture steps. However, currently available RFID technology is practically unsuitable for this application: tags are still relatively expensive and much bulkier than microcarriers, and there are problems reading large numbers of tags when these are in close proximity owing to mutual interference of signals.

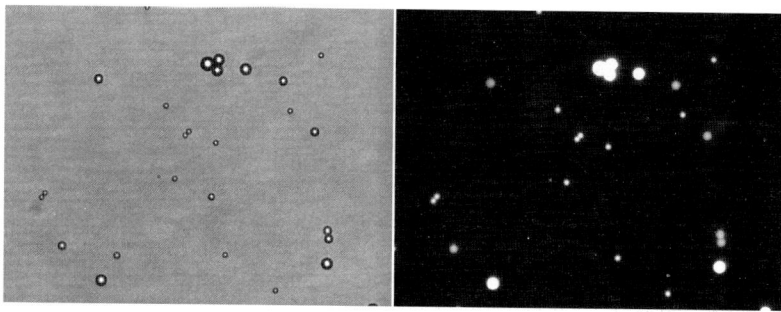

Fig. 13.4 Example of the analysis of coded microsphere tags. Fluorescent microsphere tags arrayed on a glass surface viewed using phase (left) and eplifluorescence (right) microscopy. The different tag flavours are coded by size (Ø 2–10 microns) and by loading with various concentrations of a given fluorophore

Alternatively, a number of optical or visual methods of tagging have been described [89], some of which are easily adapted for Combinatorial Cell Culture. In a number of these a pattern or bar code is encoded onto a substrate and recognised using pattern recognition technology [90–92], however most of these systems are not yet widely available and are often too complicated for large numbers of tags to be synthesised in the typical life science laboratory.

More common visual tagging systems comprise populations of monodisperse beads produced from a variety of polymeric materials and loaded or externally labeled with fluorescent organic dyes to produce distinct populations. Fluorescent microsphere arrays are in widespread use for multiplexed analysis of biomolecules [93] and such encoded beads can be easily adapted for the labeling of cell units. A well-known system is that produced by Luminex Corporation (Austin, TX) in which beads are loaded with different ratios of two dyes, producing an assortment of 100 distinguishable bead types. A further example is the QuantumPlex system (Bangs Laboratories, Fishers, IN) in which a single dye is loaded in microspheres of varying size and at different concentrations, producing a different type of array in which members are distinguished by bead size and fluorescence intensity (Fig. 13.4).

13.5.2.4 Screening of Differentiated Cell Units

Following each round of Combinatorial Cell Culture, or after a defined number of rounds, the cell units are assayed to determine whether there are members bearing large numbers of correctly differentiated cells.

This can be achieved by a variety of techniques, most obviously by detecting a marker product that is characteristic of the differentiated cell, such as a cell surface antigen that is recognised by a ligand or antibody (Fig. 13.5). Alternatively, stem cells can be engineered with an exogenous marker, such as GFP under the control

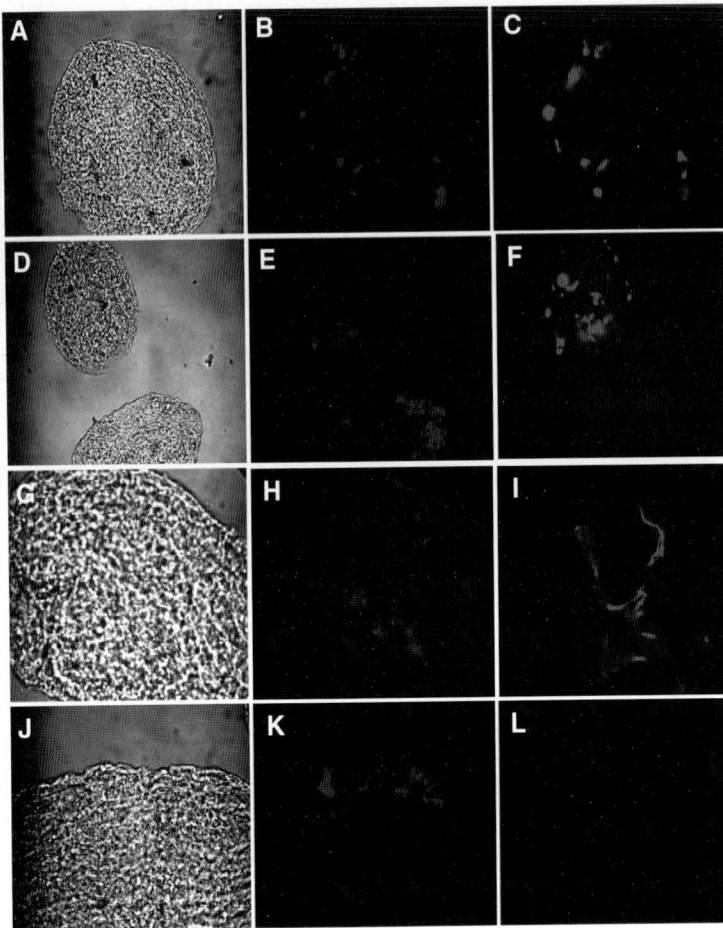

Fig. 13.5 Examples of phenotype detection using cell type-specific antibodies. Cultispher G gelatin microcarriers (Percell Biolytica) were seeded with mESCs and subjected to combinatorial cell culture to obtain neuronal lineages. Left panels show phase micrographs of the beads (under various magnifications) while the middle and right panels respectively show staining with DAPI (showing cell nuclei) and various neuron-specific primary antibodies. Panel C shows staining of dopaminergic neurons (using anti-tyrosine hydroxylase antibody); Panel F shows staining of GABA-ergic cells (anti-GABA antibody); Panel I shows astrocytes (anti-GFAP antibody). Panel L shows the secondary antibody control (*See Color Plates*)

of a cell type-specific promoter, to follow differentiation without the need to stain the cell units (Fig. 13.6). Additional advantages of integrated real time reporters are that they allow continuous monitoring of cell differentiation and unlike phenotypic screens, which are limited by the availability of a specific antibody, genetic markers can be applied to any differentially expressed gene. Reporter genes have been integrated into hESCs using phiC31 phage integrase to target genomic hotspots that

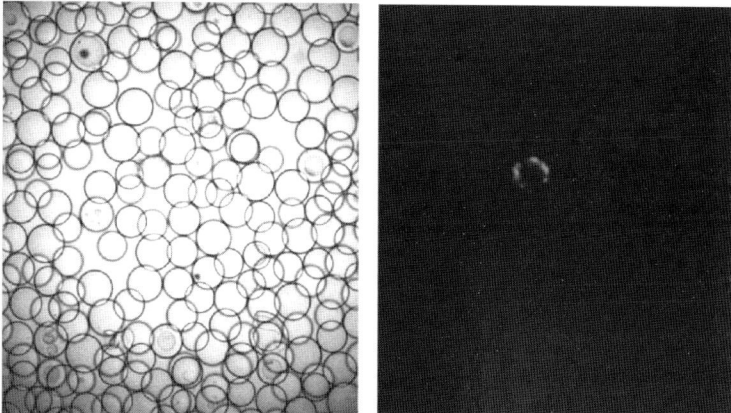

Fig. 13.6 Example of a cell unit screen to isolate a 'positive' bead. A population of Cytodex 3 microcarriers (GE Healthcare) viewed using phase (left) and epifluorescence (right) microscopy reveals a unit bearing cells that express GFP. The 'positive' bead can be isolated manually using a pipette, or using an automated bead sorter (see text) (*See Color Plates*)

support gene expression before and after cell differentiation [94] and it is likely that hESC lines modified with such reporters will become commonplace. Finally, it is possible to carry out functional screening of cell units, for instance to detect a characteristic enzyme activity (e.g. cytochrome P450 activity in hepatocytes) or other cell-specific function (e.g. phagocytosis by macrophages).

Cell units displaying large numbers of correctly differentiated cells can be isolated by a variety of techniques, but most straightforwardly by manual sorting of the cell units (under a microscope) using a pipette. Automated sorting is also possible, for instance by techniques similar to fluorescence activated bead sorting but conventional fluorescence activated cell sorting (FACS) instruments are not normally suitable owing to the large size of microcarriers. The COPAS™ instrument (Union Biometrica), devised for sorting live samples (typically embryos or small model organisms) that are too large for conventional cytometers, is capable of sorting objects including beads up to 1 mm in size based on size and fluorescence parameters.

13.5.2.5 Determining Cell Culture History of Cell Units

The absolute number of cell units to be processed for analysis depends firstly on the frequency of 'hits' and also on the level of background that can result in a certain proportion of false positives (i.e. beads which score positive in the screen but the cells have not acquired the phenotype as a result of directed differentiation). Besides false positives which occur as a result of screening artifacts, false positives may arise as a result of the interaction (signaling) of two separate cell units during any of the experimental steps, or as a result of spontaneous differentiation of cell units that pass through a series of culture conditions that are permissive for differentiation but do not necessarily reliably direct differentiation. Both these types of differentiation are difficult to reproduce. Such false positives occur more frequently when: (i) the target cell type lies in an 'easy-to-obtain' lineage; (ii) the experimental matrix is comprised predominantly of conditions which result in differentiation towards the lineage of interest; or (iii) when the media contain a general inducer of differentiation such as serum. The implication is that Combinatorial Cell Culture is practically more useful for determining conditions that lead to extremely rare events. In these cases there will presumably be a small number of 'hits' and many fewer if any false positives.

The precise method of determining the cell culture history of a cell unit depends largely on the type of tags used in the Combinatorial Cell Culture experiment, for instance whether the tags are read during or after the experiment. Our lab generally uses either microsphere or optically-encoded, nanomaterial tags, both of which are processed at the end of an experiment in a rather similar manner. Both tags attach to the microcarrier substrate generally within the pores and so must be recovered by total digestion of the cell unit (Fig. 13.3). Following digestion, tags become arrayed on a glass surface and are imaged *in situ* using an epifluorescence microscope equipped with appropriate filter sets (Fig. 13.4) or alternatively using FACS instruments. It is often not necessary to image and categorise all tags from a cell unit in order to be able to deduce the cell culture history, however it can be the case (depending on the efficiency of tagging) that certain tagging data are scarce or even absent, or that there are excess flavours of tags present (indicating tag 'hopping' between units) and in this case fuller analysis of tagging may be required. An automated image acquisition system is desirable and image recognition software is almost certainly absolutely necessary to classify the different tags.

13.5.2.6 Validation of Pathway and Cell Phenotype

Following tag analysis and determination of the cell culture history it is necessary to repeat and validate the putative differentiation protocols in order to quantify and rank the efficiency of each and eliminate irreproducible 'false positives'. Individual protocols are typically assayed by exposing a few thousand cell units to a single series of media – these conditions are not exactly equivalent to those which originally gave rise to the 'hit' since cell units in the two different experiments will almost certainly secrete different types and quantities of growth factors which condition the culture media and therefore influence cell growth and differentiation. Nevertheless this type of experiment, followed by detailed phenotypic analysis of the target cell type, will indicate whether the protocol is reproducible, providing a starting point for further development and optimisation.

Finally, an advantage of using microcarriers in Combinatorial Cell Culture is that the protocol may be adapted for the production of large quantities of differentiated tissue through straightforward scale up of the microculture.

Acknowledgements I would like to gratefully acknowledge John Girdlestone, Nadire Ali, Fraser Hornby, Ying Chen, Marina Tarunina, Bettina Huhse and Chris Johnson who at various times (in the order in which they are listed) contributed to the development of Combinatorial Cell Culture methods at Plasticell Ltd., and (in alphabetical order) Chris Adam, Nick Allen, Hugh Cochrane, Martin Evans, Danny Green, Andrew Griffiths and Aaron Klug for their help and support in this project. I am thankful to N Allen, BH, TM and CJ for their comments and suggestions of improvements to the text and to CJ for help in preparing the manuscript.

References

1. Scrip's Complete Guide to Transplantation (1998) PJB Publications, New York, USA
2. McNeish J (2004) Embryonic stem cells in drug discovery. Nat Rev Drug Discov 3:70–80
3. Pouton CW, Haynes JM (2007) Embryonic stem cells as a source of models for drug discovery. Nat Rev Drug Discov 6:605–616
4. Takahashi K, Tanabe K, Ohnuki M, et al. (2007) Induction of pluripotent stem cells from adult human fibroblasts by defined factors. Cell 131:861–872
5. Evans MJ, Kaufman MH (1981) Establishment in culture of pluripotential cells from mouse embryos. Nature 292:154–156
6. Martin GR (1981) Isolation of a pluripotent cell line from early mouse embryos cultured in medium conditioned by teratocarcinoma stem cells. Proc Natl Acad Sci U S A 78:7634–7638
7. Thomson JA, Itskovitz-Eldor J, Shapiro SS, et al. (1998) Embryonic stem cell lines derived from human blastocysts. Science 282:1145–1147
8. Guhr A, Kurtz A, Friedgen K, et al. (2006) Current state of human embryonic stem cell research: an overview of cell lines and their use in experimental work. Stem Cells 24:2187–2191
9. Adewumi O, Aflatoonian B, Ahrlund-Richter L, et al. (2007) Characterization of human embryonic stem cell lines by the International Stem Cell Initiative. Nat Biotechnol 25:803–816
10. Thomson H (2007) Bioprocessing of embryonic stem cells for drug discovery. Trends Biotechnol 25:224–230
11. Keller G (2005) Embryonic stem cell differentiation: emergence of a new era in biology and medicine. Genes Dev 19:1129–1155
12. Hewitt ZA, Amps KJ, Moore HD (2007) Derivation of GMP raw materials for use in regenerative medicine: hESC-based therapies, progress toward clinical application. Clin Pharmacol Ther 82(4):448–452
13. Fletcher JM, Ferrier PM, Gardner JO, et al. (2006) Variations in humanized and defined culture conditions supporting derivation of new human embryonic stem cell lines. Cloning Stem Cells 8:319–334
14. Mallon BS, Park KY, Chen KG, et al. (2006) Toward xeno-free culture of human embryonic stem cells. Int J Biochem Cell Biol 38:1063–1075
15. Terstegge S, Laufenberg I, Pochert J, et al. (2007) Automated maintenance of embryonic stem cell cultures. Biotechnol Bioeng 96:195–201
16. Thomson H (2007) Bioprocessing of embryonic stem cells for drug discovery. Trends Biotechnol 25:224–230
17. Xu C, Inokuma MS, Denham J, et al. (2001) Feeder-free growth of undifferentiated human embryonic stem cells. Nat Biotechnol 19:971–974
18. Stacey GN, Cobo F, Nieto A, et al. (2006) The development of 'feeder' cells for the preparation of clinical grade hESC lines: challenges and solutions. J Biotechnol 125:583–588
19. Mallon BS, Park K-Y, Chen KG, et al. (2006) Toward xeno-free culture of human embryonic stem cells. Int J Biochem Cell Biol 38:1063–1075
20. Joannides A, Fiore-Heriche C, Westmore K, et al. (2006) Automated mechanical passaging: a novel and efficient method for human embryonic stem cell expansion. Stem Cells 24:230–235

21. Ellerstrom C, Strehl R, Noaksson K, et al. (2007) Facilitated expansion of human embryonic stem cells by single-cell enzymatic dissociation. Stem Cells 25:1690–1696

22. Watanabe K, Ueno M, Kamiya D, et al. (2007) A ROCK inhibitor permits survival of dissociated human embryonic stem cells. Nat Biotechnol 25:681–686

23. Terstegge S, Pochert J, Brustle O (2004) Hamilton's new cellhost system for full automation of embryonic stem cell cultures. Nat Meth 1:271–272

24. Hewitt ZA, Amps KJ, Moore HD (2007) Derivation of GMP raw materials for use in regenerative medicine: hESC-based therapies, progress toward clinical application. Clin Pharmacol Ther 82:448–452

25. Rao M (2008) Scalable human ES culture for therapeutic use: propagation, differentiation, genetic modification and regulatory issues. Gene Ther 15(2):82–88

26. Kurosawa H (2007) Methods for inducing embryoid body formation: *in vitro* differentiation system of embryonic stem cells. J Biosci Bioeng 103:389–398

27. Rideout WM, 3rd, Eggan K, Jaenisch R (2001) Nuclear cloning and epigenetic reprogramming of the genome. Science 293:1093–1098

28. Blyszczuk P, Czyz J, Kania G, et al. (2003) Expression of Pax4 in embryonic stem cells promotes differentiation of nestin-positive progenitor and insulin-producing cells. Proc Natl Acad Sci U S A 100:998–1003

29. Miyazaki S, Yamato E, Miyazaki J-i (2004) Regulated expression of pdx-1 promotes *in vitro* differentiation of insulin-producing cells from embryonic stem cells. Diabetes 53:1030–1037

30. Kim J-H, Auerbach JM, Rodriguez-Gomez JA, et al. (2002) Dopamine neurons derived from embryonic stem cells function in an animal model of Parkinson's disease. Nature 418:50–56

31. Martinat C, Bacci J-J, Leete T, et al. (2006) Cooperative transcription activation by Nurr1 and Pitx3 induces embryonic stem cell maturation to the midbrain dopamine neuron phenotype. Proc Natl Acad Sci U S A 103:2874–2879

32. Woods NB, Bottero V, Schmidt M, et al. (2006) Gene therapy: therapeutic gene causing lymphoma. Nature 440:1123

33. de-Leon SB-T, Davidson EH (2007) Gene regulation: gene control network in development. Annu Rev Biophys and Biomol Struct 36:191–212

34. Keller GM (1995) *In vitro* differentiation of embryonic stem cells. Curr Opin Cell Biol 7:862–869

35. Trounson A (2006) The production and directed differentiation of human embryonic stem cells. Endocr Rev 27:208–219

36. D'Amour KA, Agulnick AD, Eliazer S, et al. (2005) Efficient differentiation of human embryonic stem cells to definitive endoderm. Nat Biotechnol 23:1534–1541

37. Ma F, Wang D, Hanada S, et al. (2007) Novel method for efficient production of multipotential hematopoietic progenitors from human embryonic stem cells. Int J Hematol 85:371–379

38. Koay EJ, Hoben GM, Athanasiou KA (2007) Tissue engineering with chondrogenically differentiated human embryonic stem cells. Stem Cells 25:2183–2190

39. Barberi T, Willis LM, Socci ND, et al. (2005) Derivation of multipotent mesenchymal precursors from human embryonic stem cells. PLoS Med 2:e161

40. Lamba DA, Karl MO, Ware CB, et al. (2006) Efficient generation of retinal progenitor cells from human embryonic stem cells. Proc Natl Acad Sci U S A 103:12769–12774

41. Xu C, He JQ, Kamp TJ, et al. (2006) Human embryonic stem cell-derived cardiomyocytes can be maintained in defined medium without serum. Stem Cells Dev 15:931–941

42. Xu C, Police S, Rao N, et al. (2002) Characterization and enrichment of cardiomyocytes derived from human embryonic stem cells. Circ Res 91:501–508

43. Laflamme MA, Chen KY, Naumova AV, et al. (2007) Cardiomyocytes derived from human embryonic stem cells in pro-survival factors enhance function of infarcted rat hearts. Nat Biotechnol 25:1015–1024

44. Leor J, Gerecht S, Cohen S, et al. (2007) Human embryonic stem cell transplantation to repair the infarcted myocardium. Heart 93:1278–1284

45. Barberi T, Bradbury M, Dincer Z, et al. (2007) Derivation of engraftable skeletal myoblasts from human embryonic stem cells. Nat Med 13:642–648

46. Flaim CJ, Chien S, Bhatia SN (2005) An extracellular matrix microarray for probing cellular differentiation. Nat Methods 2:119–125

47. Anderson DG, Levenberg S, Langer R (2004) Nanoliter-scale synthesis of arrayed biomaterials and application to human embryonic stem cells. Nat Biotechnol 22:863–866

48. Mei Y, Goldberg M, Anderson D (2007) The development of high-throughput screening approaches for stem cell engineering. Curr Opin Chem Biol 11:388–393

49. Wichterle H, Lieberam I, Porter JA, et al. (2002) Directed differentiation of embryonic stem cells into motor neurons. Cell 110:385–397

50. Reubinoff BE, Itsykson P, Turetsky T, et al. (2001) Neural progenitors from human embryonic stem cells. Nat Biotechnol 19:1134–1140

51. Zhang SC, Wernig M, Duncan ID, et al. (2001) *In vitro* differentiation of transplantable neural precursors from human embryonic stem cells. Nat Biotechnol 19:1129–1133

52. Li XJ, Du ZW, Zarnowska ED, et al. (2005) Specification of motoneurons from human embryonic stem cells. Nat Biotechnol 23:215–221

53. Perrier AL, Tabar V, Barberi T, et al. (2004) From the Cover: derivation of midbrain dopamine neurons from human embryonic stem cells. Proc Natl Acad Sci U S A 101:12543–12548

54. Yan Y, Yang D, Zarnowska ED, et al. (2005) Directed differentiation of dopaminergic neuronal subtypes from human embryonic stem cells. Stem Cells 23:781–790

55. Roy NS, Cleren C, Singh SK, et al. (2006) Functional engraftment of human ESC-derived dopaminergic neurons enriched by coculture with telomerase-immortalized midbrain astrocytes. Nat Med 12:1259–1268

56. Ohyama K, Ellis P, Kimura S, et al. (2005) Directed differentiation of neural cells to hypothalamic dopaminergic neurons. Development 132:5185–5197

57. Salero E, Hatten ME (2007) Differentiation of ESCs into cerebellar neurons. Proc Natl Acad Sci U S A 104:2997–3002

58. Mizuseki K, Sakamoto T, Watanabe K, et al. (2003) Generation of neural crest-derived peripheral neurons and floor plate cells from mouse and primate embryonic stem cells. Proc Natl Acad Sci U S A 100:5828–5833

59. Rathjen J, Haines BP, Hudson KM, et al. (2002) Directed differentiation of pluripotent cells to neural lineages: homogeneous formation and differentiation of a neurectoderm population. Development 129:2649–2661

60. Motohashi T, Aoki H, Chiba K, et al. (2007) Multipotent cell fate of neural crest-like cells derived from embryonic stem cells. Stem Cells 25:402–410

61. Keirstead HS, Nistor G, Bernal G, et al. (2005) Human embryonic stem cell-derived oligodendrocyte progenitor cell transplants remyelinate and restore locomotion after spinal cord injury. J Neurosci 25:4694–4705

62. Brustle O, Jones KN, Learish RD, et al. (1999) Embryonic stem cell-derived glial precursors: a source of myelinating transplants. Science 285:754–756

63. Aubert J, Stavridis MP, Tweedie S, et al. (2003) Screening for mammalian neural genes via fluorescence-activated cell sorter purification of neural precursors from Sox1-gfp knock-in mice. Proc Natl Acad Sci U S A 100:11836–11841

64. Klug MG, Soonpaa MH, Koh GY, et al. (1996) Genetically selected cardiomyocytes from differentiating embronic stem cells form stable intracardiac grafts. J Clin Invest 98:216–224

65. Li M, Pevny L, Lovell-Badge R, et al. (1998) Generation of purified neural precursors from embryonic stem cells by lineage selection. Curr Biol 8:971–974

66. Laflamme MA, Chen KY, Naumova AV, et al. (2007) Cardiomyocytes derived from human embryonic stem cells in pro-survival factors enhance function of infarcted rat hearts. Nat Biotechnol 25:1015–1024

67. Joannides AJ, Fiore-Heriche C, Battersby AA, et al. (2007) A scaleable and defined system for generating neural stem cells from human embryonic stem cells. Stem Cells 25:731–737

68. Bouhon IA, Kato H, Chandran S, et al. (2005) Neural differentiation of mouse embryonic stem cells in chemically defined medium. Brain Res Bull 68:62–75

69. Watanabe K, Kamiya D, Nishiyama A, et al. (2005) Directed differentiation of telencephalic precursors from embryonic stem cells. Nat Neurosci 8:288–296

70. Conti L, Pollard SM, Gorba T, et al. (2005) Niche-independent symmetrical self-renewal of a mammalian tissue stem cell. PLoS Biol 3:e283

71. Yasunaga M, Tada S, Torikai-Nishikawa S, et al. (2005) Induction and monitoring of definitive and visceral endoderm differentiation of mouse ESCs. Nat Biotechnol 23:1542–1550

72. D'Amour KA, Agulnick AD, Eliazer S, et al. (2005) Efficient differentiation of human embryonic stem cells to definitive endoderm. Nat Biotechnol 23:1534–1541

73. Itskovitz-Eldor J, Schuldiner M, Karsenti D, et al. (2000) Differentiation of human embryonic stem cells into embryoid bodies comprising the three embryonic germ layers. Mol Med 6:88–95

74. Chen S, Hilcove S, Ding S (2006) Exploring stem cell biology with small molecules. Mol Biosyst 2:18–24

75. Takahashi T, Lord B, Schulze PC, et al. (2003) Ascorbic acid enhances differentiation of embryonic stem cells into cardiac myocytes. Circulation 107:1912–1916

76. Wu X, Ding S, Ding Q, et al. (2004) Small molecules that induce cardiomyogenesis in embryonic stem cells. J Am Chem Soc 126:1590–1591

77. Chen S, Do JT, Zhang Q, et al. (2006) Self-renewal of embryonic stem cells by a small molecule. Proc Natl Acad Sci 103:17266–17271

78. Karen H. Chang, Peter W. Zandstra (2004) Quantitative screening of embryonic stem cell differentiation: endoderm formation as a model. Biotechnol Bioeng 88:287–298

79. Arnold FH (1998) Design by directed evolution. Acc Chem Res 31:125–131

80. Smith GP (1985) Filamentous fusion phage: novel expression vectors that display cloned antigens on the virion surface. Science 228:1315–1317

81. Tawfik DS, Griffiths AD (1998) Man-made cell-like compartments for molecular evolution. Nat Biotechnol 16:652–656

82. Choo Y (2002) Cell Culture. GB0222846.8, 3 Oct 2002

83. GE (http://www6.gelifesciences.com/aptrix/upp00919.nsf/Content/WD:Microcarrier + ce(148896581-B345)) Microcarrier cell culture - principles and methods.

84. Nicolaou KCE, Hanko RE, Hartwig WE (2002) Handbook of Combinatorial Chemistry: Drugs, Catalysts, Materials. Wiley-VCH, Weinheim, Germany

85. Terrett NK (1998) Combinatorial Chemistry (Oxford Chemistry Masters). Oxford University Press

86. Braeckmans K, De Smedt SC, Leblans M, et al. (2002) Encoding microcarriers: present and future technologies. Nat Rev Drug Discov 1:447–456

87. Walton CA (1983) Portable radio frequency emitting identifier. US Patent 4,384,288, 17 May 1983

88. Cardullo MW, Parks WL (1973) Transponder apparatus and system. US Patent 3,713,148, 23 Jan 1973

89. Finkel NH, Lou XH, Wang CY, et al. (2004) Barcoding the microworld. Anal Chem 76:353A–359A

90. Nicewarner-Pena SR, Freeman RG, Reiss BD, et al. (2001) Submicrometer metallic barcodes. Science 294:137–141

91. Gudiksen MS, Lauhon LJ, Wang J, et al. (2002) Growth of nanowire superlattice structures for nanoscale photonics and electronics. Nature 415:617–620

92. Matthias S, Schilling J, Nielsch K, et al. (2002) Monodisperse diameter-modulated gold microwires. Adv Mater 14:1618–1621

93. Probst MCO, Rothe G, Schmitz G (2003) Bead-based multiplex analysis. Bead-basierte multiplexanalyse. Laboratoriums Medizin 27:182–187

94. Thyagarajan B, Liu Y, Shin S, et al. (2008) Creation of engineered human embryonic stem cell lines using phiC31 integrase. Stem Cells 26:119–126

Chapter 14
Adult Stem Cell Therapies for Tissue Regeneration: *Ex Vivo* Expansion in an Automated System

Kristin L. Goltry[1]*, Douglas M. Smith[1], James E. Dennis[2], Jon A. Rowley[1], and Ronnda L. Bartel[1]

Abstract Cell therapy is an emerging field whose technology is being investigated for the treatment of a variety of injuries and diseases affecting multiple tissue types. Many questions exist in the field of cell therapy, from understanding the basic mechanisms of action, to the optimal methods for preparing and administering cells to the patient. Answers to these questions will help determine the best cell source, optimal protocols for *ex vivo* manipulation of cells, and the best methods for delivery of cells. This chapter details one experience in the development of an *ex vivo* cultured autologous cell therapy for tissue repair, in this case the healing of non-union bone fractures. Methods were developed to expand a population of bone marrow mononuclear cells in culture resulting in a mixed population of cells with greatly enhanced bone-forming potential. These Tissue Repair Cells (TRCs) have been shown to possess multi-lineage potential both *in vitro* and *in vivo* in animal models. A manufacturing platform has been designed to culture and harvest the cell product in an automated closed fashion. After mixing TRCs with a bone scaffold material, cells maintained their ability to proliferate, secrete cytokines, and differentiate into the desired cell lineage. Preliminary results have demonstrated that TRCs can be successfully implanted and heal bone fractures in the clinic.

Keywords *Ex vivo* expansion, adult stem cells, tissue regeneration

[1] Aastrom Biosciences, Inc., Ann Arbor, MI, USA

[2] Department of Orthopaedics, Case Western Reserve University, Cleveland, OH, USA

*Corresponding Author:
24 Frank Lloyd Wright Dr. Lobby K, Ann Arbor, MI 48105
e-mail: kgoltry@aastrom.com

Y. Shi, D.O. Clegg (eds.) *Stem Cell Research and Therapeutics*,
© Springer Science+Business Media B.V. 2008

14.1 Introduction

14.1.1 Approaches to Cell Therapy

There are many clinical situations in which cell therapies are being explored as an opportunity to treat diseases or heal injuries. Indications in which cell therapy is being investigated as a treatment range from diabetes, muscular dystrophy, Parkinson's disease, autism, peripheral arterial disease, cardiovascular disease, heart failure, and trauma, including spinal cord injury and bone fractures [1–11]. Institutes are being established around the world with a focus on regenerative medicine, combining biology and engineering expertise to address issues surrounding cell therapy and tissue regeneration. Many questions remain unanswered in the realm of cell therapy: What is the best source of cells for specific indications? How many cells are required? Are multiple cell types required? Should they be differentiated into specific lineages or be more "stem-like"? What is the mechanism of action? Answers to these questions are the focus of intense investigation and will certainly differ based on the therapeutic indication.

14.1.2 Cell Sources

One of the first examples of stem cell therapy was bone marrow transplantation [12]. Donor bone marrow was shown to reconstitute the hematopoietic system of the host, leading to complete or mixed chimaerism. Since then, bone marrow has been shown to be a rich source of stem and progenitor cells capable of regenerating a variety of non-hematopoietic tissues including vascular, bone, cartilage, fat, and muscle [13, 14].

In addition to bone marrow, there are other sources of stem and progenitor cells from adult non-embryonic tissues, including peripheral blood [15, 16], umbilical cord blood [17–19], and specific tissues such as adipose [20, 21], liver, skin, muscle, and brain [22, 23]. Cells from these sources are being used in both pre-clinical and clinical studies.

Embryonic stem cells are being investigated as another source of cells for therapy, although work is still in the pre-clinical phase [24]. It is thought that the potential of embryonic stem cells is greater than that of adult stem cells for regenerating all tissue types. However, issues which need to be addressed include the use of allogeneic cells with respect to immune rejection and the potential for teratoma formation with their enhanced proliferative potential.

Autologous cells come directly from the patient so there is little chance of rejection. Furthermore, new methods of reprogramming suggest that autologous cells might be converted to pluripotency for a wide variety of applications. However, there are logistical difficulties for the isolation, culturing, and delivery of an autologous cell product that must remain sterile and whose procedures must adhere to strict FDA rules and Good Manufacturing Practices (GMP). Additionally, if the underlying indication is a genetic defect, or there are age-related issues affecting the stem cells, allogeneic transplantation may be more beneficial. Allogeneic cells have the benefit of being "off-the-shelf" but with concomitant issues of immune reactivity and rejection which need to be addressed as far as safety and long-term benefits.

14.1.3 Cell Purity

Many cell therapies are utilizing purified cell populations derived from bone marrow, including CD34+ cells, CD133+ cells, or mesenchymal stem cells (MSC) [25–29]. Cells are purified by direct or indirect selection methods or by culture purifying. Purified populations may be beneficial when the exact mechanism of action is known, or if other cell types are thought to hinder repair. However, mixed cell populations contain multiple cell lineages with the potential to provide multi-lineage repair of complex organs and tissues. Organs and tissues are, by definition, made up of more than one cell type, and complete regeneration in many cases will mean regeneration of multiple cell types.

14.1.4 Mechanism of Action

The mechanism of action of cell therapies can differ, and in many cases is largely unknown. In some cases, cells may directly contribute to regeneration of the target tissue by differentiation and integration into the tissue cell type, while in other cases the therapeutic cells do not make a significant direct contribution of functional end-stage cells, but instead contribute to overall tissue healing. For example, it is known that cells secrete factors that can promote or stimulate tissue repair or regeneration, may regulate the inflammatory response to favor tissue repair over tissue destruction, and may contribute to revascularization, diminish scarring and inhibit apoptosis [30–33]. The mechanism of action will certainly differ by the cell type used, the delivery mechanism (local vs. systemic), and the indication. Until the mechanism of action for tissue repair or regeneration is known, it will be difficult to optimize cell therapy approaches.

14.1.5 Ex Vivo Culture

Some autologous therapies utilize cells directly after harvest from the patient, or manipulate cells only minimally prior to delivery to the patient [34–36]. However, when there are not enough regenerative cells in the initial harvest, *ex vivo* culturing has been employed. Culturing has potential advantages, not only increasing the number of cells, but also by using conditions that may lead to purification, activation, differentiation or functional enhancement of stem and progenitor cells. However, conditions must be optimized and extensively tested to ensure the regenerative potential of the cells is maintained during the culture period.

One of the biggest challenges of *ex vivo* cell therapy, particularly an autologous approach, is the transfer of cell-based products from *ex vivo* culture to the patient in a clinically and commercially viable way. While autologous cell therapy provides significant advantages including safety to the patient, it presents a unique manufacturing challenge.

14.1.6 Implementation and Commercialization of Cell Therapy

The regulatory environment and requirements are very different when comparing minimally manipulated cell products and *ex vivo* cultured cell therapeutics. If *ex vivo* expansion is required to increase numbers of cells, a consistent and scalable cell manufacturing is required. The practical delivery of an *ex vivo* cell therapy requires a comprehensive GMP-compliant cell manufacturing process that integrates: (1) the biological process that drives production of functional cells in sufficient numbers; (2) the culture device capable of supporting the biological process; (3) an automated support system which provides reliability and reproducibility of the process in a closed system environment; and (4) post-manufacturing processing of the cell product to prepare for patient administration. Release criteria including identity, purity and potency must be defined for each lot of cells produced. There are very few cell products that have been commercialized to date, and none have had to go through the regulatory pathways now in place for cell therapies.

The remainder of this chapter will focus on one approach to deliver an *ex vivo* cultured autologous cell therapy for the regeneration of bone. This includes the manufacturing and characterization of the cell product, formulation of the product for delivery to patient, and potential mechanisms of action for tissue regeneration using this cell product.

14.2 Automated Cell Manufacturing Platform

Ex vivo autologous cell therapy presents a unique manufacturing challenge as the dose of cells for each patient must be produced and released as its own unique manufacturing lot. Manual methods of generating cells in flasks or other culture devices have been used clinically, but these methods require many resources, more manual steps, technician time with associated costs, and open steps which introduce potential sources for errors or contamination. Thus, there is an increased need for an automated system to minimize the number of manual steps and increase safety while reliably producing functional cell products.

An automated closed system has previously been developed for the *ex vivo* expansion bone marrow mononuclear cells (BM MNCs) from a small volume bone marrow aspirate [37]. This cell manufacturing system embodies a modular, closed-system process comprised of a pre-sterilized, single-use disposable cell cassette operated by automated instruments. The bioreactor within the cell cassette implements single-pass perfusion (SPP) for optimal cell growth.

14.2.1 Single Pass Perfusion

Single pass perfusion is a unique method for replacement of consumed medium components and removal of metabolic byproducts while decoupling the rate of gas exchange from medium exchange. For example, slow continuous medium perfusion rates can be implemented to provide fresh medium and optimal exchange of nutrients without disturbance or removal of adherent or non-adherent cell types. This method maintains the bone-marrow-like microenvironment provided by the interaction of multiple cellular subpopulations together with endogenous secretion of extracellular matrix components, cytokines and other growth factors.

Previous work has shown the importance of medium perfusion, not only on the productivity and longevity of BM cultures [38], but also on the metabolic activity and growth factor production rates of marrow stromal cells [39]. Monocyte-derived dendritic cells have demonstrated enhanced antigen presentation and maturation with increased medium perfusion (Smith DM, Gorgas GC, Hastie KR et al. unpublished data 2001). Similarly, continuous SPP in human T-lymphocyte cultures yielded very high density cultures and cells with superior replicative potential and enhanced biological function, as measured by release of GM-CSF and TNF-α in response to anti-CD3 [41]. Thus, single pass medium perfusion may enhance the critical cellular microenvironment necessary for optimal expansion and biological function of both stem and progenitor cells as well as more mature and lineage-committed cell types required for many different types of tissue repair.

In more recent work, the beneficial effect of frequent medium exchange on BM MNC culture output was evaluated in small-scale cultures over a range of inoculum densities. The absolute number of marrow stromal cells, as defined by the expression of the cell surface marker CD90, was enhanced with increasing rate of medium exchange when evaluated at harvest on day 12 or day 19 of culture (Fig. 14.1). The CD90 surface antigen has been established as one of several key mesenchymal markers for bone-forming progenitors that correlates closely with colony forming unit – fibroblast (CFU-F) activity and osteogenesis in a murine xenogeneic model [42]. CFU-F formation is also an indicator of cellular proliferative potential. As shown in Fig. 14.2, CFU-F output in 12 day bone marrow cultures was also increased with increasing rate of medium exchange.

In addition to cell output, frequent medium exchange strikingly enhances endogenous cytokine secretion during the course of a 12 day culture (Fig. 14.3). Interleukin-6 (IL-6) is a pleiotrophic cytokine with hematopoietic and immunomodulatory

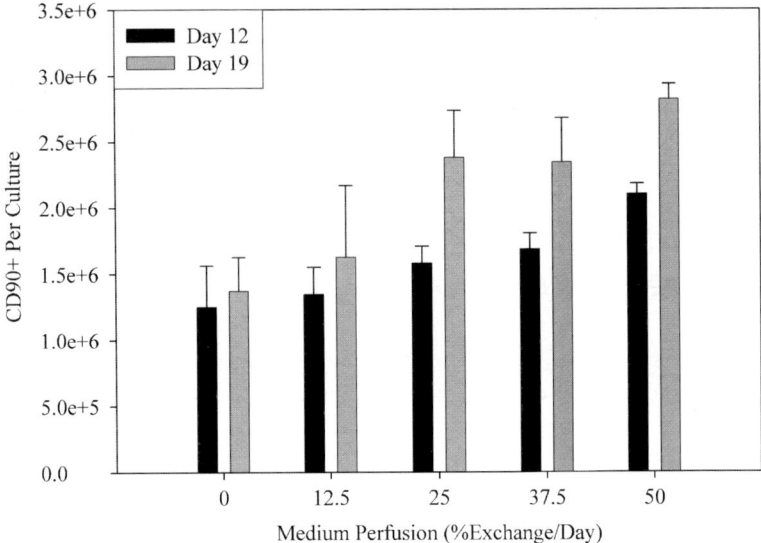

Fig. 14.1 Frequent medium exchange enhances the output of CD90+ marrow stromal progenitors. BM MNC (3×10^5 cells/cm^2) were inoculated in replicate cultures on day 0 and maintained in LTBMC medium for 12 or 19 days over a range of medium exchange rates. The average number of CD-90-positive cells are indicated, with error bars indicating the range from two experiments. Similar results were observed for both low (1.5×10^5 cells/cm^2) or high (6×10^5 cells/cm^2) inoculum density cultures (data not shown)

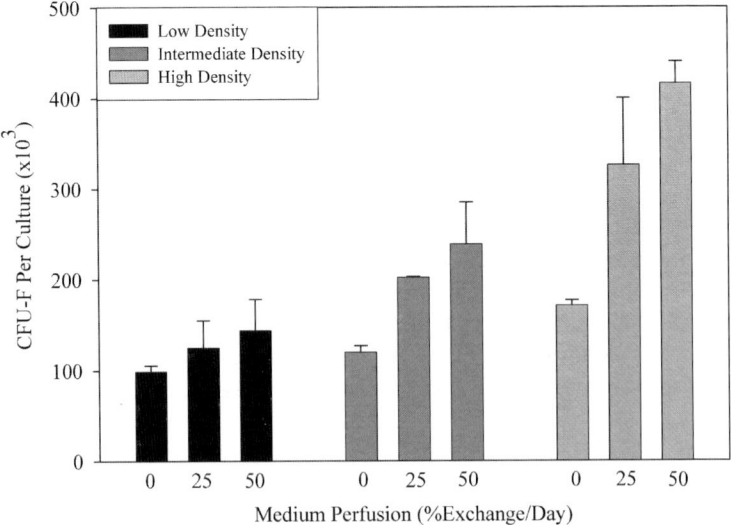

Fig. 14.2 Frequent medium exchange enhances CFU-F output. BM MNCs were cultured in LTBMC medium for 12 days. The number of CFU-Fs at harvest is shown for low (1.5×10^5 cells/ cm^2), intermediate (3×10^5 cells/cm^2) and high (6×10^5 cells/cm^2) inoculum density cultures maintained over a range of perfusion rates. The average and range from two experiments is shown (*See Color Plates*)

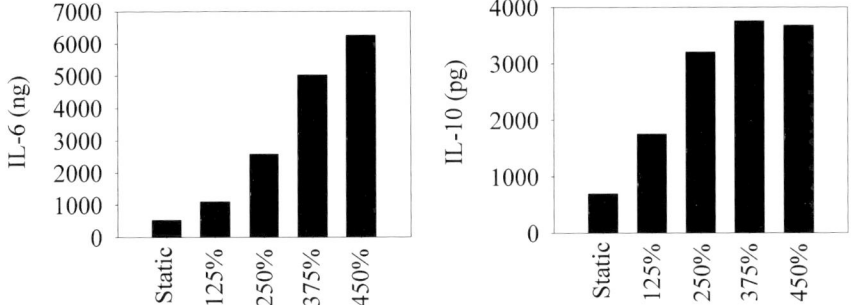

Fig. 14.3 Medium perfusion enhances the endogenous secretion of cytokines in cultures. BM MNCs were cultured in LTBMC medium for 12 days. Total cytokine production was measured by Luminex. Results are presented as total cytokine production vs. total medium exchange (%vol/vol) over the 12 day culture process

activities secreted by multiple populations including the stromal cell component, while interleukin-10 (IL-10) is an anti-inflammatory cytokine characteristically produced by alternatively-activated macrophages within the cell mixture. Lower production of these cytokines in cultures with less frequent medium exchange may be the result of some type of feedback inhibition. These observations suggest that continuous medium perfusion may provide a unique microenvironment for cellular expansion and differentiation of bone marrow derived cells when compared to conventional static culture conditions such as traditional Dexter type cultures.

14.2.2 Cell Manufacturing System

Standardization of SPP technology led to the development of the automated perfused bioreactor system which supports the production of a unique mixture of highly functional patient-specific stem and progenitor cells with multiple tissue regenerative capabilities.

One component of the automated system is the cell cassette, which provides a functionally closed, sterile environment which supports SPP technology and provides a surface for cell attachment and growth (Fig. 14.4). The incorporation of a gas-permeable and liquid-impermeable membrane within the bioreactor design enables continuous medium replacement while simultaneously providing uniform oxygen diffusion as necessary for cell expansion over a wide range of medium exchange rates. The fluid pathway in the cell cassette includes the cell culture vessel (bioreactor), a medium supply container, a waste container, and a container for harvested cells. Gases are exchanged through a membrane above the medium. All components are interconnected with sterile barrier elements throughout, to protect the culture from contamination during use.

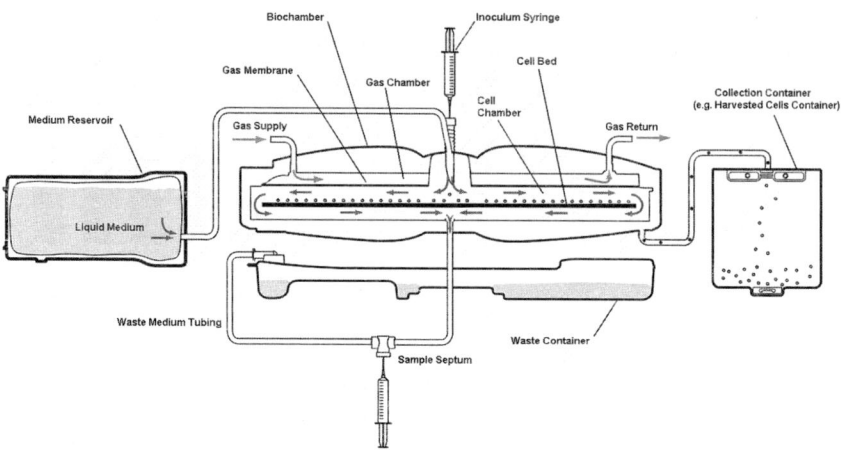

Fig. 14.4 Schematic of bioreactor cassette. Single-pass medium perfusion occurs from the center port of the bioreactor and continues radially over an 850 cm² tissue-culture-treated plastic growth surface. Uniform oxygen delivery is achieved independently of medium exchange through a gas-permeable, liquid-impermeable membrane separating the gas and liquid sides of the bioreactor cassette

The instrumentation components of the manufacturing platform, described previously [37], include a set of incubator units and a cell processor unit, along with a computer-based system manager (Fig. 14.5). Each incubator can control the flow of medium to the growth chamber, the temperature of the growth medium supply compartment, the temperature of the cell growth chamber, and the concentration of gases (O_2, CO_2 and N_2) independently. The cell processor performs the priming of the bioreactor with growth medium, the inoculation and distribution of cells, and is used at the end of culture to harvest the cells. A semiconductor memory device and clock is attached to each cell cassette and provides reliable identification of the cell product, instructs the instruments during cell production process, prevents mix-ups and operator error, and stores the primary data for a complete process history record-effectively a "manufacturing batch record" for the cell product.

This manufacturing platform has proven successful in the automated expansion of a variety of cell types. Protocols have been developed for the production of hematopoietic stem and progenitor cells from BM [43, 44], and umbilical cord blood (UCB) [45–47] for use in stem cell transplants. This platform also supports the expansion of mesenchymal components of BM and is currently being used in clinical trials for bone regeneration [48]. Protocols for the production of dendritic cells and T-cells have been developed for use in cancer vaccines [49].

Automation of the cell culture process has resulted in reliable and reproducible cell production while limiting the amount of cell manipulation. In total, this manufacturing

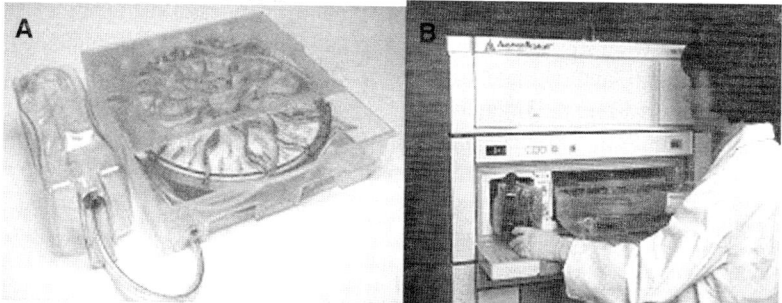

Fig. 14.5 Bioreactor cassette and incubator from the automated system. Pictured is a single use cell cassette with medium reservoir (**A**) and an incubator being loaded with a cell cassette containing BM MNC (**B**). The incubator holds up to four individual cassettes that can be controlled independently for flow rate, temperature and gas levels (*See Color Plates*)

system has supported more than 625 *ex-vivo* cell production lots for over 250 patients. The current manufacturing capacity is approximately 500 doses of cells per year, with cells being produced in a centralized GMP manufacturing facility.

14.2.3   Post-culture Processing

A critical step in the cell production process is preparing the cells for patient administration. This entails the removal of medium residuals (such as serum proteins), achieving an appropriate product volume, and, depending on the application, mixing cells with delivery vehicles such as scaffolds or injectable matrices, prior to implantation. Many of these post-culture processing steps are not currently automated or easily integrated into the manufacturing process, so they remain inefficient and result in cell loss and decreased cell viability. As a result, the post-culture phase remains a relatively time-consuming process, subject to increased risks of variability, operator error, contamination, and excessive holding times. Although these issues have been managed for limited patient capacity, development of an automated unit process that leads to high recovery and viability of the cell product is critical for manufacturing scale-up of an autologous product.

14.3   Tissue Repair Cell (TRC) Biology

Currently, the manufacturing platform is being used to produce a BM derived cell mixture referred to here as Tissue Repair Cells (TRCs). BM MNCs are cultured for 12 days with SPP in a long term bone marrow culture medium (LTBMC) consisting of IMDM with 10% horse serum, 10% fetal bovine serum, and 5 μM hydrocortisone [42]. The harvested TRC cell product is a unique mixture of cells from hematopoietic, mesenchymal, and endothelial lineages. Overall, the culture process results in a significant increase in the frequency of key stem and progenitor cell lineages with an overall decrease in total nucleated cell numbers.

One method employed to characterize this mixture of cells is flow cytometry to determine the presence of cells with specific surface markers. Markers for hematopoietic, mesenchymal, and endothelial lineages have been examined. Average results from four experiments comparing starting BM MNC and TRC product are shown in Fig. 14.6.

Most hematopoietic lineage cells, including CD11b$^+$ myeloid, CD34$^+$ progenitor, and CD3$^+$ lymphoid are decreased slightly. The CD14$^+$ population is separated into autofluorescent positive (auto+) macrophages and autofluorescent negative (auto−) monocytic populations. While CD14$^+$ auto- monocytes are slightly decreased during culture, the CD14$^+$ auto+ macrophages are expanded 81-fold. The mesenchymal cells, defined by CD90$^+$ and CD14$^-$ or CD105$^+$/166$^+$ and CD45$^-$/14$^-$ were expanded up to 373-fold. Cells that may be involved in vascularization, including mature vascular endothelial cells (CD144$^+$/146$^+$) and CXCR4$^+$/VEGFR1$^+$ supportive cells [50] are expanded from 6- to 21-fold. Although most hematopoietic lineage cells do not

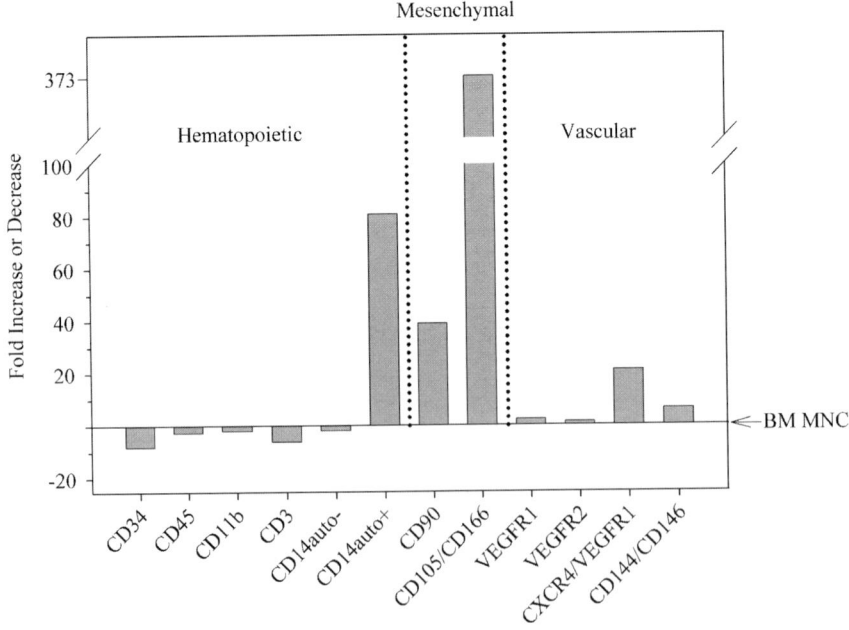

Fig. 14.6 Fold change in cell lineages after ex vivo culture. BM MNC were cultured for 12 days in LTBMC medium. After harvest, cells were counted and analyzed by flow cytometry. The absolute number of different cell types was measured in TRCs and compared to BM MNC. The average fold increase or decrease in cell type from four experiments is shown

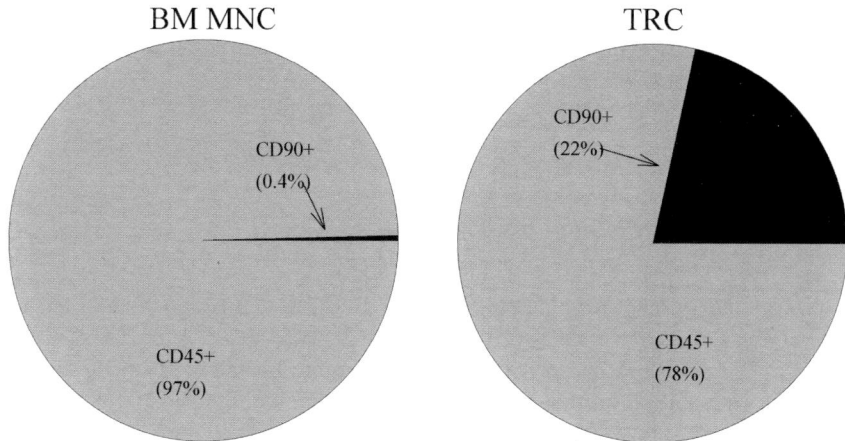

Fig. 14.7 Frequency of hematopoietic and mesenchymal elements in BM MNC and TRC. A pie chart illustrates the frequency (%) as measured by flow cytometry of cells expressing the CD45 and CD90 antigens in BM MNCs and TRCs

Table 14.1 Average colony forming ability of TRCs

| Colon type | BM MNC | | TRC Product | | Fold |
	%	Total #	%	Total #	Expansion
CFU-F	0.01	2.42E + 04	3.77	3.77E + 06	283
CFU-GM	0.63	1.59E + 06	0.56	1.06E + 06	0.71

Results are the average ± SEM from eight clinical-scale experiments.

expand in these cultures, the final product still contains close to 80% CD45$^+$ hematopoietic cells and approximately 20% CD90+ mesenchymal cells (Fig. 14.7).

The ability of cells within TRCs to form colonies was also measured. Both hematopoietic (CFU-GM) and mesenchymal (CFU-F) colonies are present (Table 14.1), and, while CFU-F were increased 280-fold, CFU-GM were slightly decreased by culturing compared to starting BM MNC.

14.4   Bone Regeneration

It is widely accepted that there are three main components required for optimal bone regeneration; (1) a scaffold material on which new bone formation will occur (osteoconductive); (2) a source of growth factors which promote bone formation (osteoinductive); and (3) cells that can differentiate and form new bone (osteogenic).

Human allograft bone and synthetic bone graft substitutes are being examined to augment bone regeneration [51–53], however these carriers do not possess osteogenic properties. Adding osteogenic cells to bone graft material may provide enhanced bone regeneration [54–59].

The frequency of osteoprogenitor cells within normal bone marrow is typically less than 1%. Increasing the number of these osteogenic cells through *ex vivo* expansion techniques offers a potentially superior approach. Therefore studies were conducted to examine the osteogenic potential of TRCs.

14.4.1   In Vitro Osteogenic Potential of TRCs

The osteogenic or bone-forming potential of TRCs was compared to that of normal BM MNCs. Cells were incubated for 14 days with osteogenic factors (dexamethasone, ascorbic acid, and beta-glycerophosphate). Figure 14.8 shows that, after induction, TRCs are able to form a calcified matrix as measured by calcium production, and have increased levels of alkaline phosphatase activity, showing their osteogenic potential. Osteo-specific genes including osteocalcin, osteopontin, and osteoprotegerin, are also increased after induction (data not shown). Importantly, the level of osteogenic potential is much greater in TRC than in normal BM MNC.

To identify which population of cells within TRCs is responsible for this osteogenic potential, cells were separated based on surface markers using fluorescence-activated cell sorting (FACS). Cell sorting experiments showed that the CFU-F and

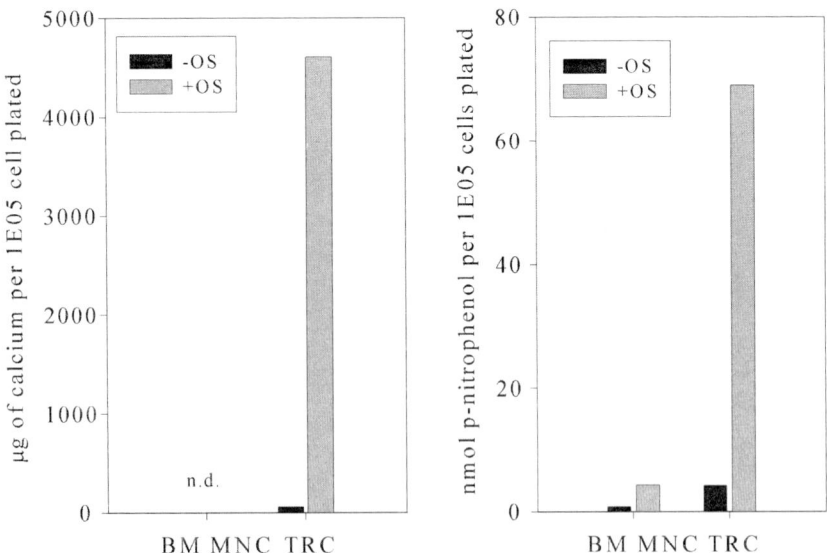

Fig. 14.8 In vitro osteogenic differentiation of TRCs. TRCs or BM MNCs were plated in medium with (+OS) or without (−OS) dexamethasone, ascorbic acid, and beta-glycerophosphate for 14–21 days. Differentiation was measured by calcium deposition (left panel) and alkaline phosphatase activity (right panel). Representative results from one experiment are shown (n.d. = none detected)

osteogenic potential are associated with a subset of cells expressing the CD90 cell surface antigen (Table 14.2).

14.4.2 In Vivo Animal Model for Bone Regeneration

Bone formation was measured by seeding human TRCs into fibronectin-coated ceramic cubes and implanting them subcutaneously in NOD/*scid* mice. Bone scores were calculated by examining histological sections of the mineralized ossicles and counting the number of pores within the matrix that contain new bone. Mineralized bone ossicles were detected after 4–6 weeks [60, 61]. When comparing TRCs to BM MNCs, TRCs showed higher levels of bone formation (Fig. 14.9) [42]. Additional studies showed that the frequency of CD90$^+$ cells within the TRC population has a strong correlation with the amount of bone formation ($r^2 = 0.91$).

14.4.3 Importance of Accessory Cells for Optimal Osteogenic Potential

Mesenchymal stem cells or stromal cells are typically cultured as a purified population of cells expressing CD90 cell surface marker among others. They are purified during the culture process by removing nonadherent cells on day 2–3 of culture. Further purification occurs with passaging of the cells. The osteogenic potential of TRCs was compared to that of typical bone marrow stromal cells (BMSCs). For BMSC, BM MNC were seeded into flasks and nonadherent cells were removed on day 3. Remaining adherent cells were cultured until day 14. Cells were assayed from this primary culture and were not passaged.

The osteogenic potential of TRCs and BMSCs was measured by culturing in osteogenic medium containing dexamethasone, β-glycerophosphate, and L-ascorbate-2-phosphate. After 2 weeks, calcium deposition and alkaline phosphatase activity were determined as a measure of osteogenic differentiation. In osteogenic cultures, nonadherent cells are removed with a 100% medium exchange on day 1 so only plastic adherent cells are measured for osteogenic potential.

Results show similar osteogenic potential between TRCs and BMSCs (Fig. 14.10, left panel) even though the frequency of CD90$^+$ cells was only 20% in TRCs compared to more than 80% in BMSCs for these experiments. Since the osteogenic

Table 14.2 CD90+ fraction has CFU-F and osteogenic potential

TRC cell population	Average CFU-F per 100 cells	Osteogenic potential Calcium deposition (μg/dish)
CD90+	3.2 ± 0.8	7,260 ± 2,118
CD90–	<1 in 12,000	13 ± 11

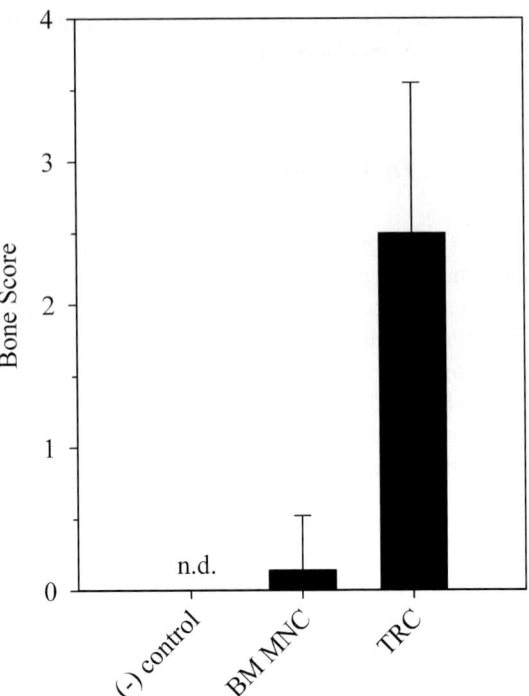

Fig. 14.9 In vivo ectopic bone formation. TRCs or BM MNCs were loaded onto fibronectin-coated ceramic cubes at 5×10^6 cells per mL then implanted subcutaneously in NOD/scid mice. The negative control (−)consisted of DMEM without cells. After 6 weeks, cubes were harvested and processed for histology. Bone scores were obtained after staining as described [73] (n.d. = none detected)

potential of TRCs resides entirely within the CD90$^+$ cell population, the results were then compared on a per CD90$^+$ cell basis (Fig. 14.10, right panel) and showed higher potential in TRCs.

TRCs were also compared to BMSC *in vivo* in an animal model for bone formation. In one initial experiment, TRC and BMSC cells were generated, loaded onto fibronectin-coated ceramic cubes and implanted subcutaneously. After 6 weeks, cubes were harvested and new bone formation was assessed by histology. The bone scores for TRC were equal to or better than those for BMSC (Fig. 14.11). In this experiment, TRCs contained 22% CD90$^+$ cells while BMSCs contained 68%. When analyzed on a per CD90$^+$ cell basis, the osteogenic potential from TRC was much greater than BMSC.

It may be that the presence of accessory cells during primary TRC culture, or perhaps during osteogenic assays themselves, results in higher osteogenic activity of this cell product. Accessory cells may produce soluble factors or provide important cell:cell communication leading to enhanced activity. These potentially critical accessory cells are removed during BMSC culture. Previous studies have shown the importance of accessory cell populations, monocyte and endothelial cells, in modulating gene expression and functional potential of MSCs [62–64]. Studies to further characterize interactions of accessory cells and mesenchymal components during TRC culture and identifying their role in enhanced functional potential are warranted.

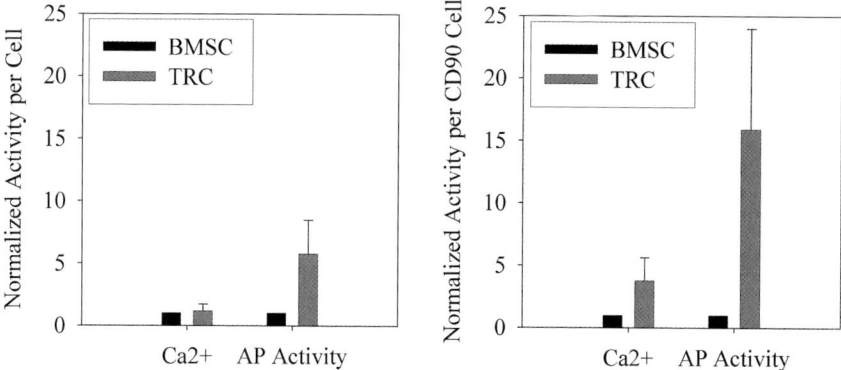

Fig. 14.10 In vitro osteogenic potential of TRCs and BMSCs. TRCs or BMSCs were plated in medium with (+OS) or without (−OS) dexamethasone, ascorbic acid, and beta-glycerophosphate for 14–21 days. Differentiation was measured by quantifying calcium deposition (Ca^{2+}) and alkaline phosphatase (AP) activity. Results were normalized to BMSCs (1.0) and are represented on a per cell basis (left panel) or per $CD90^+$ cell basis (right panel). The average from five experiments ± SEM is presented

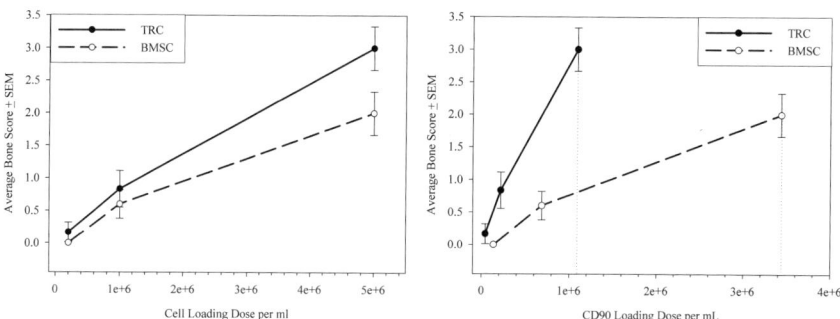

Fig. 14.11 In vivo osteogenic potential of TRCs and BMSCs. TRCs or BMSCs were loaded onto fibronectin coated ceramic cubes at 0.2, 1, and 5×10^6 cells per mL then implanted subcutaneously in NOD/scid mice. After 6 weeks, cubes were harvested and processed for histology. Bone scores were obtained after staining as described [73]. The left graph shows bone scores based on total cells loaded. The right graph shows bone scores based on total $CD90^+$ cells loaded

14.4.4 Vascular Potential of TRCs

To get complete regeneration of bone tissue, there must be a concomitant vascular component formed within the tissue [65]. Cotransplantation of endothelial cells with bone marrow stromal cells has been shown to enhance orthotopic bone regeneration [64]. Bone marrow-derived cells are known to enhance neovascularization in models of myocardial and peripheral ischemia. Cultured cells can incorporate into sites of neovascularization in ischemic tissues, preserving left ventricular function in the ischemic heart [66] and enhancing blood flow in ischemic limbs [67, 68].

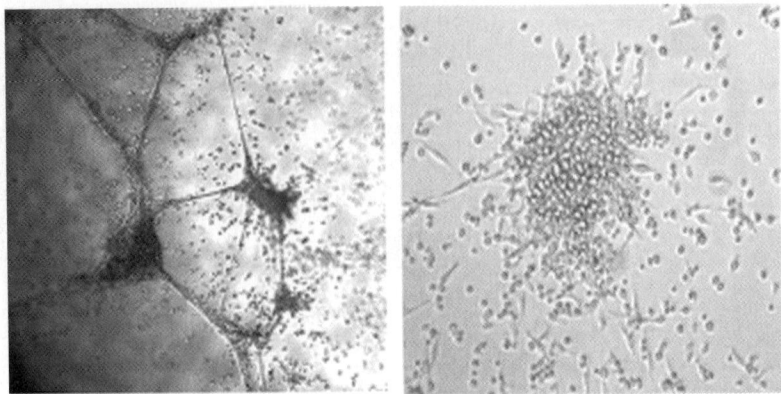

Fig. 14.12 Vascular potential of TRCs in vitro. TRCs were plated in matrigel for up to 24 hours and assessed microscopically for tube formation. For endothelial progenitor colony assays, the CFU-Hill procedure was followed (Stem Cell Technologies, Vancouver, BC). Photomicrographs of tube formation (left) and an endothelial colony (right) are shown

As TRCs are a mixed population of cells, it was of interest to examine their potential for regeneration of vascular tissues either through the production of soluble factors, or in vitro functional assays. Results from these studies have shown upregulation of numerous angiogenic factors compared to native BM, including vascular endothelial growth factors (VEGFs A, B, and C), Leptin, IL-6, Neuropilin 1 (NRP1), and G-CSF measured by targeted microarrays. Results in Fig. 14.12 show that cells within TRCs can form tube-like structures in Matrigel in the presence of endothelial growth factors. TRCs also contain endothelial progenitors that can generate endothelial cell colonies.

14.5   Delivery of Cell Products

For bone regeneration, a suspension of cells must be loaded onto a scaffold material to fill the void space in the damaged bone and provide a structural matrix within which the transplanted cells can engraft, proliferate and produce new bone. Mixing procedures have been developed and *in vitro* studies performed to ensure the viability and functionality of the formulated TRC product is maintained during the procedure. Cells have been evaluated on both ceramic matrices and on human demineralized allograft particles using human plasma as a binder. Cell function was examined *in situ* in the matrix/plasma material, by assessing metabolic activity and cytokine production. Additionally, after placing the cell/matrix composite in medium to induce differentiation into the osteogenic lineage, the production of osteogenic markers such as alkaline phosphatase, osteocalcin and osteopontin was measured.

Results presented in Figs. 14.13 and 14.14 show that TRCs: (1) survive the matrix mixing process, (2) proliferate extensively on matrix material, (3) differentiate

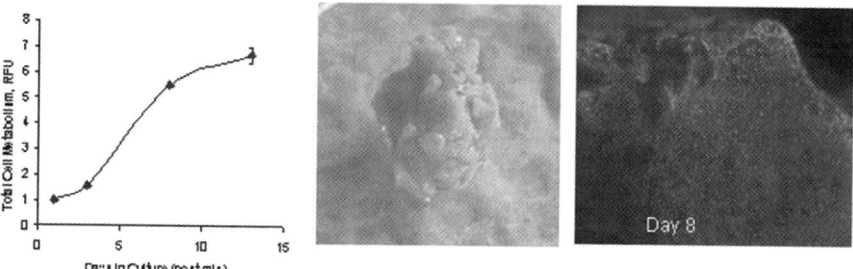

Fig. 14.13 Growth of TRCs on bone matrix material. TRCs were combined with allograft bone matrix material and plasma, and then cultured for up to 14 days in LTBMC medium. Metabolic activity of cells was measured using the cell titer blue assay (left panel). The middle panel is a gross picture of TRC-loaded matrix material after culture. The right panel is a photomicrograph of cells on the matrix after live-dead staining on day 8 of culture. The fluorescent image shows live cells as green and nonviable cells as red (*See Color Plates*)

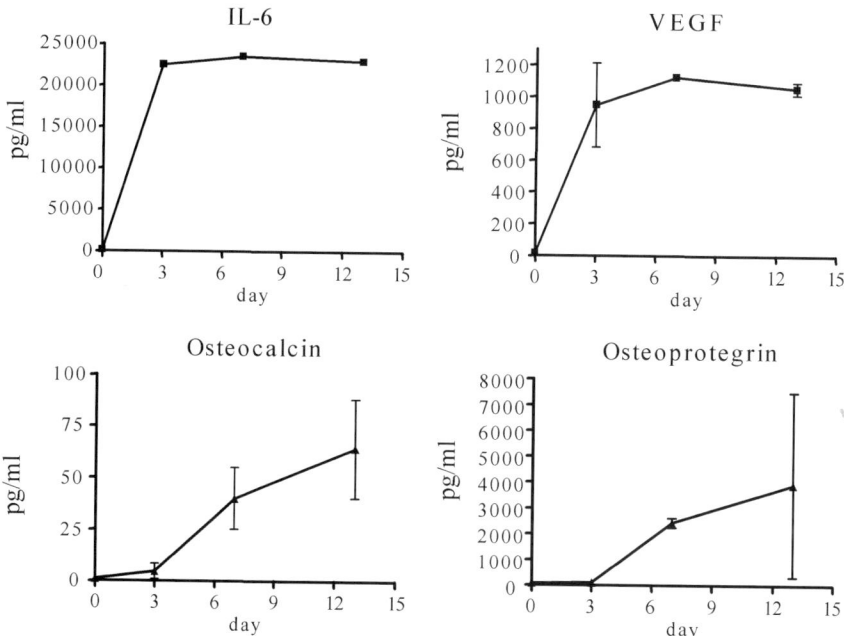

Fig. 14.14 *In vitro* secretion of factors by TRCs on bone matrix. TRCs were combined with allograft bone matrix material and plasma, then cultured for up to 14 days in either LTBMC medium (top panel) or osteogenic medium (+OS; bottom panel). At several timepoints, supernatant was collected from LTBMC cultures and the presence of IL-6 and VEGF were determined using Luminex technology. Supernatant was collected from the +OS cultures and the presence of the osteogenic specific factors osteocalcin and osteoprotegrin were determined

into bone on matrices, and (4) secrete a variety of osteogenic, angiogenic and hematopoietic regulatory cytokines while cultured on matrix material.

Feasibility clinical trials have been conducted involving over 40 patients in which TRCs formulated with matrix material with or without plasma were used in the treatment of long bone non-union fractures. Autoradiographic images show that almost all patients exhibited fracture healing with no cell-related adverse events [48, 69]. In addition to bone healing, reduced post-operative inflammation and swelling at the surgical site was observed for many patients.

14.6   Mechanism(s) of Action

After administration of TRCs in bone matrix, new bone has been observed both in the animal models described above (Fig. 14.9) and in clinical trials, however the mechanism of this new bone formation was not determined. Several preliminary studies now suggest that there are multiple mechanisms of action of TRCs in bone formation.

14.6.1   Direct Incorporation of TRCs into Developing Bone

Bone formation was measured by seeding human TRCs into a gelatin sponge (Gelfoam) and implanting them subcutaneously in *scid* mice. Prior to implantation, TRCs were transfected with a lentivirus carrying GFP under the Col 2.3 kb promoter [70]. This promoter limits expression of GFP to only mature osteoblasts. Therefore, if cells derived from TRCs differentiate into mature osteoblasts and incorporate into new bone, that bone would be fluorescent. At 4 weeks, ossicles formed by GFP-col 2.3-labelled cells could be detected in frozen sections. Figure 14.15 shows new bone formation fluorescently stained, demonstrating that it was derived from TRCs (P. Liu, D. Yin, Z. Wang, and P. Krebsbach, 2006).

14.6.2   Involvement of TRCs in Formation of Vasculature

In another *scid* mouse model, the ability of TRCs to generate bone in a calvarial defect was established. TRCs were loaded into a gelatin sponge (Gelfoam) and implanted into a calvarial defect as previously described [64]. After 7 weeks, samples were collected and processed for histology. Along with the detection of new bone (not shown), sections were stained with human-specific antibodies to detect vascular endothelium. In one example shown in Fig. 14.16, human cells expressing VEGFR2 were detected in many areas, including surrounding putative blood vessels. VEGFR2 is typically expressed in all vessel-derived endothelial cells. These results suggest that TRCs are a source of cells capable of contributing to vasculature within newly formed bone.

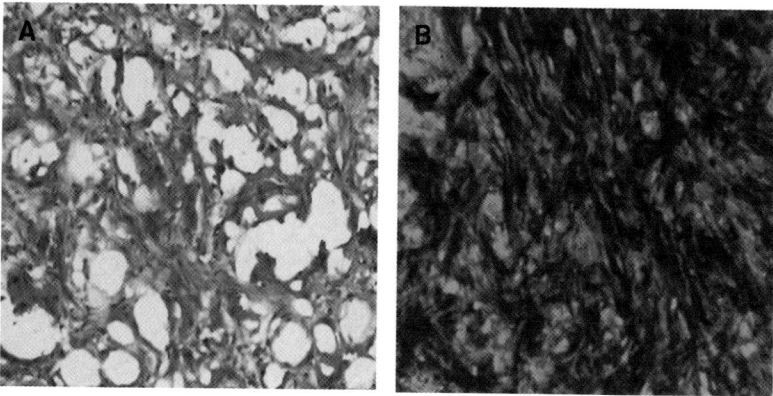

Fig. 14.15 TRCs differentiate into bone in vivo. GFP-transfected TRCs were loaded onto a gelatin matrix (Gelfoam) and implanted subcutaneously into *scid* mice. At 4 weeks, ossicles were sectioned and new bone formation was detected by staining with hematoxylin-eosin (**A**) or by fluorescence microscopy (**B**). Photomicrographs were taken at 400X magnification (**A**) or 40X magnification (**B**) (*See Color Plates*)

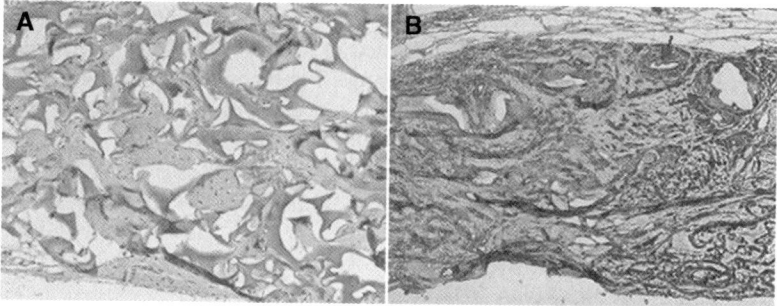

Fig. 14.16 Vascular components in new bone. TRCs were loaded onto a gelatin matrix (Gelfoam) and implanted into a calvarial defect model in *scid* mice. At 7 weeks, samples were processed for immunohistochemistry. (**A**) No primary antibody control. (**B**) Human specific VEGFR2 antibody. Arrows points to vasculature present within new bone. Photomicrographs were taken at 200X magnification (*See Color Plates*)

14.6.3 Potential Modulation of Inflammatory Response by TRCs

As mentioned above, in clinical trials, inflammation and swelling were reduced or absent after surgery when TRCs were implanted to heal non-union fractures [69], suggesting some modulation of the inflammatory response. Additional pre-clinical studies have focused on characterization of the immunomodulatory properties of the TRC mixture by examining the production of a variety of cytokines and their ability to suppress T-cell proliferation. Results of these studies show that TRCs

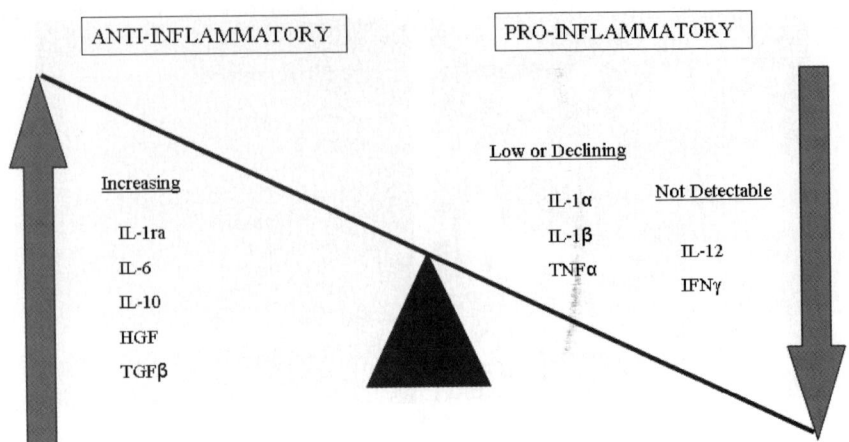

Fig. 14.17 Summary of *in vitro* secretion of immunomodulatory factors by TRCs (*See Color Plates*)

express immunomodulatory factors that strongly polarize or bias the host response away from the tissue-destructive inflammation and toward wound repair with more rapid healing of injured tissues (summarized in Fig. 14.17). Bone marrow-derived MSCs have previously been shown to suppress T-cell activation and T-cell proliferation [71, 72]. This suppression requires the activation of MSCs by CD14+ monocytes [63], both of which are present in TRCs.

14.7 Summary

Many questions remain unanswered in the field of cell therapy. However, there is intense investigation into the use of cell therapy for many clinical indications involving the treatment of tissue injuries and diseases. Understanding and optimizing cell therapy for each indication is a major undertaking. Additionally, the translation to the clinic and commercialization of cell therapy are significant, although not insurmountable, hurdles. In the end, any treatment modality that includes stem or progenitor cells is going to have to be developed in a manner that meets FDA regulations for safety, including GMPs. To this end, the SPP system described here allows for the production of cells under strictly definable conditions in a closed system that minimizes handling and automates the tracking and documentation of each individual cell product. This method can serve as a paradigm for development of procedures for growth of other autologous cells for therapy, including reprogrammed cells. As issues surrounding cell therapies are resolved, the use of stem and progenitor cells for the regeneration of tissues and/or treatment of diseases will most certainly lead to improvements in patient treatments and clinical practice.

Acknowledgements This work was supported in part by a grant from the National Institute of Diabetes and Digestive and Kidney Diseases (R44 DK074201).

References

1. Lindvall O, Kokaia Z (2006) Stem cells for the treatment of neurological disorders. Nature 441:1094–1096
2. Kobayashi N (2006) Cell therapy for diabetes mellitus. Cell Transplant. 15:849–854
3. Grounds MD, Davies KE (2007) The allure of stem cell therapy for muscular dystrophy. Neuromuscul. Disord. 17:206–208
4. Sohn RL, Gussoni E (2004) Stem cell therapy for muscular dystrophy. Expert. Opin. Biol. Ther. 4:1–9
5. Ichim TE, Solano F, Glenn E et al. (2007) Stem cell therapy for autism. J. Transl. Med. 5:30
6. Kinnaird T, Stabile E, Burnett MS et al. (2004) Bone-marrow-derived cells for enhancing collateral development: mechanisms, animal data, and initial clinical experiences. Circ. Res. 95(4):354–363
7. Caplice NM, Gersh BJ, Alegria JR (2005) Cell therapy for cardiovascular disease: what cells, what diseases and for whom? Nat. Clin. Pract. Cardiovasc. Med. 2:37–43
8. Ott HC, McCue J, Taylor DA (2005) Cell-based cardiovascular repair–the hurdles and the opportunities. Basic Res. Cardiol. 100:504–517
9. Goldman S (2005) Stem and progenitor cell-based therapy of the human central nervous system. Nat. Biotechnol. 23:862–871
10. Samadikuchaksaraei A (2007) An overview of tissue engineering approaches for management of spinal cord injuries. J. Neuroengineering. Rehabil. 4:15
11. Bruder SP, Kurth AA, Shea M et al. (1998) Bone regeneration by implantation of purified, culture-expanded human mesenchymal stem cells. J. Orthop. Res. 16:155–162
12. Thomas ED, Blume KG, Forman SJ (eds) (1999) Hematopoietic Cell Transplantation. Blackwell Science, Malden, MA
13. Pittenger MF, Mackay AM, Beck SC et al. (1999) Multilineage potential of adult human mesenchymal stem cells. Science 284:143–147
14. Reyes M, Lund T, Lenvik T et al. (2001) Purification and ex vivo expansion of postnatal human marrow mesodermal progenitor cells. Blood 98:2615–2625
15. Zhao Y, Glesne D, Huberman E (2003) A human peripheral blood monocyte-derived subset acts as pluripotent stem cells. Proc. Natl. Acad Sci. U S A 100:2426–2431
16. Mayani H, varado-Moreno JA, Flores-Guzman P (2003) Biology of human hematopoietic stem and progenitor cells present in circulation. Arch. Med. Res. 34:476–488
17. Weiss ML, Troyer DL (2006) Stem cells in the umbilical cord. Stem Cell Rev. 2:155–162
18. Kogler G, Sensken S, Wernet P (2006) Comparative generation and characterization of pluripotent unrestricted somatic stem cells with mesenchymal stem cells from human cord blood. Exp. Hematol. 34:1589–1595
19. Mayani H, Lansdorp PM (1998) Biology of human umbilical cord blood-derived hematopoietic stem/progenitor cells. Stem Cells 16:153–165
20. Guilak F, Lott KE, Awad HA et al. (2006) Clonal analysis of the differentiation potential of human adipose-derived adult stem cells. J. Cell Physiol. 206:229–237
21. Zuk PA, Zhu M, Ashjian P et al. (2002) Human adipose tissue is a source of multipotent stem cells. Mol. Biol. Cell 13:4279–4295
22. Sell S (ed) (2004) Stem Cells Handbook. Humana, Totowa, NJ
23. Turksen K (ed) (2004) Adult Stem Cells. Humana, Totowa, NJ
24. Biswas A, Hutchins R (2007) Embryonic stem cells. Stem Cells Dev. 16:213–222
25. Koc ON, Day J, Nieder M et al. (2002) Allogeneic mesenchymal stem cell infusion for treatment of metachromatic leukodystrophy (MLD) and Hurler syndrome (MPS-IH). Bone Marrow Transplant. 30:215–222

26. Shake JG, Gruber PJ, Baumgartner WA et al. (2002) Mesenchymal stem cell implantation in a swine myocardial infarct model: engraftment and functional effects. Ann. Thorac. Surg 73:1919–1925

27. Yanovich S, Mitsky P, Cornetta K et al. (2000) Transplantation of CD34+ peripheral blood cells selected using a fully automated immunomagnetic system in patients with high-risk breast cancer: results of a prospective randomized multicenter clinical trial. Bone Marrow Transplant. 25:1165–1174

28. Stamm C, Kleine HD, Choi YH et al. (2007) Intramyocardial delivery of CD133+ bone marrow cells and coronary artery bypass grafting for chronic ischemic heart disease: safety and efficacy studies. J. Thorac. Cardiovasc. Surg 133:717–725

29. Manginas A, Goussetis E, Koutelou M et al. (2007) Pilot study to evaluate the safety and feasibility of intracoronary CD133(+) and CD133(−) CD34(+) cell therapy in patients with non-viable anterior myocardial infarction. Catheter. Cardiovasc. Interv. 69:773–781

30. Kan I, Melamed E, Offen D (2007) Autotransplantation of bone marrow-derived stem cells as a therapy for neurodegenerative diseases. Handb. Exp. Pharmacol.:219–242

31. Shepler SA, Patel AN (2007) Cardiac cell therapy: a treatment option for cardiomyopathy. Crit. Care Nurs. Q. 30:74–80

32. Grigoropoulos NF, Mathur A (2006) Stem cells in cardiac repair. Curr. Opin. Pharmacol. 6:169–175

33. Caplan AI, Dennis JE (2006) Mesenchymal stem cells as trophic mediators. J Cell Biochem. 98:1076–1084

34. Tateishi-Yuyama E, Matsubara H, Murohara T et al. (2002) Therapeutic angiogenesis for patients with limb ischaemia by autologous transplantation of bone-marrow cells: a pilot study and a randomised controlled trial. Lancet 360:427–435

35. Muschler GF, Matsukura Y, Nitto H et al. (2005) Selective retention of bone marrow-derived cells to enhance spinal fusion. Clin. Orthop. Rel. Res. 432:242–251

36. Ishida A, Ohya Y, Sakuda H et al. (2005) Autologous peripheral blood mononuclear cell implantation for patients with peripheral arterial disease improves limb ischemia. Circ. J. 69:1260–1265

37. Mandalam R, Koller MR, Smith A (1999) Ex vivo hematopoietic cell expansion for bone marrow transplantation. In: Schindhelm K, Nordon R (eds) Ex Vivo Cell Therapy. Academic, San Diego, CA

38. Schwartz RM, Palsson BØ, Emerson SG (1991) Rapid medium perfusion rate significantly increases the productivity and longevity of human bone marrow cultures. Proc. Natl. Acad. Sci. U S A 88(15):6760–6764

39. Caldwell J, Palsson BO, Locey B et al. (1991) Culture perfusion schedules influence the metabolic activity and granulocyte-macrophage colony-stimulating factor production rates of human bone marrow stromal cells. J. Cell. Physiol. 147:344–353

40. Smith DM, Gorgas GC, Hastie KR et al. (2001) Enhanced yield and antigen presenting function of human dendritic cells produced under perfusion culture conditions in a unique clinicalscale bioreactor system. Keystone Symposia: Dendritic Cells: Interfaces with Immunobiology and Medicine (abstract)

41. Armstrong RD, Smith D, Mandalam R et al. (1997) Continuous medium perfusion during ex vivo expansion of human CD8+ T-cells produces high density cultures and enhances proliferation potential and lymphokine release. Exp Hematol 25:s886

42. Dennis JE, Esterly K, Awadallah A et al. (2007) Clinical-scale expansion of a mixed population of bone marrow derived stem and progenitor cells for potential use in bone tissue regeneration. Stem Cells 25:2575–2582

43. Stiff P, Chen B, Franklin W et al. (2000) Autologous transplantation of ex vivo expanded bone marrow cells grown from small aliquots after high-dose chemotherapy for breast cancer. Blood 95:2169–2174

44. Pecora AL, Stiff P, LeMaistre CF et al. (2001) A phase II trial evaluating the safety and effectiveness of the AastromReplicell System for augmentation of low-dose blood stem cell transplantation. Bone Marrow Transplant. 28:295–303

45. Koller MR, Manchel I, Maher RJ et al. (1998) Clinical-scale human umbilical cord blood cell expansion in a novel automated perfusion culture system. Bone Marrow Transplant. 21:653–663
46. Pecora AL, Stiff P, Jennis A et al. (2000) Prompt and durable engraftment in two older adult patients with high risk chronic myelogenous leukemia (CML) using ex vivo expanded and unmanipulated unrelated umbilical cord blood. Bone Marrow Transplant. 25:797–799
47. Jaroscak J, Goltry K, Smith A et al. (2003) Augmentation of umbilical cord blood (UCB) transplantation with ex vivo-expanded UCB cells: results of a phase I trial using the AastromReplicell System. Blood 101(12):5061–5067
48. Jimenez ML, Lyon T, Nowinski G et al. (2007) Stem and progenitor cell therapy for management of refractory long bone nonunions: a multicenter clinical feasibility study. American Academy of Orthopaedic Surgeons Annual Meeting (abstract)
49. Guardino AE, Rajapaksa R, Ong KH et al. (2006) Production of myeloid dendritic cells (DC) pulsed with tumor-specific idiotype protein for vaccination of patients with multiple myeloma. Cytotherapy 8:277–289
50. Kopp HG, Ramos CA, Rafii S (2006) Contribution of endothelial progenitors and proangiogenic hematopoietic cells to vascularization of tumor and ischemic tissue. Curr. Opin. Hematol. 13:175–181
51. Bauer TW, Muschler GF (2000) Bone graft materials: an overview of the basic science. Clin. Orthop. Relat. Res. 371:10–27
52. Giannoudis PV, Dinopoulos H, Tsiridis E (2005) Bone substitutes: an update. Injury 36 Suppl 3:S20–S27
53. Stevenson S (1998) Enhancement of fracture healing with autogenous and allogeneic bone grafts. Clin. Orthop. Relat. Res. 355S:S239–S246
54. Lindsey RW, Wood GW, Sadasivian KK et al. (2006) Grafting long bone fractures with demineralized bone matrix putty enriched with bone marrow: pilot findings. Orthopedics 29:939–941
55. Skoff HD (1995) Bone marrow/allograft component therapy. A clinical trial. Am. J. Orthop. 24:40–47
56. Tiedeman JJ, Garvin KL, Kile TA et al. (1995) The role of a composite, demineralized bone matrix and bone marrow in the treatment of osseous defects. Orthopedics 18:1153–1158
57. Kelly CM, Wilkins RM, Gitelis S et al. (2001) The use of a surgical grade calcium sulfate as a bone graft substitute: results of a multicenter trial. Clin. Orthop. Relat. Res. 382:42–50
58. Chapman MW, Bucholz R, Cornell C (1997) Treatment of acute fractures with a collagen-calcium phosphate graft material. A randomized clinical trial. J. Bone Joint Surg. Am. 79:495–502
59. Betz RR (2002) Limitations of autograft and allograft: new synthetic solutions. Orthopedics 25:s561–s570
60. Dennis JE, Renshaw K, Awadallah A et al. (2004) In vivo bone formation of bone marrow-derived cells correlates with CD105, CD166, and Thy1 cell surface markers. J. Bone Min. Res. 19 Suppl:S266
61. Dennis JE, Renshaw K, Awadallah A et al. (2005) Optimizing bone marrow-derived osteogenic progenitor cell expansion using the replicell bioreactor system. J. Bone Miner. Res. 20 Suppl:S247
62. Pillai MM, Iwata M, Awaya N et al. (2006) Monocyte-derived CXCL7 peptides in the marrow microenvironment. Blood 107:3520–3526
63. Groh ME, Maitra B, Szekely E et al. (2005) Human mesenchymal stem cells require monocyte-mediated activation to suppress alloreactive T cells. Exp. Hematol. 33:928–934
64. Kaigler D, Krebsbach PH, Wang Z et al. (2006) Transplanted endothelial cells enhance orthotopic bone regeneration. J. Dent. Res. 85:633–637
65. Carano RAD, Filvaroff EH (2003) Angiogenesis and bone repair. Drug Discov. Today 8(21):980–989
66. Kawamoto A, Gwon H-C, Iwaguro H et al. (2001) Therapeutic potential of ex vivo expanded endothelial progenitor cells for myocardial ischemia. Circulation 103:634–637
67. Murohara T, Ikeda H, Duan J et al. (2000) Transplanted cord blood-derived endothelial precursor cells augment postnatal neovascularization. J. Clin. Invest. 105:1527–1536

68. Kalka C, Masuda H, Takahashi T et al. (2000) Transplantation of ex vivo expanded endothe-lial progenitor cells for therapeutic neovascularization. Proc. Natl. Acad. Sci. U S A 97:3422–3427

69. Solano C, Rodriguez L, Torrico C et al. (2006) Clinical feasibility study. The use of cultured enriched autologous bone marrow cells to treat refractory atrophic and hypotrophic nonunion fractures. Annual Meeting International Society for Cell Therapy (abstract)

70. Kalajzic I, Kalajzic Z, Kaliterna M et al. (2002) Use of type I collagen green fluorescent pro-tein transgenes to identify subpopulations of cells at different stages of the osteoblast lineage. J. Bone Min. Res. 17:15–25

71. Maitra B, Szekely E, Gjini K et al. (2004) Human mesenchymal stem cells support unrelated donor hematopoietic stem cells and suppress T-cell activation. Bone Marrow Transplant. 33:597–604

72. Bartholomew A, Sturgeon C, Siatskas M et al. (2002) Mesenchymal stem cells suppress lym-phocyte proliferation in vitro and prolong skin graft survival in vivo. Exp. Hematol. 30:42–48

73. Dennis JE, Konstantakos EK, Arm D et al. (1998) *In vivo* osteogenesis assay: a rapid method for quantitative analysis. Biomaterials 19:1323–1328

Chapter 15
The Hair Follicle Stem Cell as the Paradigm Multipotent Adult Stem Cell

Robert M. Hoffman

Abstract Our laboratory has discovered that the hair follicle is an abundant, easily accessible source of actively growing multipotent adult stem cells that can form non-follicular cell types. We observed that nestin, a protein marker for neural stem cells, is also expressed in follicle stem cells and their immediate, differentiated progeny. The green fluorescent protein (GFP), whose expression is driven by the nestin regulatory element in transgenic mice (ND-GFP mice), served to mark hair follicle stem cells and could be used to trace their fate. The ND-GFP hair-follicle stem cells are positive for the stem cell marker CD34 but negative for keratinocyte marker keratin 15, suggesting their relatively undifferentiated state. We have shown that these hair follicle stem cells can differentiate into neurons, glia, keratinocytes, smooth muscle cells and melanocvytes in vitro. In vivo studies show the hair follicle stem cells can differentiate into blood vessels and neural tissue after transplantation to the subcutis of nude mice. Hair follicle stem cells implanted into the gap region of severed sciatic or tibial nerves greatly enhance the rate of nerve regeneration and the restoration of nerve function. When transplanted to the severed nerves of the mice, the follicle cells transdifferentiate largely into Schwann cells, which are known to support neuron regrowth. The transplanted mice regain the ability to walk normally. Thus, hair follicle stem cells are multipotent and provide an effective, accessible, autologous source of stem cells for treatment of peripheral nerve injury and appear to be a paradigm for adult stem cells.

Keywords Hair follicle, stem cells, nestin, GFP, multipotency

AntiCancer, Inc., 7917 Ostrow Street, San Diego, CA 92111, USA and Department of Surgery, University of California, San Diego, CA 92103-8220, USA
e-mail: all@anticancer.com

Y. Shi, D.O. Clegg (eds.) *Stem Cell Research and Therapeutics*,
© Springer Science+Business Media B.V. 2008

15.1   The Hair Follicle as a "Mini-Organ"

The hair follicle produces a terminally differentiated keratinized end product, the hair shaft, which is eventually shed. The follicle undergoes cyclical regeneration with at least 10 different epithelial and mesenchymal cell lineages [1]. Hair is formed by rapidly proliferating matrix keratinocytes in the bulb located at the base of the growing (anagen) follicle. The duration of anagen varies greatly between hairs of differing lengths. Nevertheless, matrix cells eventually stop proliferating, and hair growth ceases at catagen when the lower follicle regresses (telogen). After telogen, the lower hair-producing portion of the follicle regenerates, starting the new anagen phase [1].

Hair follicle stem cells, located in the hair follicle bulge, possess stem cell characteristics, including multipotency, high proliferative potential, and ability to enter quiescence. Lineage analysis has demonstrated that all epithelial layers within the adult follicle and hair originated from bulge cells [1, 2]. The hair follicle stem cells appear to be responsible for regenerating the hair follicle in each hair cycle.

Very recent studies have shown that, after wounding, hair follicles form de novo in adult mice. The nascent follicles arise from epithelial cells outside of the hair follicle stem cell niche, suggesting that epidermal cells in the wound assume a hair follicle stem cell phenotype. The newly generated hair follicles establish a stem cell population, express known molecular markers of follicle differentiation, produce a hair shaft, and progress through all stages of the hair follicle cycle [3].

15.2   Tracking Hair Follicle Stem Cells *In Vivo*

The insufficiency of markers to identify and track hair follicle stem cells in the bulge area has hindered the study of hair follicle stem cells. CD34 expression as first defined by Trempus et al. [4] is a marker for hair follicle stem cells. Antibodies recognizing CD34 were used to collect viable bulge cells by fluorescent activated cell sorting [4, 5]. K15 is expressed at high levels in the bulge, but lower levels of expression can be present in the basal layers of the lower follicle outer-root sheath (ORS) and the epidermis [6, 7]. A K15 promoter used for generation of transgenic mice was active only in the bulge in the adult mouse [8].

A breakthrough occurred with the use of transgenic mice in which the neural stem cell marker, nestin, drives the expression of green fluorescent protein (GFP) (ND-GFP cells). We observed in these mice that nestin was also a marker for hair follicle stem cells which suggested that hair follicle stem cells could form neurons and were multipotent [9]. The hair follicle stem cells could then be tracked by their green fluorescence. These relatively small, oval-shaped, ND-GFP-expressing cells surround the hair shaft and are interconnected by short dendrites. In mid- and late anagen, the ND-GFP-expressing cells are located in the upper outer-root sheath as well as in the bulge area but not in the hair matrix bulb (Figs. 15.1, 15.2). These observations show that the ND-GFP-expressing cells form the outer-root sheath. Following our report that ND-GFP can serve as a marker for hair follicle stem cells to track them in the live animal, Morris et al. [10] subsequently used GFP to isolate hair follicle stem cells in transgenic mice. Fuchs' group also subsequently used GFP to identify hair follicle stem cells and possibly other skin stem cells in transgenic mice [11, 12]. Yu et al. [13] showed that nestin was present in human hair follicle stem cells confirming our original observation [9].

Li et al. [14] have reported that nuclei from hair follicle stem cells can be successfully used as nuclear transfer (NT) donors, resulting in live cloned mice. Thus, the nuclei of hair follicle stem cells can be reprogrammed to the pluripotent state by exposure to the cytoplasm of unfertilized oocytes. These results confirm our earlier results demonstrating the pluripotency of hair follicle stem cells [9].

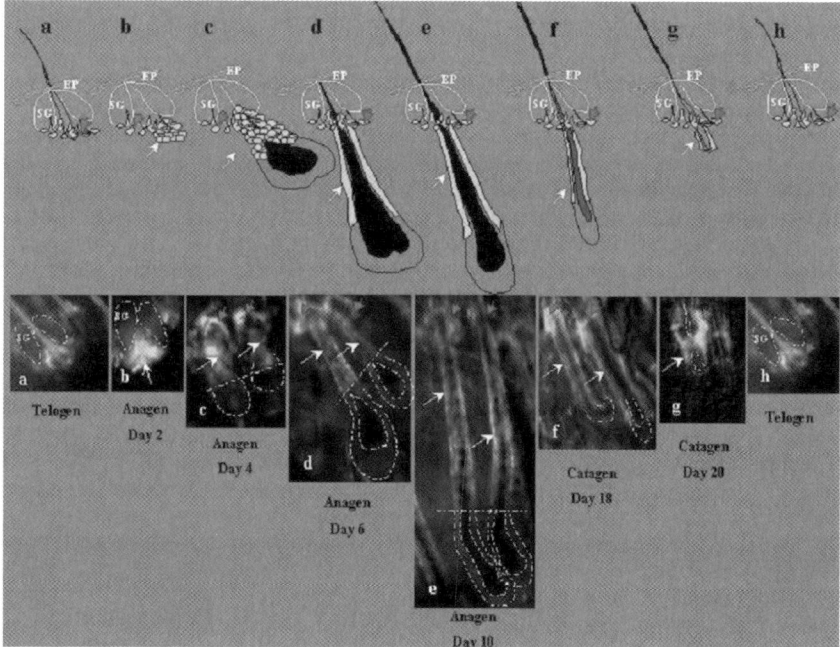

Fig. 15.1 Hair follicle stem cells in the hair-growth cycle [9]. (*Upper*) Cartoon showing position of ND-GFP stem cells at each stage of the hair follicle cycle. SG, sebaceous gland; EP, epidermis. (*Lower* **a**) ND-GFP-expressing hair follicle stem cells (red arrow) located near the hair follicle bulge area in telogen phase. (**b**) Day 2 after anagen induction by depilation. Note the new hair follicle cells (white arrow) formed directly from the ND-GFP-expressing stem cells. (**c–e**) Day 4 (**c**), day 6 (**d**), and day 10 (**e**) after anagen induction by depilation. Note the ND-GFP-expressing outer-root sheath cells (white arrows) in the upper two-thirds of the hair follicle. (**f** and **g**) Day 19 (**f**) and day 20 (**g**) after depilation. Note in f and g that the hair follicles are in the catagen phase and are undergoing regression and degeneration, including the ND-GFP-expressing cells in the outer-root sheath. The ND-GFP-expressing stem cells remain. (**h**) Hair follicle cycling in telogen phase (*See Color Plates*)

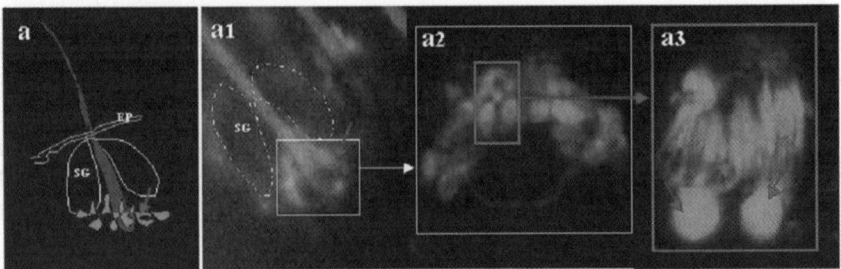

Telogen   Nestin-GFP-expressing stem cells in telogen hair follicle

Fig. 15.2 Hair follicle ND-GFP-expressing cells in the telogen phase of ND-GFP transgenic mouse skin [9]. The skin sample was prepared freshly right after excision from the back skin of a ND-GFP transgenic mouse. The skin sample then was directly observed by fluorescence or confocal microscopy with the dermis side up after s.c. tissue was dissected out. (**a**) Cartoon of telogen hair follicle showing position of ND-GFP-expressing hair follicle stem cells. (**a1**) Low-magnification fluorescence microscopy image showing the ring of ND-GFP-expressing stem cells (small white box, see **a**). (**a2**) High-magnification confocal microscopy image reflecting the small white box in **a1**. Note the small round- or oval-shaped ND-GFP-expressing cells near the bulge area of the hair follicle (small red box). (**a3**) High-magnification fluorescence microscopy image showing two individual ND-GFP-expressing stem cells reflecting the red box in **a2**. Note the unique morphology of the hair follicle stem cells and multiple dendrite-like structures of each cell. Red arrows indicate the cell body, and red arrowheads show the multiple dendritic structure of each cell (Original magnifications: **a1** × 100; **a2** × 400; **a3** × 1,600.) (SG, sebaceous gland; EP, epidermis) (*See Color Plates*)

The evidence that nestin-expressing cells are hair follicle stem cells rather than a population of stem cells that reside in the hair follicle whose purpose is to regenerate the neuronal and endothelial components associated with the pilosebaceous unit is that the nestin-expressing (and GFP-expressing) cells have been imaged over time to regenerate a large portion of the hair follicle as described above [9]. The ND-GFP marker may have enabled the identification and isolation of the most puripotent cells in the hair follicle.

15.3   The Ability of Hair Follicle Stem Cells to Differentiate to Follicular and Non-follicular Cell Types

Hair follicle stem cells from adult mice, when combined with neonatal dermal cells, formed hair follicles after injection into immunodeficient mice [5, 10]. Cultured, individually cloned bulge cells from adult mice also were shown to form hair follicles in skin reconstitution assays [5].

Taylor et al. [15] reported that hair follicle bulge stem cells are potentially bipotent because they can give rise to not only cells of the hair follicle but also to epidermal cells. However, hair follicle stem cells may form epidermal stem cells only when the epidermis is wounded [16]. Other experiments [17] also have provided new evidence that the upper outer-root sheath of vibrissal (whisker) follicles of adult mice contains pluripotent stem cells, which can differentiate into hair follicle matrix cells, sebaceous gland basal cells, and epidermis. Toma et al. [18] reported that pluripotent adult stem cells isolated from enzyme-digested mammalian skin dermis, termed skin-derived precursors, can proliferate and differentiate in culture to produce neurons, glia, smooth muscle cells, and adipocytes. However, the exact location of these stem cells in skin is unknown, and their functions are still unclear.

15.4 Blood Vessels Derived from Hair-Follicle Stem Cells

We observed that in ND-GFP mice, skin blood vessels express ND-GFP and appear to originate from hair follicles and form a follicle-linking network. This was seen most clearly by transplanting ND-GFP-labeled vibrissa (whisker) hair follicles to unlabeled nude mice. New vessels grew from the transplanted follicle, and the number of vessels increased when the local recipient skin was wounded. The ND-GFP-expressing blood vessels display the characteristic endothelial-cell-specific markers CD31 and von Willebrand factor [19] (Figs. 15.3, 15.4).

15.5 Differentiation of Hair Follicle Stem Cells to Neural and Other Cell Types

ND-GFP hair follicle stem cells can differentiate into neurons, glia, keratinocytes, smooth muscle cells, and melanocytes *in vitro*. These pluripotent ND-GFP stem cells are positive for the stem cell marker CD34, and negative for keratin 15, suggesting their relatively undifferentiated state as mentioned above. The apparent primitive state of the ND-GFP stem cells is compatible with their pluripotency. The ND-GFP hair follicle stem cells may be more primitive than those hair follicle stem cells previously isolated [2]. Furthermore, we showed that the hair follicle stem cells differentiated into neurons after transplantation to the subcutis of nude mice [20] (Figs. 15.5, 15.6).

15.6 Hair Follicle Stem Cells Can Effect Nerve Repair

When the GFP hair follicle stem cells were implanted into the gap region of a severed sciatic nerve they greatly enhanced the rate of nerve regeneration and the restoration of nerve function. After transplantation to severed nerves, the hair follicle stem cells differentiated largely into Schwann cells, which are known to support neuron regrowth. Function of the rejoined sciatic nerve was measured by contraction of the gastrocnemius muscle upon electrical stimulation. The transplanted mice recovered the ability to walk normally [21] (Figs. 15.7, 15.8).

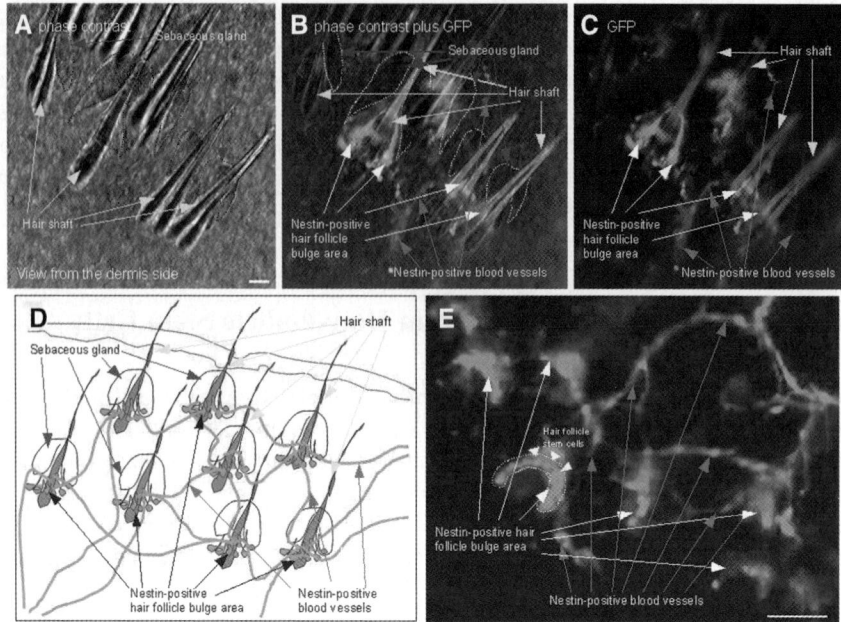

Fig. 15.3 View from the dermis side of the dorsal skin in ND-GFP transgenic mice [19]. (**a**) Phase-contrast microscopy. Sebaceous glands (blue arrows) are located around the hair shaft (yellow arrows). (**b**) Phase-contrast microscopy plus GFP fluorescence. ND-GFP cells are visualized near the follicular bulge area (white arrows) and blood vessels (red arrows). The follicular bulge area is located beneath the sebaceous gland. (**c**) GFP fluorescence. The ND-GFP blood vessels (red arrows) are connected to ND-GFP hair follicles (white arrows). (**d**) Schematic of telogen hair follicle showing position of ND-GFP hair-follicle stem cells (black arrows) and blood vessel network (red arrows). (**e**) GFP fluorescence. The ND-GFP blood vessels (red arrows) are associated with ND-GFP hair-follicle stem cells (white arrows) (Scale bars, 100 μm) (*See Color Plates*)

15.7 Conclusions

We have shown that the hair follicle bulge area is an abundant easily accessible source of actively growing pluripotent adult stem cells that could serve as a clinical source in humans. The availability of the ND-GFP mice has enabled the identification,

→

Fig. 15.4 Transplantation of an ND-GFP vibrissa follicle into the subcutis of a nude mouse [19]. (**a**) Phase-contrast micrograph of follicle 28 days after transplantation. (**b**) Phase-contrast micrograph plus GFP fluorescence. (**c**) GFP fluorescence. In **b** and **c**, ND-GFP blood vessels (arrows) are seen growing from the transplanted ND-GFP hair follicle and associating with preexisting blood vessels in the nude-mouse skin. (**d** and **e**) Higher magnification of the ND-GFP vessels of **b** and **c**, respectively. (**f** and **g**) Colocalization of GFP and the endothelial cell marker CD31 (arrows). **f** is a fluorescent image, and **g** shows the same field air-dried and immunohistochemically stained with CD31 (Scale bars, 100 μm) (*See Color Plates*)

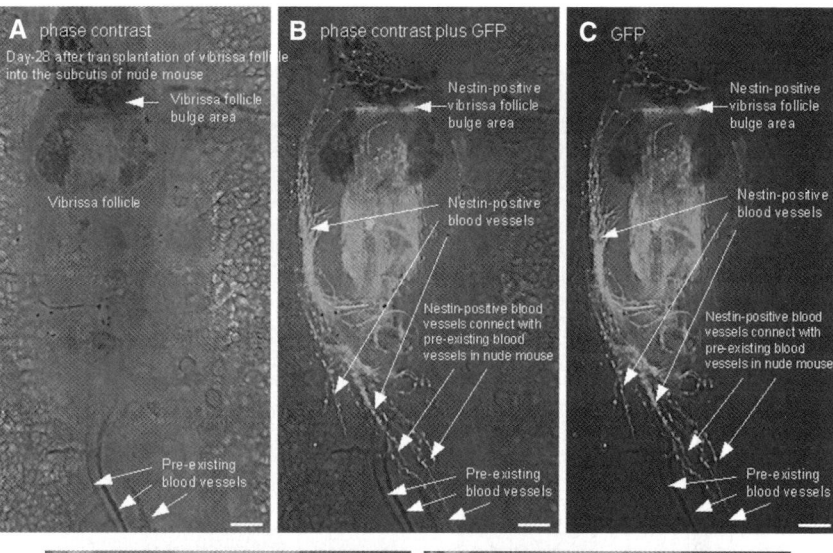

A phase contrast

Day-28 after transplantation of vibrissa follicle into the subcutis of nude mouse

Vibrissa follicle bulge area

Vibrissa follicle

Pre-existing blood vessels

B phase contrast plus GFP

Nestin-positive vibrissa follicle bulge area

Nestin-positive blood vessels

Nestin-positive blood vessels connect with pre-existing blood vessels in nude mouse

Pre-existing blood vessels

C GFP

Nestin-positive vibrissa follicle bulge area

Nestin-positive blood vessels

Nestin-positive blood vessels connect with pre-existing blood vessels in nude mouse

Pre-existing blood vessels

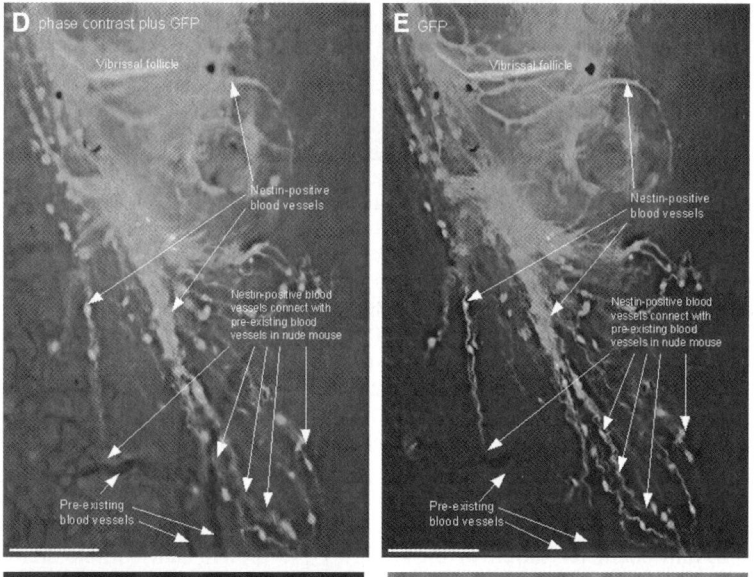

D phase contrast plus GFP

Vibrissal follicle

Nestin-positive blood vessels

Nestin-positive blood vessels connect with pre-existing blood vessels in nude mouse

Pre-existing blood vessels

E GFP

Vibrissal follicle

Nestin-positive blood vessels

Nestin-positive blood vessels connect with pre-existing blood vessels in nude mouse

Pre-existing blood vessels

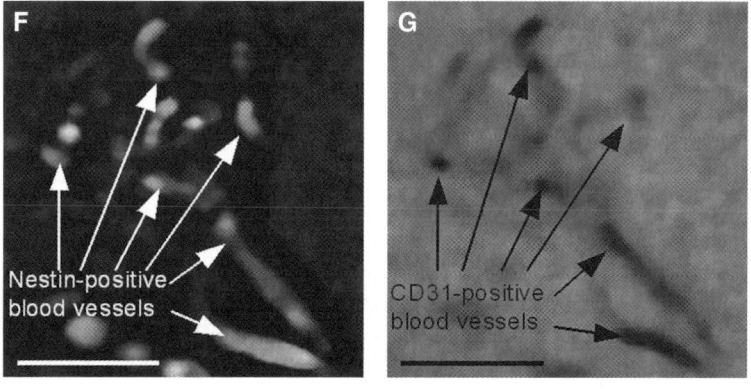

F

Nestin-positive blood vessels

G

CD31-positive blood vessels

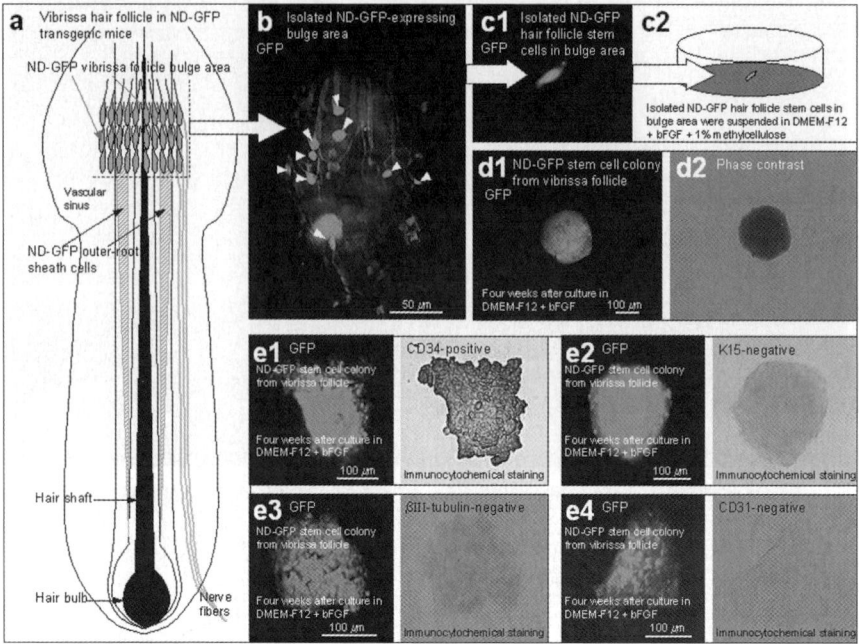

Fig. 15.5 Isolation, culture, and characterization of ND-GFP hair follicle stem cells [20]. (**a**) Schematic representation of a vibrissa hair follicle in ND-GFP transgenic mice showing the position of the ND-GFP-expressing vibrissa follicular stem cells (red arrows) and ND-GFP-expressing outer-root sheath cells (black arrows). (**b**) Isolated ND-GFP-expressing vibrissa follicular stem cells (white arrow heads). (**c1** and **c2**) The ND-GFP-expressing hair-follicle stem cells in the vibrissa were isolated and suspended in DMEM-F12 containing B-27 and 1% methylcellulose supplemented with bFGF every 2 days. (**d1** and **d2**) After 4 weeks, ND-GFP-expressing hair-follicle stem cells from the vibrissa area formed the ND-GFP-expressing cell colony. (**e**) ND-GFP-expressing cells within the colony were CD34-positive (**e1**), and the ND-GFP-expressing cells within the colony were K15- (**e2**), III β-tubulin- (**e3**), and CD31-negative (**e4**) (*See Color Plates*)

isolation, and characterization of these highly pluripotent hair follicle stem cells. These hair follicle stem cells express the stem cell marker CD34 and nestin but are negative for the keratinocyte marker keratin 15, indicating their relatively undifferentiated state. The hair follicle stem cells can differentiate into neurons, glia, keratinocytes, smooth muscle cells and melanocytes in vitro. In vivo studies show the nestin-driven GFP hair follicle stem cells can differentiate into blood vessels and neural tissue after transplantation to the subcutis of nude mice. Hair follicle stem cells implanted into the gap region of a severed sciatic or tibial nerve greatly enhanced the rate of nerve regeneration and the restoration of nerve function. After transplantation to the severed nerve, the follicle cells transdifferentiated largely into Schwann cells, which are known to support neuron regrowth. The transplanted mice regain the ability to walk normally. Thus, hair follicle stem cells provide an effective, accessible, autologous source of stem cells for treatment of peripheral nerve injury.

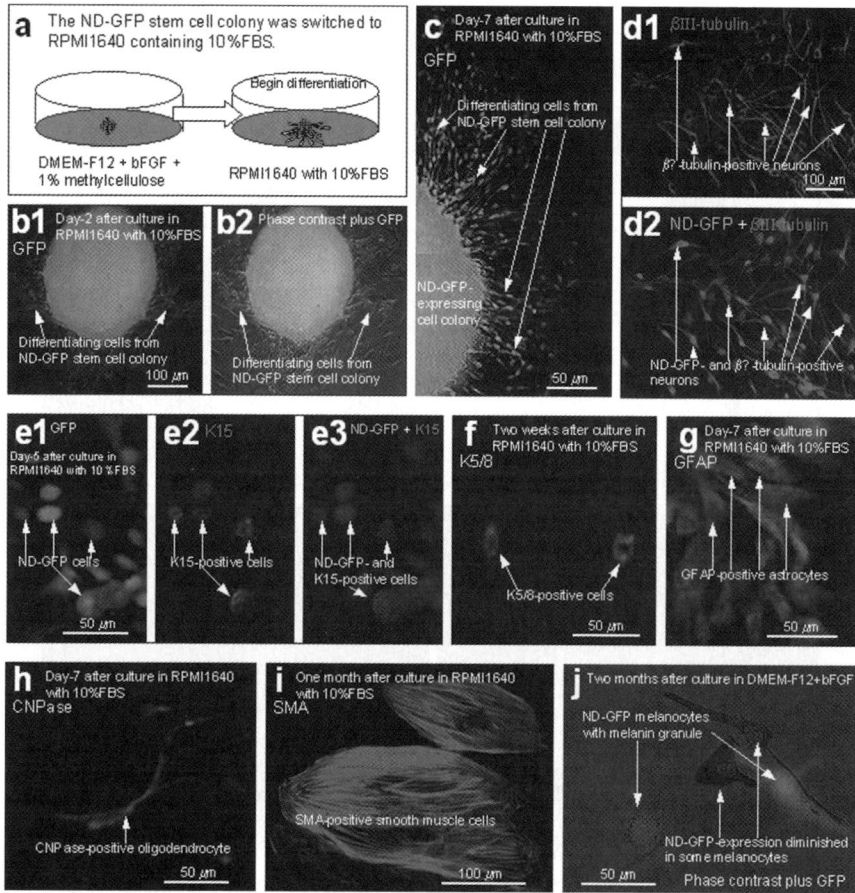

Fig. 15.6 Differentiation of ND-GFP hair follicle stem cells *in vitro* [20]. (**a**) The ND-GFP-expressing cell colony was switched to RPMI medium 1640 containing 10% FBS from DMEM-F12 containing B-27 and 1% methylcellulose supplemented with bFGF every 2 days. (**b1** and **b2**) At 2 days after switching into RPMI medium 1640 containing 10% FBS, differentiating cells migrated out of the ND-GFP-expressing cell colony. (**c**) At 7 days after switching to RPMI medium 1640, many differentiating cells migrated out of the ND-GFP-expressing cell colony. (**d1** and **d2**) ND-GFP-expressing cells differentiated to III β-tubulin-positive neurons which maintain ND-GFP-expression. (**e1–e3**) At 5 days after switching to RPMI medium 1640, ND-GFP-expressing cells differentiated to K15-positive cells (red fluorescence, arrows) (**e2**). The K15-positive cells still expressed ND-GFP. (**f**) ND-GFP-expressing cells differentiated to K5/8-positive cells 2 weeks after switching to RPMI medium 1640. (**g**) At 7 days after switching to RPMI medium 1640, ND-GFP-expressing cells differentiated to GFAP-positive astrocytes. (**h**) At 7 days after switching to RPMI medium 1640, ND-GFP-expressing cells differentiated to 2`,3`-cyclic nucleotide 3'-phosphodiesterase (CNPase)-positive oligodendrocytes. (**i**) At 1 month after culture in RPMI medium 1640 containing 10% FBS, ND-GFP-expressing cells differentiated to SMA-positive smooth muscle cells. (**j**) At 2 months after culture in DMEM-F12 containing B-27 and 1% methylcellulose supplemented with bFGF every 2 days, ND-GFP-expressing cells differentiated to melanocytes containing melanin. Some melanocytes still expressed ND-GFP (*See Color Plates*)

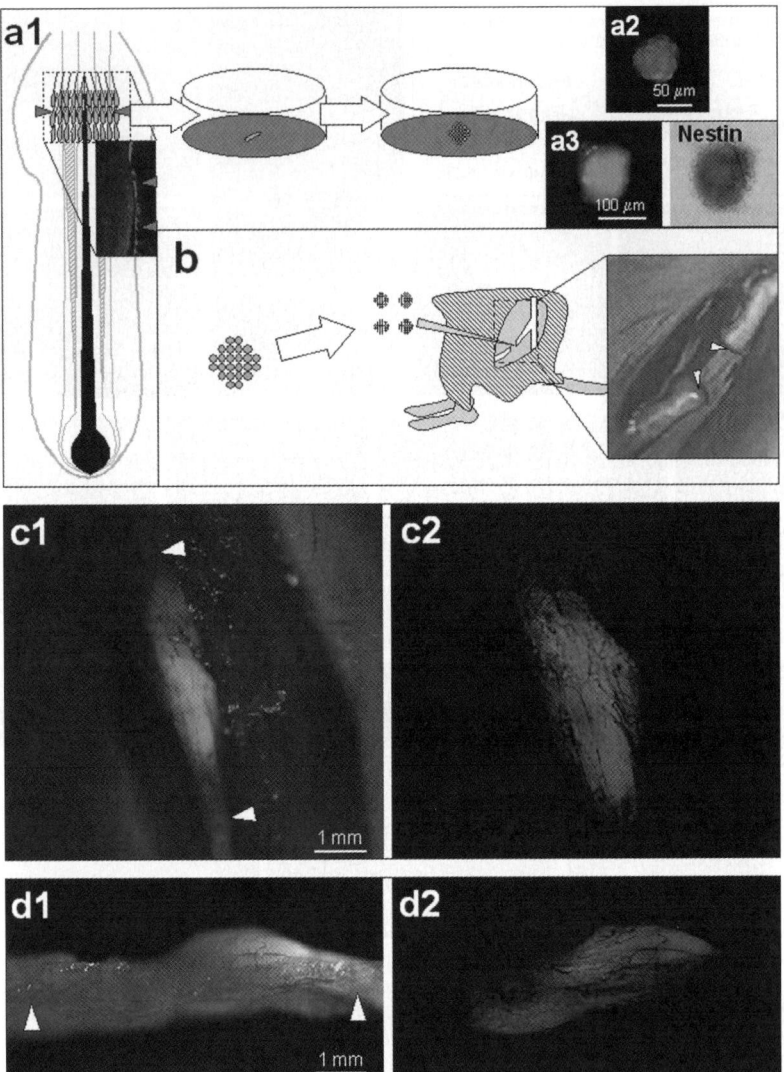

Fig. 15.7 Rejoining severed sciatic nerve with hair follicle stem cells [21]. (**a1**) Schematic of vibrissa follicle of GFP transgenic mice showing the position of GFP- and nestin-expressing vibrissa follicle stem cells (red arrowheads). (**a2**) Colony formed from GFP-expressing hair follicle stem cells from the vibrissa after 2 months in culture. (**a3**) GFP-expressing cells within the colony were nestin-positive. (**b**) GFP-expressing hair follicle stem cells grown for 2 months in DMEM-F12 containing B-27, 1% methylcellulose, and basic FGF were transplanted between the severed sciatic nerve fragments in C57BL/6 immunocompetent mice (white arrowheads). (**c1** and **c2**) Fluorescence images from a live mouse. Two months after transplantation between the severed sciatic nerve, the GFP-expressing cells joined the severed sciatic nerve. **c2** shows higher magnification of *c1*. (**d1** and **d2**) Brightfield (**d1**) and fluorescence (**d2**) images of an excised sciatic nerve. The preexisting sciatic nerve is denoted by white arrowheads (*See Color Plates*)

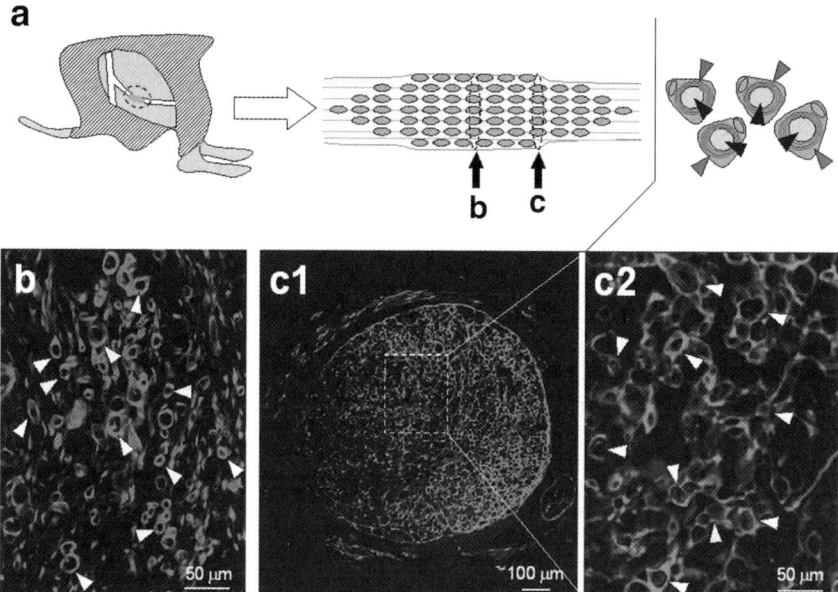

Fig. 15.8 Cell types growing in area of sciatic nerve joined by hair follicle stem cells [21]. (**a**) GFP-expressing vibrissa hair follicle stem cells were growing in the joined sciatic nerve. Most of the GFP-expressing vibrissa hair follicle stem cells differentiated to Schwann cells and formed myelin sheaths surrounding axons (red arrowheads). The axons are denoted by black arrowheads. (**b**) Transverse section of joined nerve. In the central area of the joined nerve, GFP-expressing cells formed many small myelin sheaths (white arrowheads). (**c1**) In the marginal area of the joined nerve, GFP-expressing cells formed many myelin sheaths (white arrowheads). (**c2**) Higher magnification of area of **c1** indicated by the white dashed box (*See Color Plates*)

Hair follicle stem cells thus have the potential as an alternative to the use of embryonal stem cells or fetal cells for regenerative medicine. The hair follicle stem cells do not have the ethical problems that embryonal or fetal stem cells have. Even more important, the hair follicle stem cells are much more easily accessible than these other stem-cell types and offer the potential for autologous treatment as they can be readily expended in culture after isolation from the patient. The fact that Yu et al. [13] have shown nestin expression and pluripotency of human hair follicle stem cells further suggests the clinical potential of hair follicle stem cells for regenerative medicine.

It is also important to note that the dermal papilla is a potential source of pluripotent stem cells that may have use in regenerative medicine. For example, Jahoda's group has demonstrated that hair follicle dermal cells repopulate the mouse hematopoietic system [22], can differentiate into adipogenic and osteogenic lineages [23] and participate in wound healing and induction [24]. Hair follicle stem cells also have great potential for hair restoration [1], but, as outlined in this chapter, they may have a much larger role in regenerative medicine.

References

1. Cotsarelis G. (2006) Epithelial stem cells: a folliculocentric view. J Invest Dermatol 126:1459–1468.
2. Cotsarelis G, Sun TT, Lavker RM. (1990) Label-retaining cells reside in the bulge area of pilosebaceous unit: implications for follicular stem cells, hair cycle, and skin carcinogenesis. Cell 61:1329–1337.
3. Ito M, Yang Z, Andl T, Cui C, Kim N, Millar SE, Cotsarelis G. (2007) Wnt-dependent de novo hair follicle regeneration in adult mouse skin after wounding. Nature 447:316–320.
4. Trempus C, Morris R, Bortner C, Cotsarelis G, Faircloth R, Reece, Tennant R. (2003) Enrichment for living murine keratinocytes from the hair follicle bulge with the cell surface marker CD34. J Invest Dermatol 120:501–511.
5. Blanpain C, Lowry WE, Geoghegan A, Polak L, Fuchs E. (2004) Self-renewal, multipotency, and the existence of two cell populations within an epithelial stem cell niche. Cell 118:635–648.
6. Lyle S, Christofidou-Solomidou M, Liu Y, Elder DE, Albelda S, Cotsarelis G. (1998) The C8/144B monoclonal antibody recognizes cytokeratin 15 and defines the location of human hair follicle stem cells. J Cell Sci 111:3179–3188.
7. Waseem A, Dogan B, Tidman N, Alam Y, Purkis P, Jackson S et al. (1999) Keratin 15 expression in stratified epithelia: downregulation in activated keratinocytes. J Invest Dermatol 112:362–369.
8. Liu Y, Lyle S, Yang Z, Cotsarelis G. (2003) Keratin 15 promoter targets putative epithelial stem cells in the hair follicle bulge. J Invest Dermatol 121:963–968.
9. Li L, Mignone J, Yang M, Matic M, Penman S, Enikolopov G, Hoffman RM. (2003) Nestin expression in hair follicle sheath progenitor cells. Proc Natl Acad Sci USA 100:9958–9961.
10. Morris RJ, Liu Y, Marles L, Yang Z, Trempus C, Li S et al. (2004) Capturing and profiling adult hair follicle stem cells. Nat Biotechnol 22:411–417.
11. Tumbar T, Guasch G, Greco V, Blanpain C, Lowry WE, Rendl M, Fuchs E. (2004) Defining the epithelial stem cell niche in skin. Science 303:359–363.
12. Rhee H, Polak L, Fuchs E. (2006) Lhx2 maintains stem cell character in hair follicles. Science 312:1946–1949.
13. Yu H, Fang D, Kumar SM, Li L, Nguyen TK, Acs G, Herlyn M, Xu X. (2006) Isolation of a novel population of multipotent adult stem cells from human hair follicles. Am J Pathol 168:1879–1888.
14. Li J, Greco V, Guasch G, Fuchs E, Mombaerts P. (2007) Mice cloned from skin cells. Proc Natl Acad Sci USA 104:2738–2743.
15. Taylor G, Lehrer MS, Jensen PJ, Sun TT, Lavker RM. (2000) Involvement of follicular stem cells in forming not only the follicle but also the epidermis. Cell 102:451–461.
16. Ito M, Liu Y, Yang Z, Nguyen J, Liang F, Morris RJ, Cotsarelis G. (2005) Stem cells in the hair follicle bulge contribute to wound repair but not to homeostasis of the epidermis. Nat Med 11:1351–1354.
17. Oshima H, Rochat A, Kedzia C, Kobayashi K, Barrandon Y. (2001) Morphogenesis and renewal of hair follicles from adult multipotent stem cells. Cell 104:233–245.
18. Toma JG, Akhavan M, Fernandes KJ, Barnabe-Heider F, Sadikot A, Kaplan DR, Miller FD. (2001) Isolation of multipotent adult stem cells from the dermis of mammalian skin. Nat Cell Biol 3:778–784.
19. Amoh Y, Li L, Yang M, Moossa AR, Katsuoka K, Penman S, Hoffman RM. (2004) Nascent blood vessels in the skin arise from nestin-expressing hair follicle cells. Proc Natl Acad Sci USA 101:13291–13295.
20. Amoh Y, Li L, Katsuoka K, Penman S, Hoffman RM. (2005) Multipotent nestin-positive, keratin-negative hair-follicle-bulge stem cells can form neurons. Proc Natl Acad Sci USA 102:5530–5534.

21. Amoh Y, Li L, Campillo R, Kawahara K, Katsuoka K, Penman S, Hoffman RM. (2005) Implanted hair follicle stem cells form Schwann cells that support repair of severed peripheral nerves. Proc Natl Acad Sci USA 102:17734–17738.
22. Lako M, Armstrong L, Cairns PM, Harris S, Hole N, Jahoda CAB. (2002) Hair follicle dermal cells repopulate the mouse haematopoietic system. J Cell Sci 115(Pt 20):3967–3974.
23. Jahoda CA, Whitehouse J, Reynolds AJ, Hole N. (2003) Hair follicle dermal cells differentiate into adipogenic and osteogenic lineages. Exp Dermatol 12(6):849–859.
24. Gharzi A, Reynolds AJ, Jahoda CA. (2003) Plasticity of hair follicle dermal cells in wound healing and induction. Exp Dermatol 12(2):126–136.

Index

Color Plates

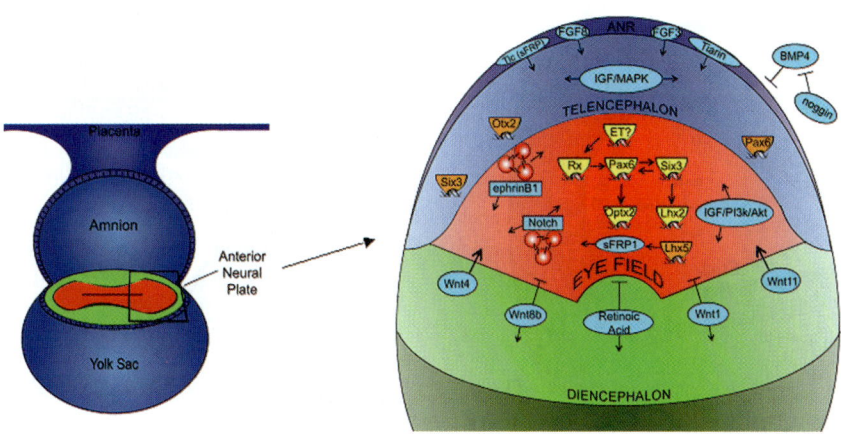

Fig. 1.1 Patterning of the eye field and anterior neural plate. The eye field is found within the anterior neural plate and bordered by the telencephalon rostrally and the diencephalon caudally. The anterior neural plate develops in a BMP-negative environment through the inhibitory action of noggin. The telencephalon and eye field are induced by suppression of the caudalizing retinoic acid and canonical Wnt/β-catenin signals whereas the diencephalon is specified by these signals (through Wnt8b/Wnt1 and RA). Wnt non-canonical signaling on the other hand specifies the eye field (through Wnt4/Wnt11). Signaling from the anterior neural ridge (ANR) specifies the telencephalon. IGF appears to activate the telencephalon and eye field through different pathways, MAPK for the telencephalon and PI3K/Akt for the eye field. Notch and ephrin cell-cell signaling guides and specifies cells to the eye field. The eye field is characterized by the overlapping expression patterns of several transcription factors, highlighted in yellow. Other important transcription factors are indicated in orange. Signaling molecules are indicated in blue

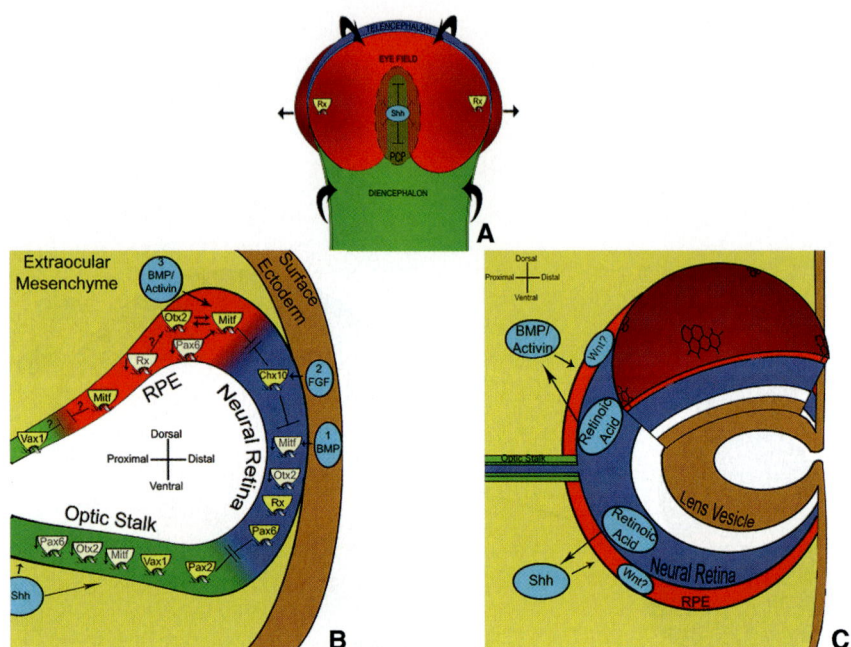

Fig. 1.2 From optic vesicle to optic cup. (**A**) *Sonic Hedgehog* (Shh) arising from the ventrally located prechordal plate (PCP) divides the eye field by down-regulating eye field transcription factors in the midline. *Rx* signaling is necessary for optic vesicle evagination towards the surface ectoderm as the neural tube folds. Arrows show morphogenetic movements. (**B**) As the optic vesicle reaches the surface ectoderm, the presumptive RPE, neural retina and optic stalk begin to differentiate. BMP signaling from the surface ectoderm induces *Mitf* expression (1). This is followed by a wave of FGF signaling from the surface ectoderm which induces *Chx10* expression (2). *Chx10* down regulates *Mitf* within the presumptive neural retina. *Mitf* is maintained/specified in the dorsal/distal optic vesicle by BMP/Activin signaling (3). Transcription factors in gray are initially expressed but eventually down-regulated. (**C**) Both the optic vesicle and the surface ectoderm invaginate to form the optic cup and lens vesicle. The RPE spreads ventrally to surround the neural retina. Many signaling molecules are thought to act at this stage, although their exact mechanisms and functions remain to be elucidated

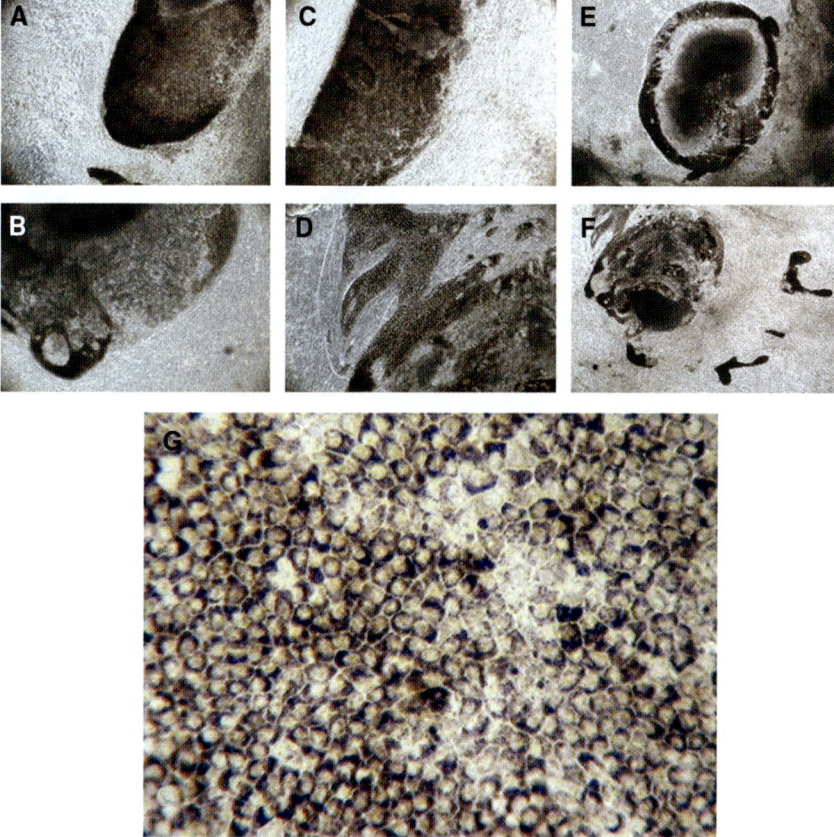

Fig. 1.3 RPE-like colonies in differentiating hESC. (**A–F**) Examples of pigmented colonies after 40 days of culture in media without bFGF are shown. (**G**) Higher magnification view of pigmented RPE-like cells (passage 1) expanded onto a 6 well plate

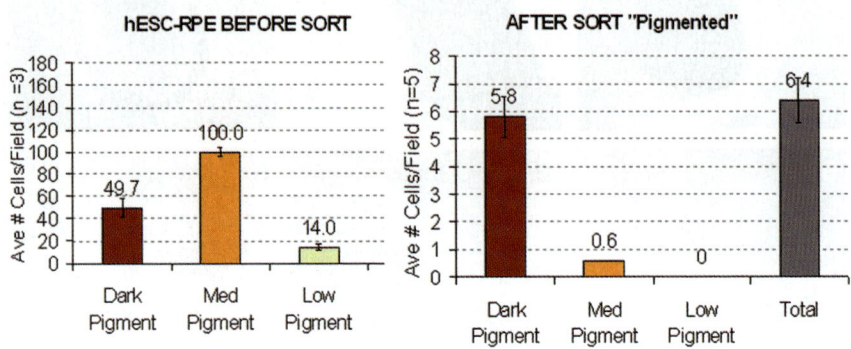

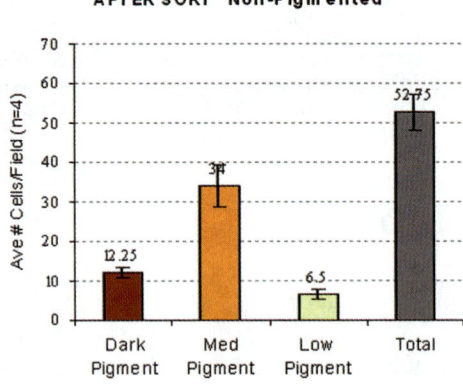

Fig. 1.4 Sorting of hESC-RPE. Shown are results of a FACS Aria sort based on light scattering. The mixed cell population contained 30.4% darkly pigmented cells before the sort and 90.6% darkly pigmented cells after the sort

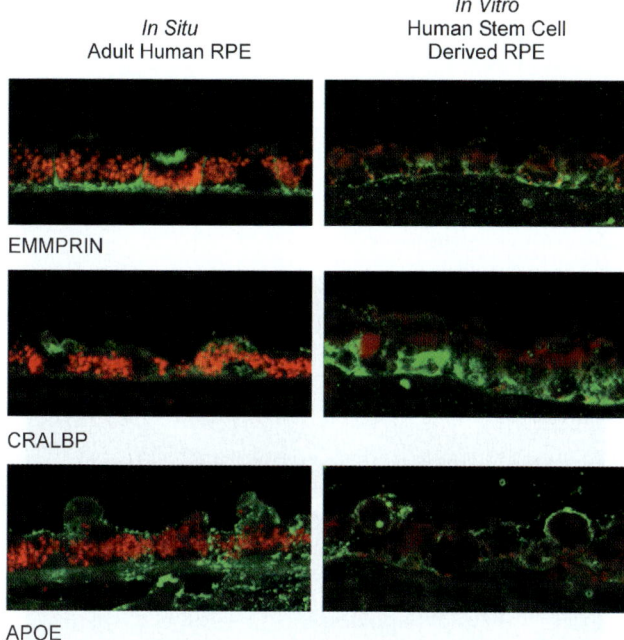

Fig. 1.5 Expression of RPE markers in hESC-RPE. The panel on the left show sections of adult human donor RPE/Choroid with staining of the marker EMPRIN indicated in green, and autofluorescent lipofuscin shown in red. The panel on the right shows a similar aspect of confluent hESC-RPE cultures

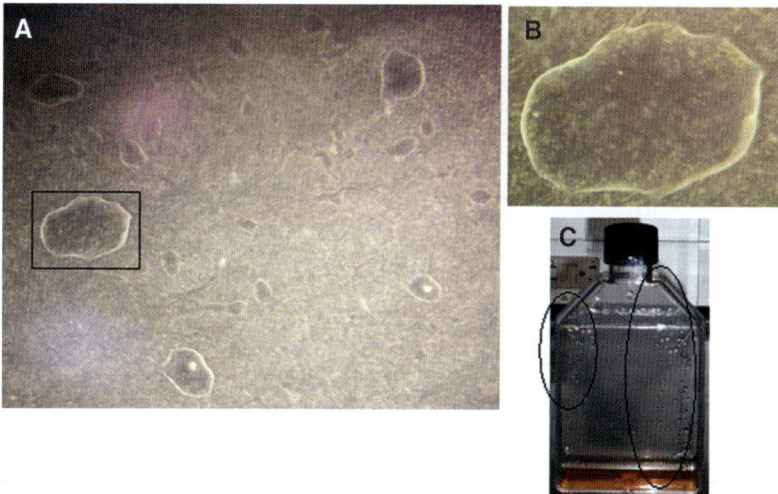

Fig. 1.6 Domes in hESC-RPE cultures. (**A**) Low magnification view of hESC-RPE after three passages. Boxed area is magnified in (**B**), showing dome. (**C**) Domes are visible to the naked eye in culture flasks

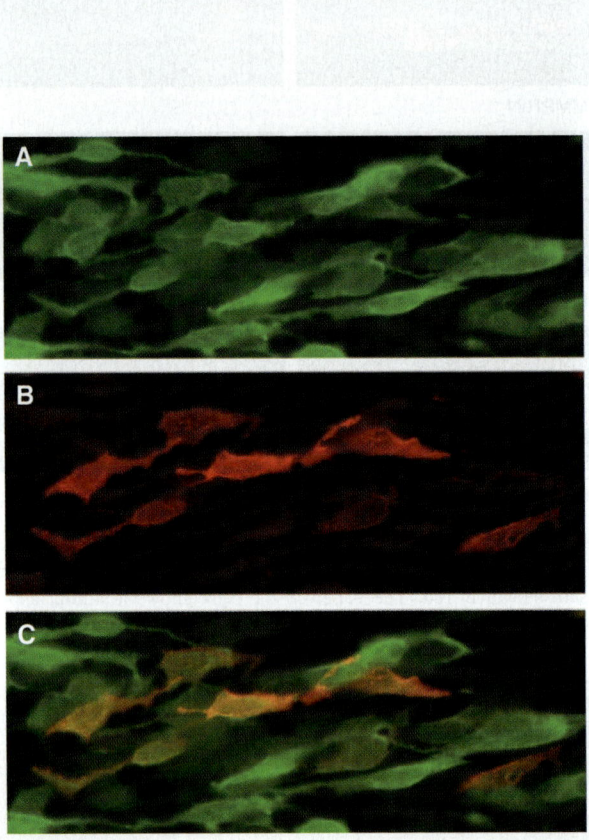

Fig. 2.2 Expression of photoreceptor markers in culture. Under differentiation conditions, porcine retinal progenitor cells expressed the photoreceptor markers recoverin (green) (**A**) and rhodopsin (red) (**B**), with co-expression of both markers in a subset of cells (**C**). Cells co-expressing rhodopsin and recoverin frequently exhibited morphologies suggestive of rod photoreceptors (From [32]; reprinted courtesy of Stem Cells)

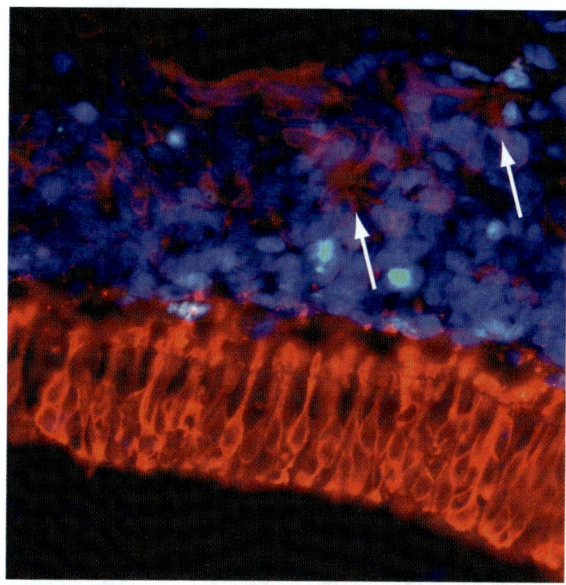

Fig. 2.3 Subretinal transplantation in allogeneic recipients. Cultured porcine retinal progenitor cells were pre-labeled with DAPI (blue) prior to transplantation. Following transplantation, many donor cells exhibited rod-like morphologies and co-expressed the photoreceptor marker rhodopsin (red). DAPI-labeled donor cells formed characteristic rosettes (arrows), suggestive of an advanced level of photoreceptor differentiation. Rhodopsin was also expressed by the DAPI-negative rods of the host (red, below) (Detail from [32]; reprinted courtesy of Stem Cells)

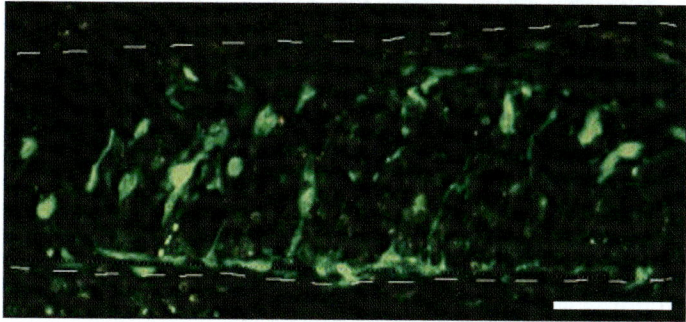

Fig. 2.4 Polymer-progenitor composite graft in the eye. GFP-transgenic mouse retinal progenitor cells were co-cultured on a sheet of PLGA followed by transplantation to the subretinal space of a pig. Note that the cells have conformed to the porous structure of the polymer by extending processes with a radial orientation. Dashed lines indicate the border of the polymer scaffold. The host RPE lies above the graft, while the host retina lies below. Scale bar 90 um. (From [50] reprinted courtesy Archives of Ophthalmology)

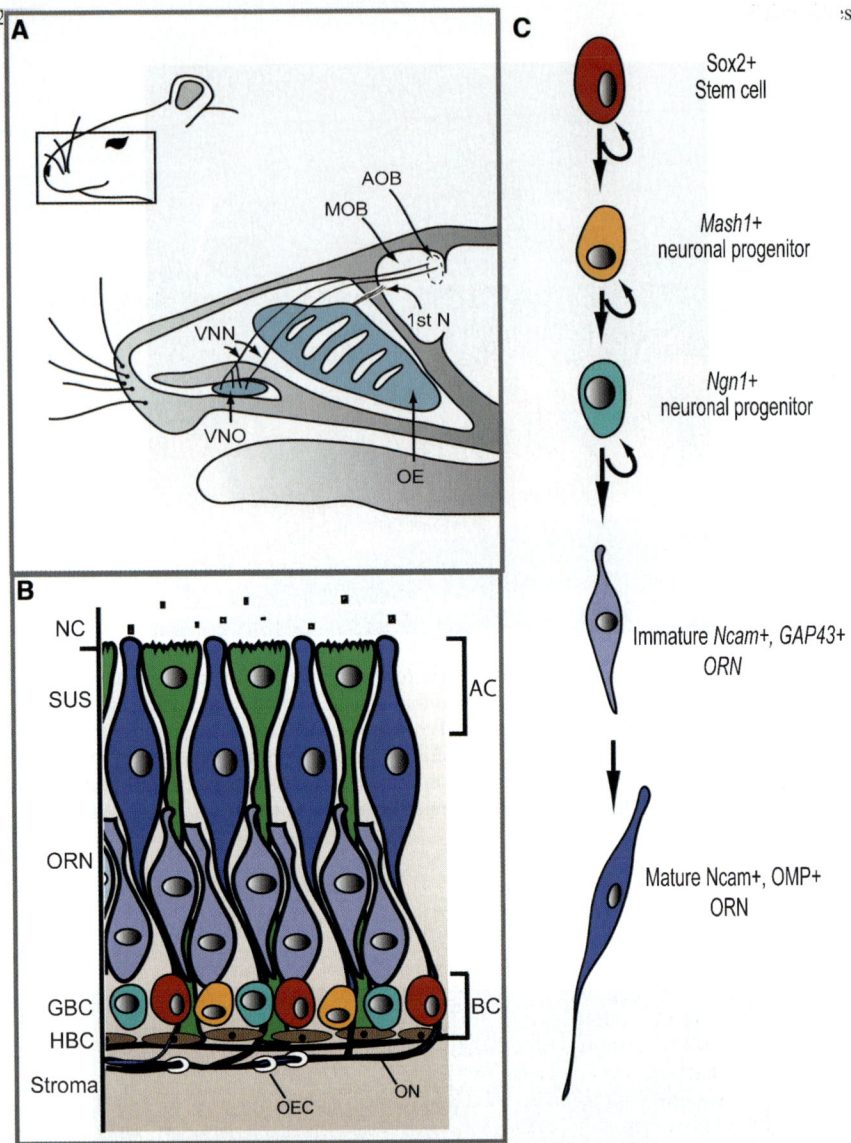

Fig. 3.1 Schematic drawings of olfactory structures and relevant developmental cell types. (**A**) Sagittal view of the nasal cavity and rostral forebrain of a mouse. The olfactory epithelium (OE) lines the nasal cavity and contains olfactory receptor neurons (ORNs), which project through the cribriform plate to glomeruli in the main olfactory bulb (MOB) within the central nervous system. Pheromone-detecting vomeronasal neurons (VNN) of the vomeronasal organ (VNO) project to the accessory olfactory bulb (AOB). (**B**) Diagram of the OE showing relative positions of cell types. From apical to basal, these include sustentacular cells (SUS; green), ORNs, and globose and horizontal basal cells (GBC; HBC). The GBCs consist of three types of neuronal progenitors: *Sox2*-expressing neuronal stem cells, *Mash1*-expressing transit amplifying progenitors, and *Ngn1*-expressing INPs. (**C**) Schematic of the neuronal differentiation pathway of OE neuronal progenitor cells. *Sox2*-expressing neuronal stem cells give rise to transit amplifying progenitors expressing *Mash1*, which produce *Ngn1*-expressing immediate neuronal precursors (INPs). INP division produces daughter cells that differentiate into immature ORNs, identified by NCAM immunoreactivity. Immature ORNs eventually mature and express NCAM and olfactory marker protein (OMP)

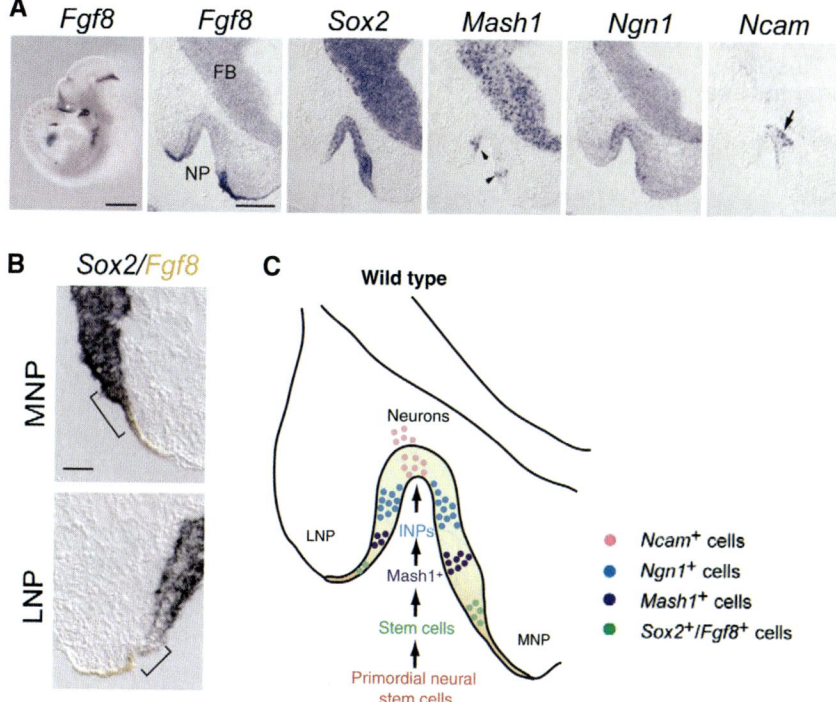

Fig. 3.2 Expression of *Fgf8* and neuronal cell markers in developing OE. (**A**) Six successive images show in situ hybridizations for *Fgf8* (full-length ORF probe) and OE neuronal lineage markers in invaginating nasal pit (NP) at E10.5. In whole-mount in situ hybridization (left-most image), *Fgf8* is detected in commissural plate and olfactory placode, branchial arches, mid-hindbrain junction, and limb and tail buds (Scale bar, 1 mm). In serial sections, locations of neuronal lineage markers within the OE are shown: arrowheads indicate *Mash1*-expressing cells, arrow indicates *Ncam1*-expressing neurons (Scale bar, 200 μm). (**B**) Double label in situ hybridization for *Fgf8* (full-length ORF probe, orange) and *Sox2* (blue) demonstrates overlap of the two markers in a small rim of surface ectoderm and adjacent invaginating neuroepithelium (brackets) (Scale bar, 50 μm). (**C**) Model of peripheral-to-central process of neuronal differentiation in developing OE and origin of *Sox2*-expressing neural stem cells from *Fgf8*-expressing ectoderm. LNP, lateral nasal pit; MNP, medial nasal pit (Adapted from [25]; reprinted courtesy of Development)

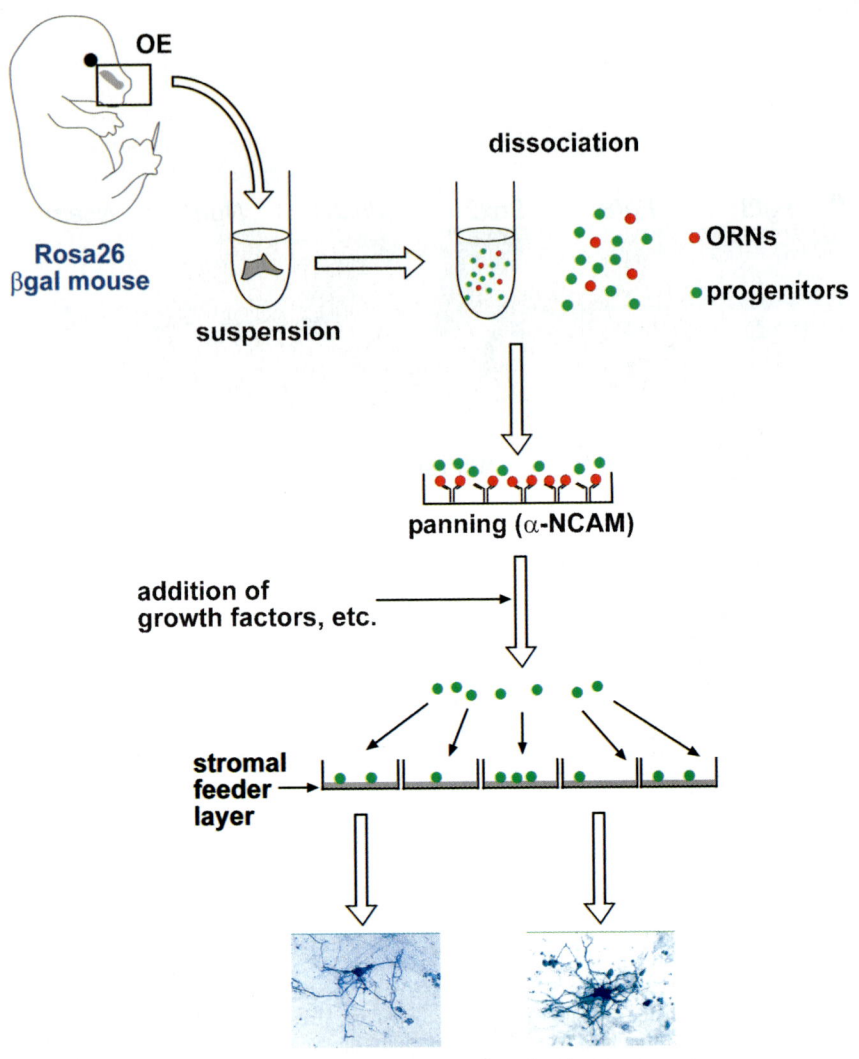

Fig. 3.3 Anti-NCAM immunological panning results in pure population of OE neuronal progenitor cells. OE neuronal cell fractions were resuspended in culture medium and incubated on panning plates for 30 minutes at room temperature in the dark, with intermittent agitation. Panning plates were prepared by coating 100-mm Petri dishes with purified culture supernatant from H28 rat anti-NCAM hybridoma cells. After 30 minutes of immunological panning, cells remaining in suspension were collected, centrifuged, resuspended in culture medium, and plated at various densities on stromal cell feeder layers. The resulting population consists of >96% pure neuronal progenitor cells

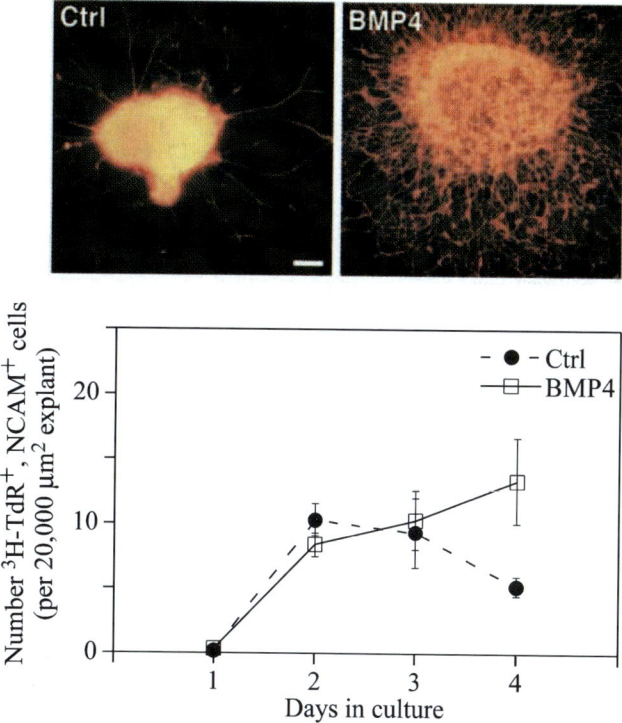

Fig. 3.6 Low-dose BMP4 has a direct effect on olfactory neurogenesis. OE explants were cultured for a total of 96 hours in the presence or absence of 0.1 ng/ml BMP4, and cultures fixed and processed for NCAM immunoreactivity. Fluorescence photomicrographs of OE explants in the two conditions, showing increased numbers of NCAM-positive ORNs surrounding the explant in the presence of BMP4 (Scale bar, 50 μm). Low-dose BMP4 also promotes survival of newly-generated ORNs, quantified from OE explant cultures treated with both BMP4 (0.1 ng/ml) and ^{3}H-TdR. A significant difference in the number of surviving ORNs was observed between control and BMP4-treated cultures after 4 days in vitro ($P = 0.02$, Student's t-test) (From [45]; reprinted courtesy of Nature Neuroscience)

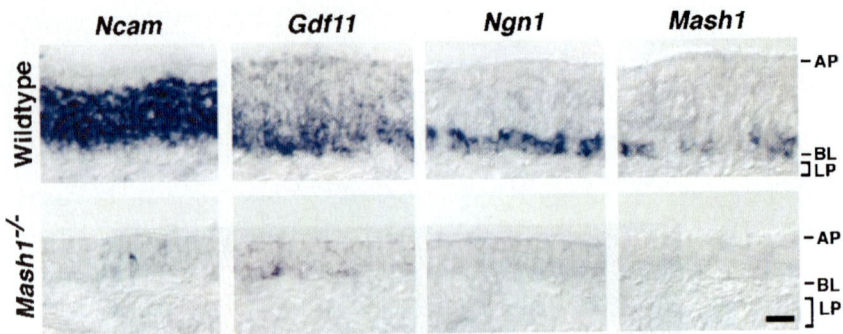

Fig. 3.7 *Gdf11* is expressed by ORNs and their progenitors. OE from E17.5 *Mash1*⁻/⁻ embryos and wild-type littermate was hybridized with probes to *Ncam*, *Gdf11*, *Ngn1*, and *Mash1*. In *Mash1*⁻/⁻ mice the ORN lineage is cut short at an early stage, as *Mash1*-expressing neuronal progenitors initially form, but then undergo apoptosis. Thus, the OE of *Mash1*⁻/⁻ mice is markedly thinner than that of wild-types, and expression of *Ngn1* and *Ncam* is drastically reduced since the epithelium lacks most ORNs and ORN progenitors. *Gdf11* expression is also essentially absent. Since sustentacular cells and horizontal basal cells are still present in *Mash1*⁻/⁻ mice, this indicates that the cells that normally express *Gdf11* must be ORNs and ORN progenitors (Scale, 20 μm; AP, apical surface; BL, basal lamina; LP, lamina propria) (From [63]; reprinted courtesy of Neuron)

Fig. 3.8 *Gdf11* mutants exhibit retinal abnormalities. (**A**) ISH for *Gdf11* and *Fst* in developing mouse retina; nbl, neuroblastic layer; gcl, ganglion cell layer. Arrow in inset indicates *Fst* expression in presumptive amacrine cells (Scale bars, 200 μm) (**B**) Left, hematoxylin-eosin-stained paraffin sections of retina. Right, ISH for *Brn3b*. Insets, higher magnification of *Brn3b*⁺ gcl (Scale bars, 100 μm) (**C**) Top, increased cell number (*P* < 0.01, student's *t*-test) in *Gdf11*-null retinas. Total cell nuclei in GCL + IPL were counted in 300 μm of central retina in P0 cryosections stained with Hoechst. Bottom, no significant change in central retina thickness. Histograms show mean ± SEM of measurements from four to five animals of each genotype. (**D**) β-galactosidase (X-gal) staining of sections of *Gdf11*-null- and *Gdf11*⁺/⁺-*Tattler-1* embryos (Scale bars, 200 μm; on, optic nerve; oc, optic chiasm) (**E**) Cross sections of dissected optic nerves stained with antibodies to neurofilament (Scale bar, 50 μm) (From [65]; reprinted courtesy of Science)

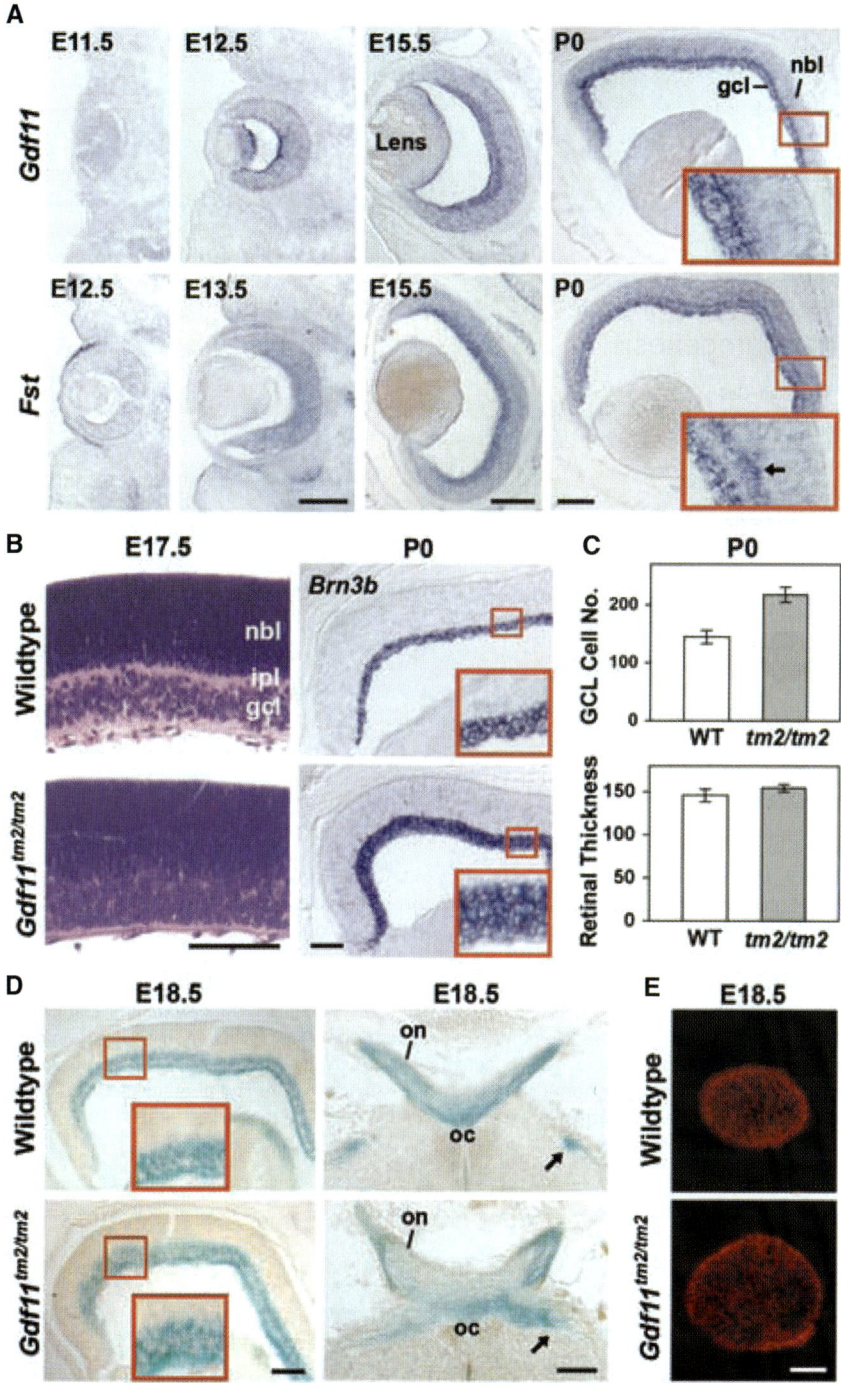

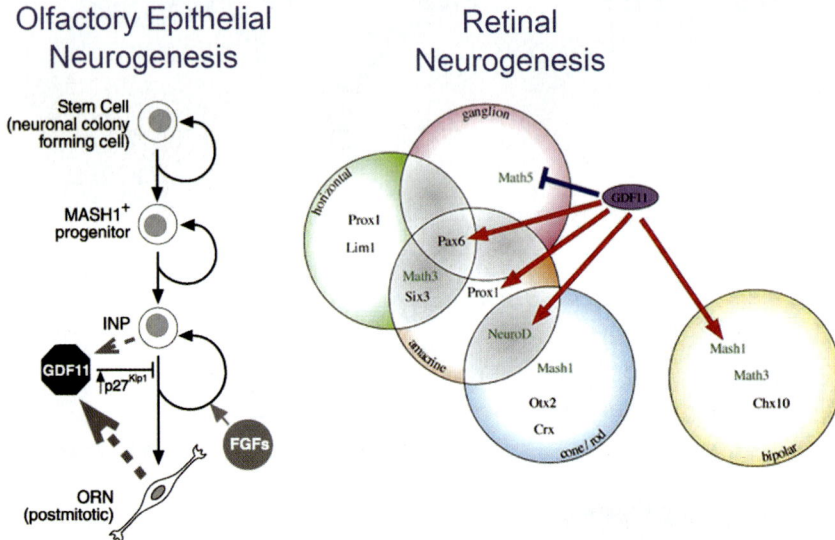

Fig. 3.9 Contrasting roles of GDF11 signaling in OE and retina neurogenesis. In developing OE, GDF11 negatively regulates neuronal production by reversibly blocking the division of *Ngn1-*expressing INPs through increased expression of the cyclin-dependent kinase inhibitor p27^{Kip1}. Loss of ORNs releases INPs from the GDF11-mediated negative regulation, allowing them to increase their proliferation until neuron number is restored. In contrast, GDF11 signaling in retinal neurogenesis specifies retinal cell type specification by regulating retinal progenitor cell competence state. GDF11 suppresses *Math5* expression, and promotes expression of various homeodomain genes such as *Pax6* and bHLH factors such as *NeuroD*, driving progenitors to acquire competence to produce later-born cell types such as amacrine cells and photoreceptors (Adapted from [63, 78] ; reprinted courtesy of Neuron and Genes and Development)

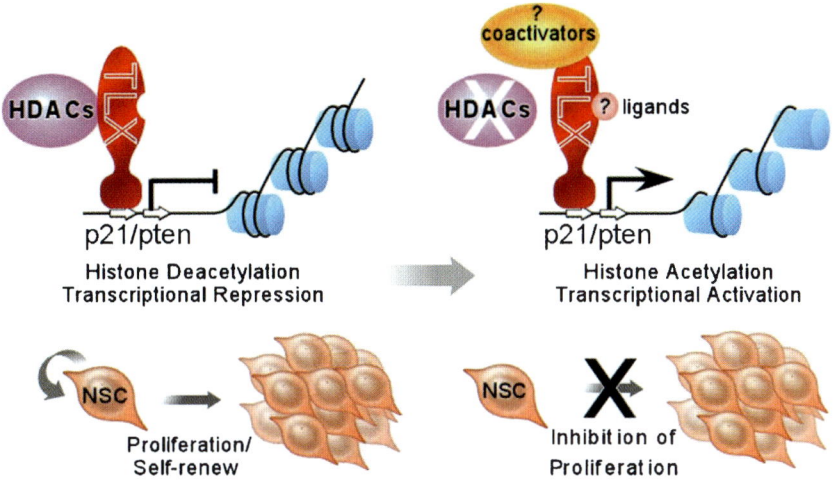

Fig. 4.2 Orphan nuclear receptor TLX partners with HDACs to regulate neural stem cell proliferation and self-renewal. Nuclear receptor TLX binds to its target genes, such as the cyclin-dependent kinase inhibitor, p21, and the tumor suppressor gene, pten. In the absence of ligand, TLX recruits the histone deacetylase complex (HDACs) to the target gene promoters and represses target gene expression. Release or inhibition of HDACs and /or recruitment of coactivator complex activates p21 and pten gene expression, which leads to inhibition of proliferation and induction of neural differentiation

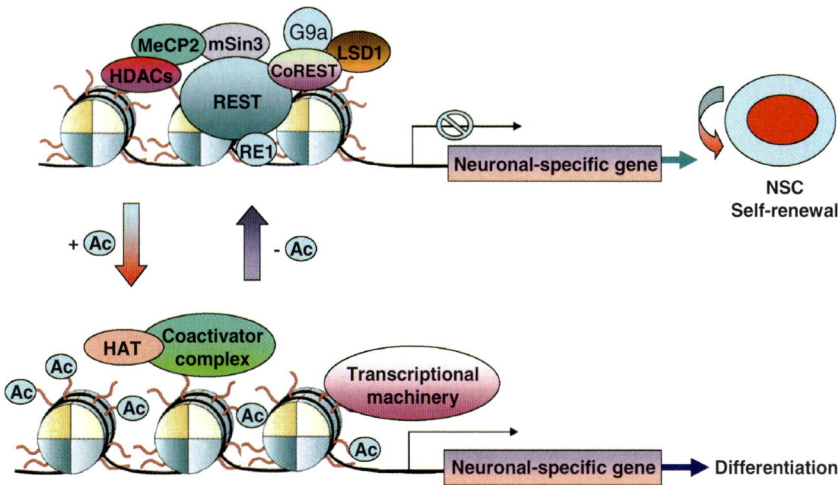

Fig. 4.3 Chromatin remodeling factors in neural stem cells. In neural stem/progenitor cells, REST (repressor element 1 silencing transcription factor) binds to a recognition site RE1 on the neuronal-specific gene promoter. REST can recruit two major complexes: mSin3 complex and CoREST complex. The mSin3 complex includes MeCP2 (methyl CpG binding protein 2) and HDACs (histone deacetylases). The CoREST complex contains HDACs, LSD1 (histone lysine specific demethylase 1) and histone H3K9 methylase G9a. Under the repressive state the neuronal gene expression is suppressed. When the complex was replaced by coactivators in neuronal-lineage cells, the neuron-specific genes are activated. Acetylations (Ac), neural stem cell (NSC)

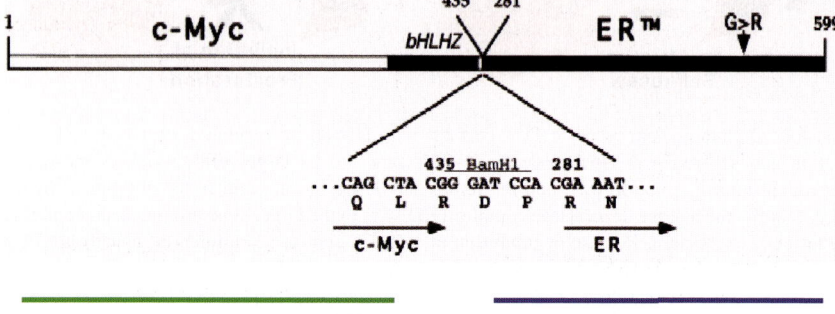

Human c-Myc   **Truncated oestrogen receptor**

c-mycER fusion protein exhibits c-Myc activities which are highly dependent upon 4-hydroxy tamoxifen

Fig. 6.2 The mycER^TAM transgene. The transgene comprises the sequence of human c-myc, fused with the ligand binding domain of the estradiol receptor but containing the point mutation to confer ligand binding selective for 4-hydroxy tamoxifen

CTX0E03
STROKE MODEL STICKY TAPE CONTACT

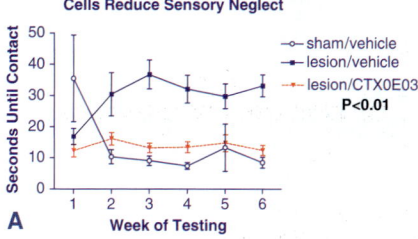

CTX0E03
STROKE MODEL STICKY TAPE REMOVAL

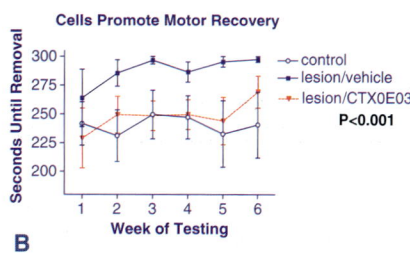

STR0C05
HUNTINGTONS MODEL: BODY SWAY TEST

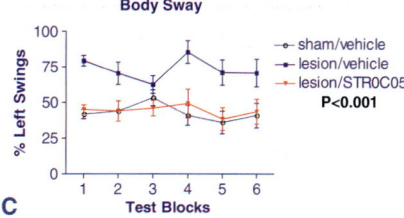

STR0C05
HUNTINGTONS MODEL : STAIRCASE TEST

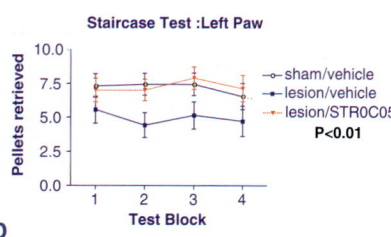

Fig. 6.4 Behavioral recovery with mycER^{TAM} cell lines. Cells were directly implanted into the CNS of rats that were given a stroke (panels **A** & **B**) or were treated with quinolinic acid (panels **C** & **D**) to emulate Huntington's disease. The ability of cells (red triangles) to normalize lesioned behavior (blue squares) back towards normal, sham (open circles) behavior, was monitored over time. A clear recovery effect with CTX0E03 is seen in both the sticky tape contact (**A**) and removal (**B**) tests in stroke. Similarly a clear recovery effect is seen with STR0C05 in the body sway test (**C**) and in the staircase test (**D**)

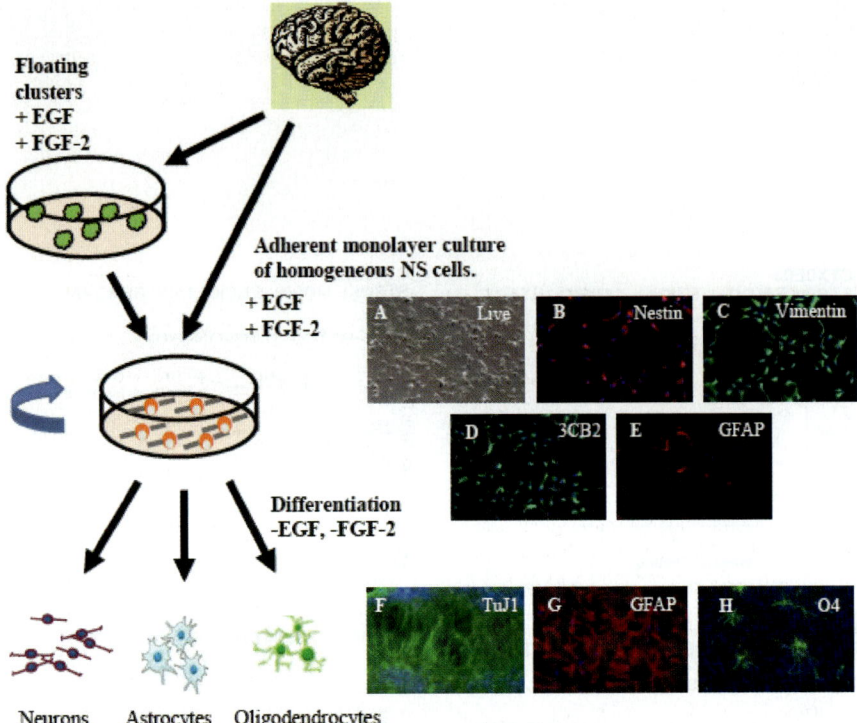

Fig. 7.1 Derivation, propagation and differentiation of human NS cells. NS cells can be derived from various regions of the fetal brain. Through the actions of EGF and FGF-2 NS cells can be expanded in monolayer conditions either from floating clusters (green) or directly in an adherent monolayer culture. (**A**) Passage 21 human NS cells in expansion media and (**B–E**) immunostained for human NS cell/radial glia markers. hNS cells can differentiate to form neurons, astrocytes and oligodendrocytes. (**F–H**) Differentiated hNS immunostained for neural (Tuj1), astrocyte (GFAP) and oligodendrocyte (O4) markers (Oligodendrocyte image courtesy of Y. Sun)

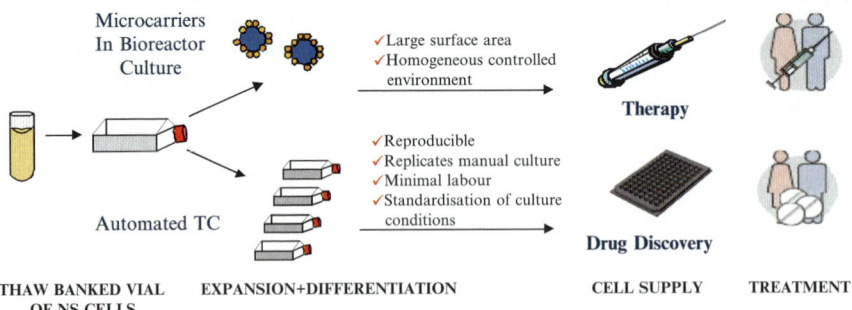

Fig. 7.2 Overview of bioprocessing of human NS cells for drug discovery and therapy. Human NS cells could be expanded and differentiated either by bioreactor culture or automated tissue culture techniques. Bioreactor culture could provide large batches of cells for transplant therapies, whereas automated tissue culture may be more suited to the generation of batches of cells in an assay ready configuration for drug discovery

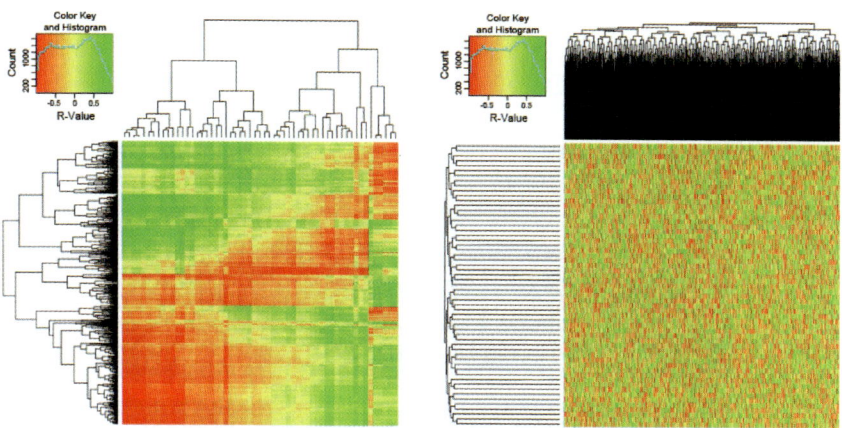

Fig. 8.1 The cross correlation matrix. Using a heatmap-like visualization technique, the correlations between microRNAs and mRNAs can be easily and readily visualized. In this experiment comparing human embryonic stem cells with embryoid bodies or embryonic carcinoma cells, regulated microRNAs (columns) are correlated to significant mRNAs (rows), and the resulting R-values are used to color the component blocks. Hierarchical clustering in both dimensions groups molecules based on their correlation across the opposing molecule type. Subclusters that are negatively correlated (red) may represent potential microRNA:mRNA target interactions resulting in degradation of the target mRNA. Regions showing strong positive correlation (green) may help to identify microRNAs and mRNAs that may have a shared functional pathway or transcriptional regulatory mechanism. The value of the biological information is seen when the connections between microRNA and mRNA are severed by randomly permuting the cross correlation matrix using the identical dataset, resulting in the complete abolition of subclusters

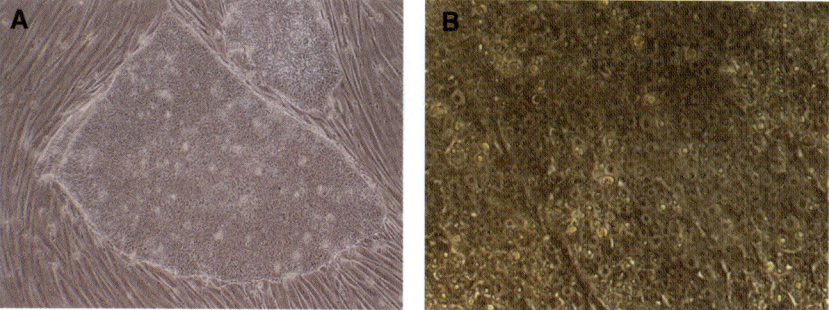

Fig. 9.1 Human ES cells grown in HEScGRO xeno-free, serum-free medium have appearance and morphology typical of human ES cells grown on human feeders. (**A**) H9 (WA09) cells, with well-defined borders and homogenous appearance within the colony. (**B**) MEL-4 cells (shown at higher magnification) display high nuclear-to-cytoplasmic ratio and visible nucleoli

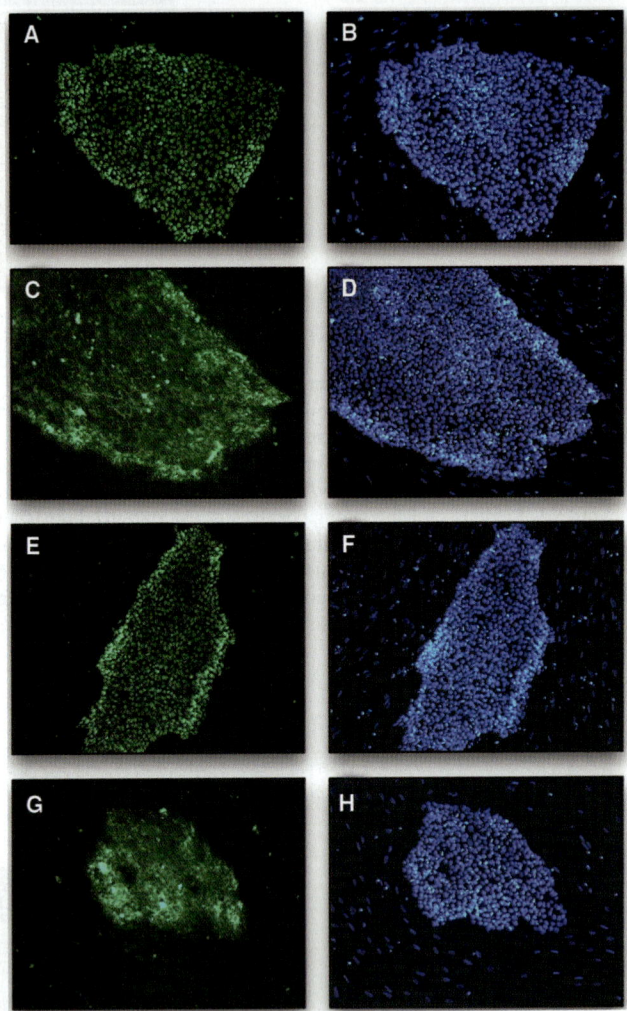

Fig. 9.2 H1 (WA01) and H9 (WA09) cells grown for multiple passages in HEScGRO continue to display markers of pluripotency. (**A–D**) H1 cells after 17 passages in HEScGRO show expression of OCT4 (**A**) and TRA-1-60 (**C**). Cells throughout each colony express these markers, as shown by comparison to the corresponding DAPI staining in **B**, **D**. (**E–H**) H9 cells after 17 passages showing expression of OCT4 (**E**) and TRA-1-60 (**G**), with corresponding DAPI images in **F**, **H**

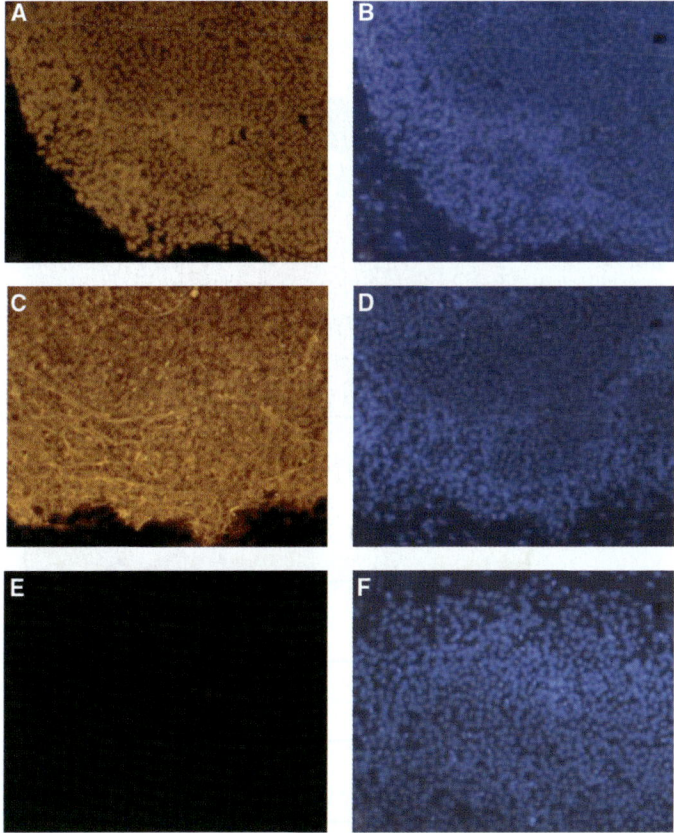

Fig. 9.3 MEL-4 human ES cells grown for 20 passages in HEScGRO have high expression of pluripotency markers and low expression of a differentiation marker. Expression of OCT4 (**A**) and TRA-1-60 (**C**) in passage 20 MEL-4 cells is high, while expression of SSEA-1 (**E**) is low. Corresponding DAPI images are shown in **B**, **D**, and **F**

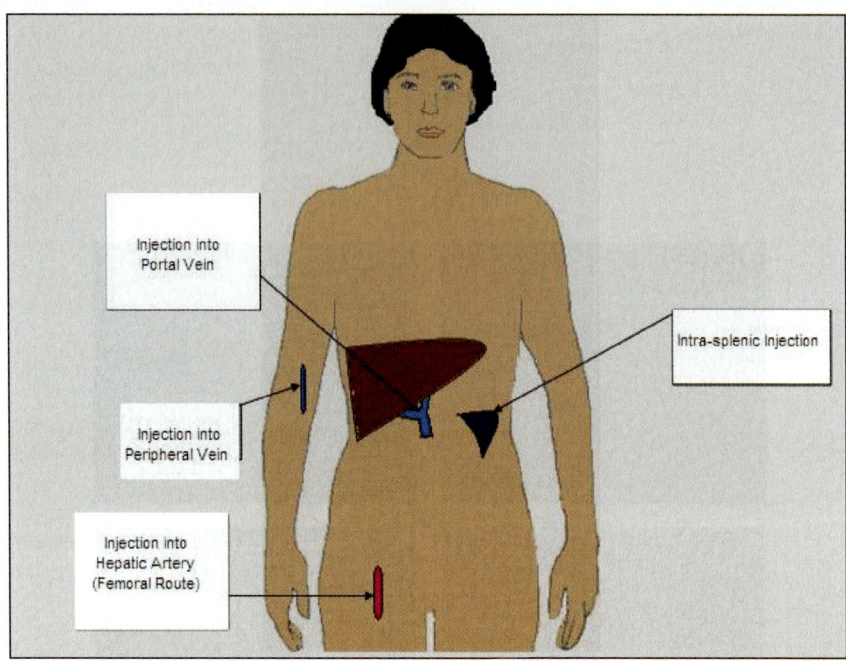

Fig. 10.1 Routes of administration of stem cells into the liver

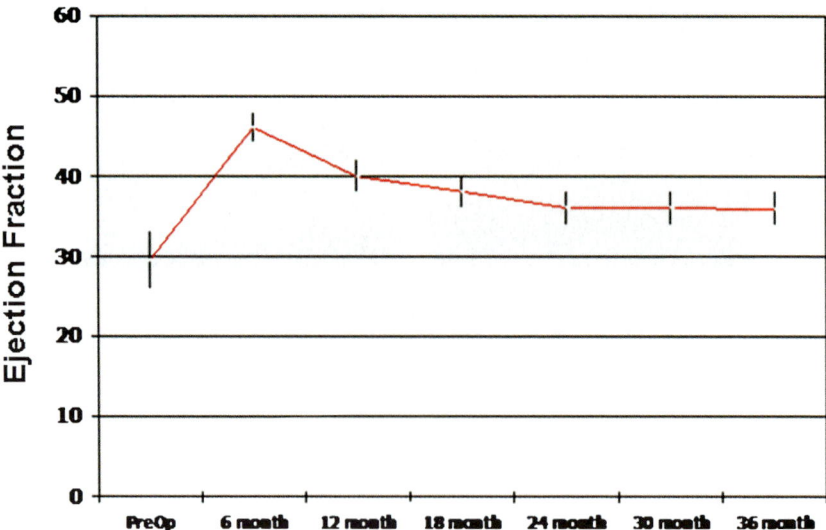

Fig. 12.1 Cardiac function in group 1 patients. These patients received a transplantation of autologous bone marrow stem cells plus coronary surgery off pump (OPCAB and MIDCAB). Ejection fraction is plotted versus time after surgery

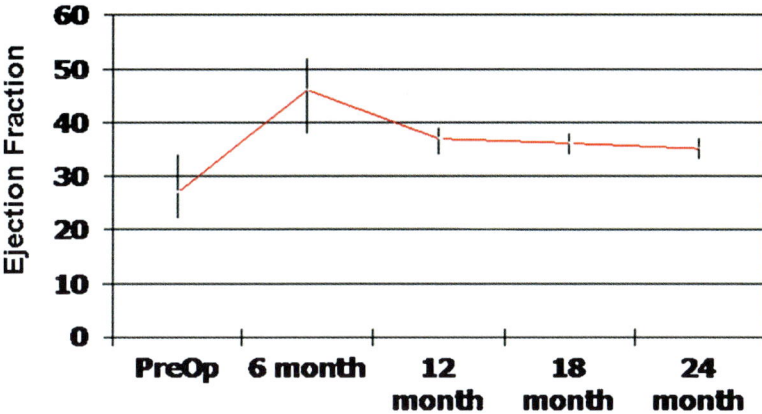

Fig. 12.2 Cardiac function in group 2 patients. Idiopathic non-ischemic cardiomyopathy patients were treated with autologous bone marrow stem cells. Ejection fraction is plotted versus time after surgery

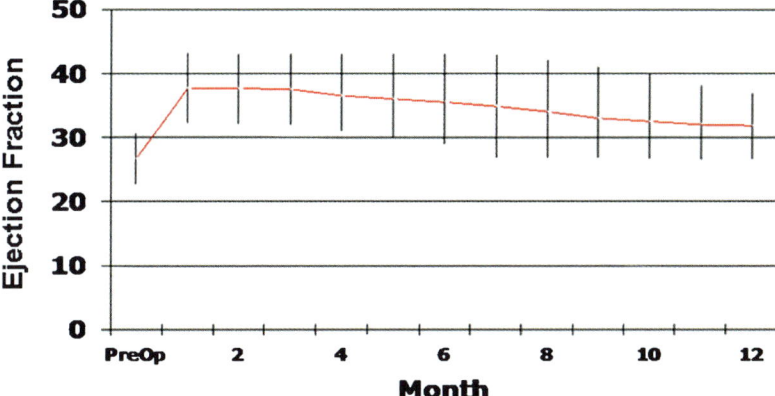

Fig. 12.3 Cardiac function in group 3 patients. Idiopathic non-ischemic cardiomyopathy patients were treated with fetal liver stem cells. Ejection fraction is plotted versus time after surgery

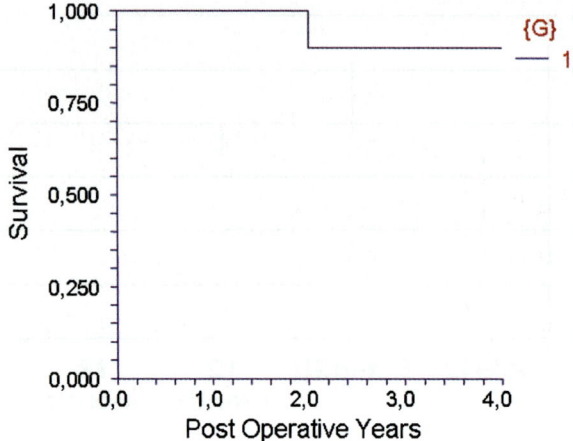

Fig. 12.4 Survival of patients treated with autologous bone marrow stem cells. The fraction surviving is plotted versus post operative time

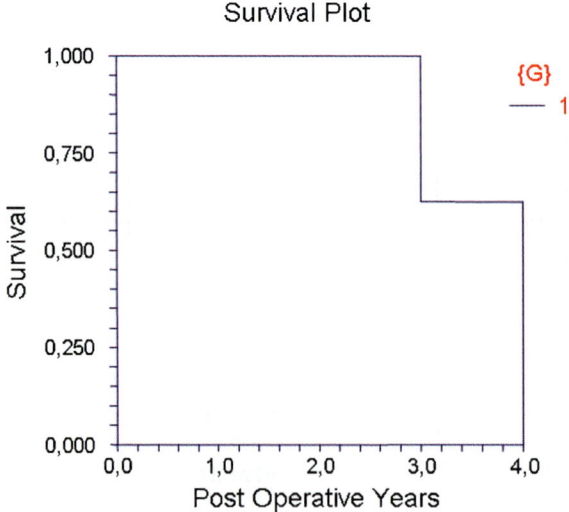

Fig. 12.5 Survival of patients treated with fetal liver stem cells. The fraction surviving is plotted versus post operative time

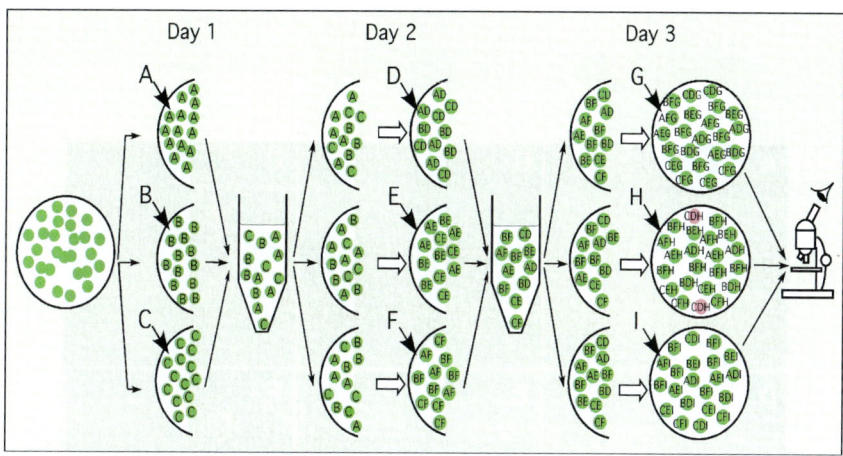

Fig. 13.1 Example of combinatorial cell culture. Cells are seeded on microcarrier beads (green). On day 1 these are split equally into three sets that are cultured under different conditions and the beads labeled using corresponding tags (A, B and C). On day 2 beads are mixed and re-partitioned into three sets that are cultured under different conditions and the beads again labeled using corresponding tags (D, E and F). On day 3 the procedure is repeated and further unique tags are added (G, H and I). At the end of the experiment, beads are screened for the desired cell type (shown as magenta) using an appropriate assay. The tags present on these 'positive' beads provide a record of the cell culture history (in this case tags C, D and H indicate cell culture in condition C on Day 1, D on Day 2 and H on Day 3) (Figure courtesy of J Green)

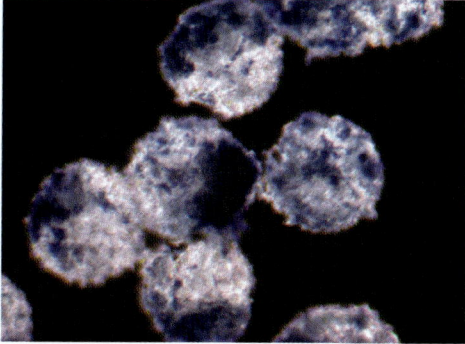

Fig. 13.2 Example of a cell unit. Macroporous, crosslinked cellulose microcarriers with a diameter of about 250 microns (Cytopore 2; GE Healthcare) seeded with mouse ESCs. Cells are stained for alkaline phosphatase activity indicating pluripotency

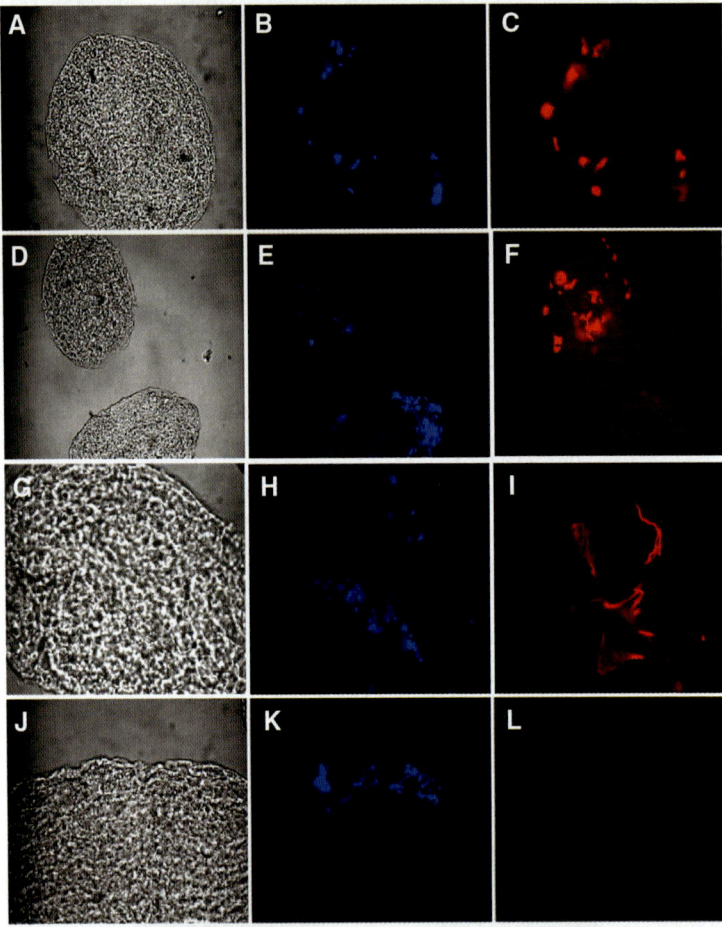

Fig. 13.5 Examples of phenotype detection using cell type-specific antibodies. Cultispher G gelatin microcarriers (Percell Biolytica) were seeded with mESCs and subjected to combinatorial cell culture to obtain neuronal lineages. Left panels show phase micrographs of the beads (under various magnifications) while the middle and right panels respectively show staining with DAPI (showing cell nuclei) and various neuron-specific primary antibodies. Panel C shows staining of dopaminergic neurons (using anti-tyrosine hydroxylase antibody); Panel F shows staining of GABA-ergic cells (anti-GABA antibody); Panel I shows astrocytes (anti-GFAP antibody). Panel L shows the secondary antibody control

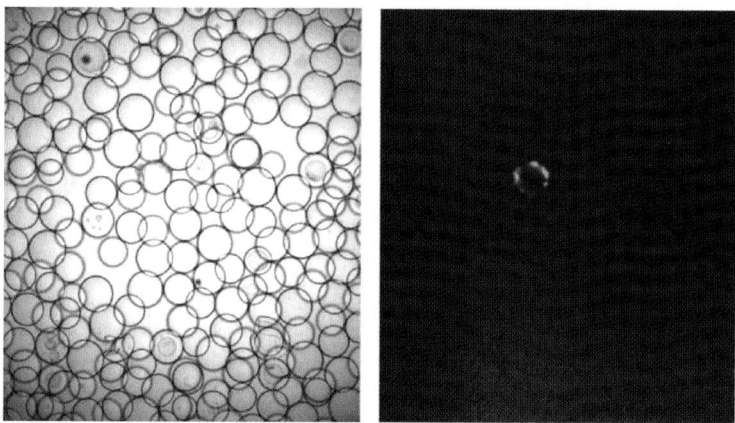

Fig. 13.6 Example of a cell unit screen to isolate a 'positive' bead. A population of Cytodex 3 microcarriers (GE Healthcare) viewed using phase (left) and epifluorescence (right) microscopy reveals a unit bearing cells that express GFP. The 'positive' bead can be isolated manually using a pipette, or using an automated bead sorter (see text)

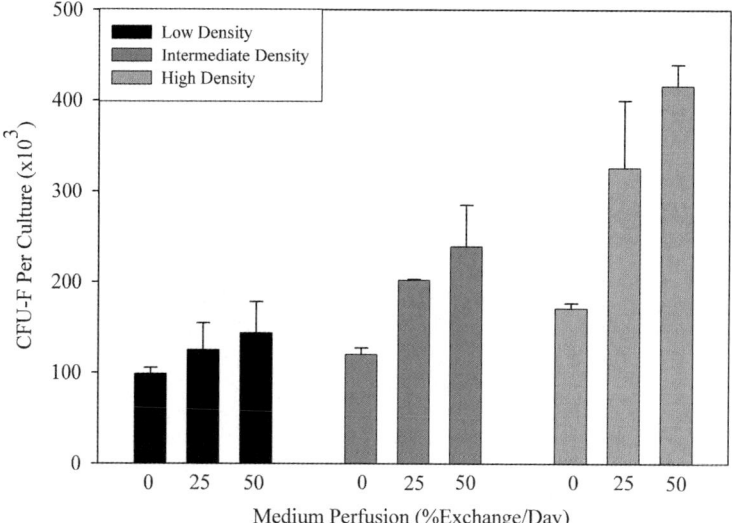

Fig. 14.2 Frequent medium exchange enhances CFU-F output. BM MNCs were cultured in LTBMC medium for 12 days. The number of CFU-Fs at harvest is shown for low (1.5×10^5 cells/cm^2), intermediate (3×10^5 cells/cm^2) and high (6×10^5 cells/cm^2) inoculum density cultures maintained over a range of perfusion rates. The average and range from two experiments is shown

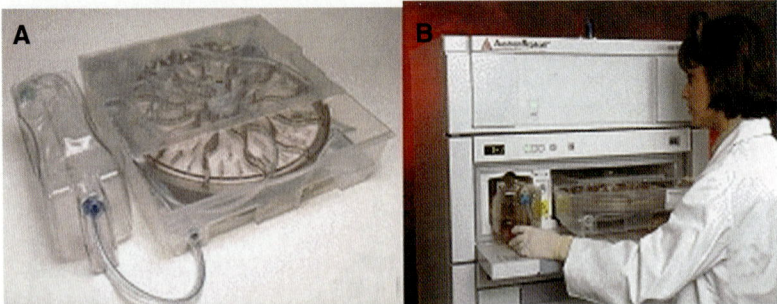

Fig. 14.5 Bioreactor cassette and incubator from the automated system. Pictured is a single use cell cassette with medium reservoir (**A**) and an incubator being loaded with a cell cassette containing BM MNC (**B**). The incubator holds up to four individual cassettes that can be controlled independently for flow rate, temperature and gas levels

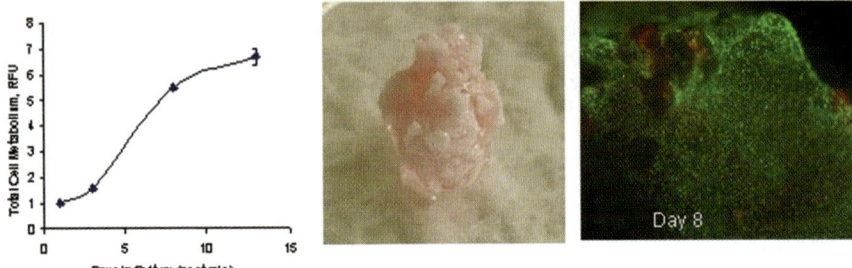

Fig. 14.13 Growth of TRCs on bone matrix material. TRCs were combined with allograft bone matrix material and plasma, and then cultured for up to 14 days in LTBMC medium. Metabolic activity of cells was measured using the cell titer blue assay (left panel). The middle panel is a gross picture of TRC-loaded matrix material after culture. The right panel is a photomicrograph of cells on the matrix after live-dead staining on day 8 of culture. The fluorescent image shows live cells as green and nonviable cells as red

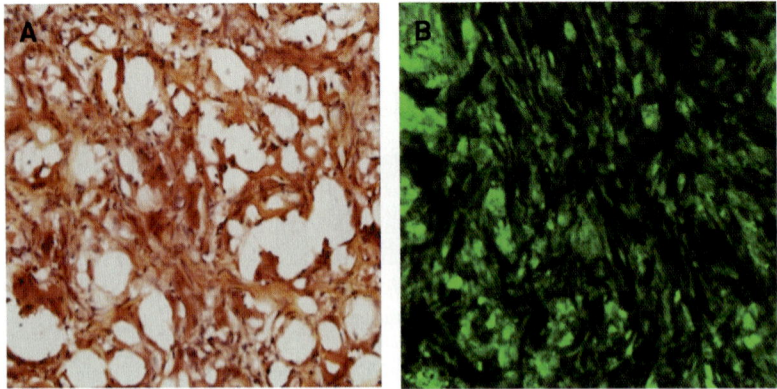

Fig. 14.15 TRCs differentiate into bone in vivo. GFP-transfected TRCs were loaded onto a gelatin matrix (Gelfoam) and implanted subcutaneously into *scid* mice. At 4 weeks, ossicles were sectioned and new bone formation was detected by staining with hematoxylin-eosin (**A**) or by fluorescence microscopy (**B**). Photomicrographs were taken at 400X magnification (**A**) or 40X magnification (**B**)

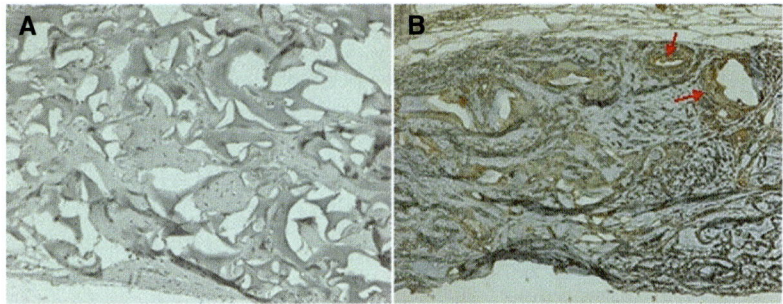

Fig. 14.16 Vascular components in new bone. TRCs were loaded onto a gelatin matrix (Gelfoam) and implanted into a calvarial defect model in *scid* mice. At 7 weeks, samples were processed for immunohistochemistry. (**A**) No primary antibody control. (**B**) Human specific VEGFR2 antibody. Arrows points to vasculature present within new bone. Photomicrographs were taken at 200X magnification

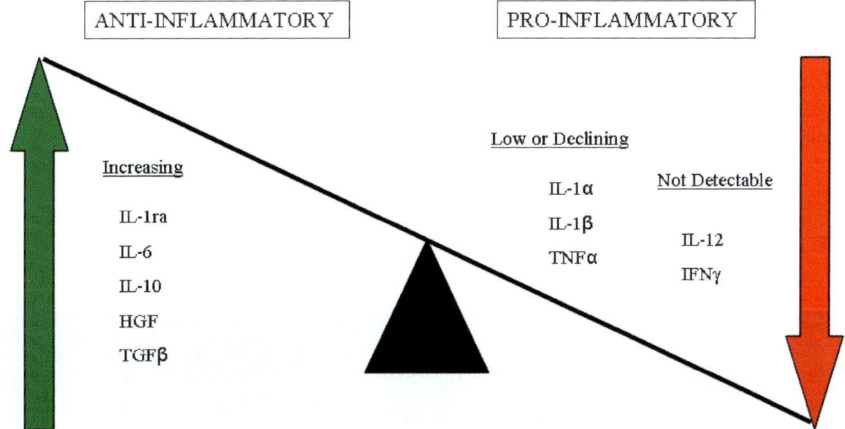

Fig. 14.17 Summary of *in vitro* secretion of immunomodulatory factors by TRCs

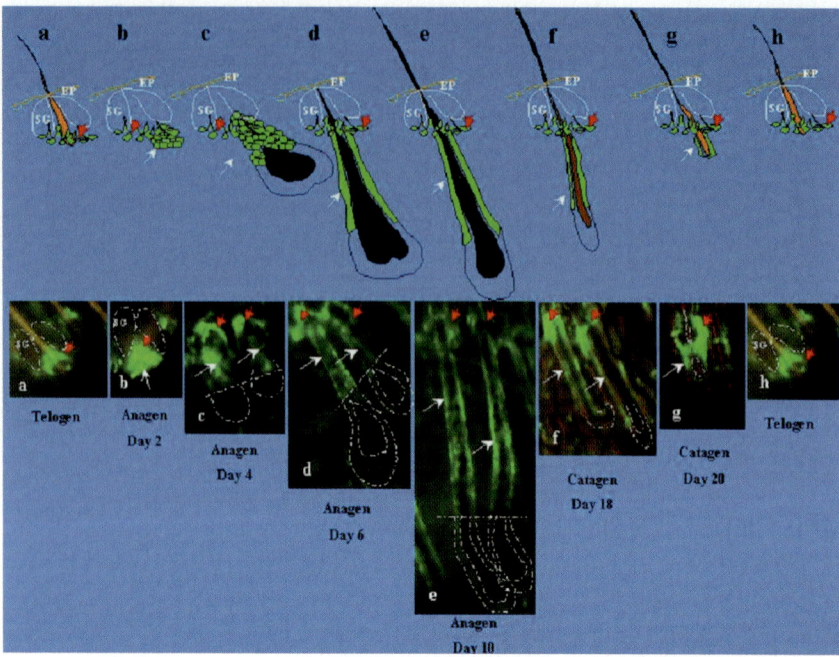

Fig. 15.1 Hair follicle stem cells in the hair-growth cycle [9]. (*Upper*) Cartoon showing position of ND-GFP stem cells at each stage of the hair follicle cycle. SG, sebaceous gland; EP, epidermis. (*Lower* **a**) ND-GFP-expressing hair follicle stem cells (red arrow) located near the hair follicle bulge area in telogen phase. (**b**) Day 2 after anagen induction by depilation. Note the new hair follicle cells (white arrow) formed directly from the ND-GFP-expressing stem cells. (**c–e**) Day 4 (**c**), day 6 (**d**), and day 10 (**e**) after anagen induction by depilation. Note the ND-GFP-expressing outer-root sheath cells (white arrows) in the upper two-thirds of the hair follicle. (**f** and **g**) Day 19 (**f**) and day 20 (**g**) after depilation. Note in f and g that the hair follicles are in the catagen phase and are undergoing regression and degeneration, including the ND-GFP-expressing cells in the outer-root sheath. The ND-GFP-expressing stem cells remain. (**h**) Hair follicle cycling in telogen phase

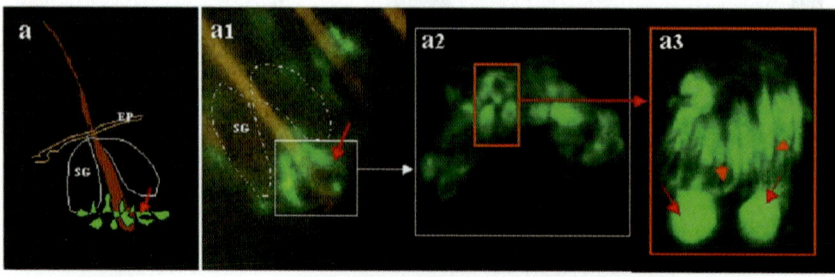

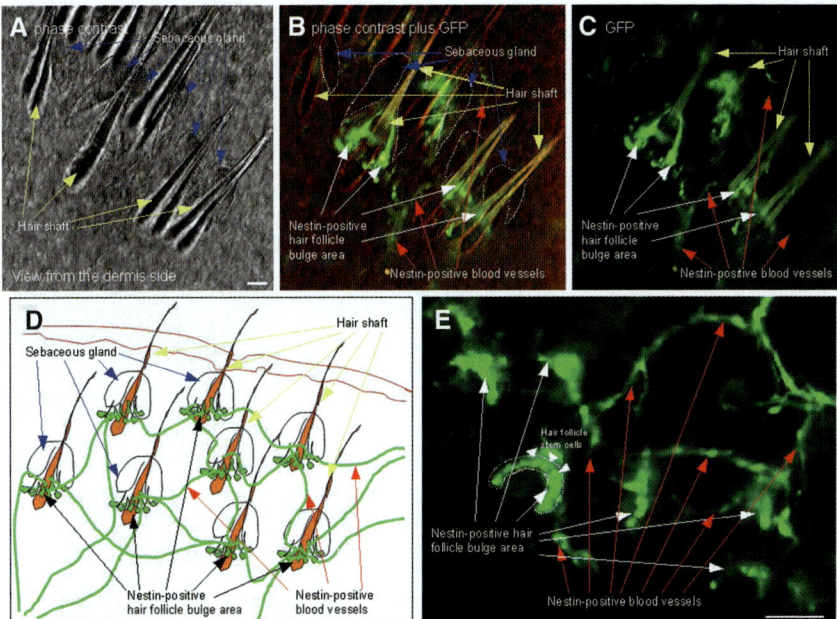

Fig. 15.3 View from the dermis side of the dorsal skin in ND-GFP transgenic mice [19]. (**a**) Phase-contrast microscopy. Sebaceous glands (blue arrows) are located around the hair shaft (yellow arrows). (**b**) Phase-contrast microscopy plus GFP fluorescence. ND-GFP cells are visualized near the follicular bulge area (white arrows) and blood vessels (red arrows). The follicular bulge area is located beneath the sebaceous gland. (**c**) GFP fluorescence. The ND-GFP blood vessels (red arrows) are connected to ND-GFP hair follicles (white arrows). (**d**) Schematic of telogen hair follicle showing position of ND-GFP hair-follicle stem cells (black arrows) and blood vessel network (red arrows). (**e**) GFP fluorescence. The ND-GFP blood vessels (red arrows) are associated with ND-GFP hair-follicle stem cells (white arrows) (Scale bars, 100 μm)

Fig. 15.2 Hair follicle ND-GFP-expressing cells in the telogen phase of ND-GFP transgenic mouse skin [9]. The skin sample was prepared freshly right after excision from the back skin of a ND-GFP transgenic mouse. The skin sample then was directly observed by fluorescence or confocal microscopy with the dermis side up after s.c. tissue was dissected out. (**a**) Cartoon of telogen hair follicle showing position of ND-GFP-expressing hair follicle stem cells. (**a1**) Low-magnification fluorescence microscopy image showing the ring of ND-GFP-expressing stem cells (small white box, see **a**). (**a2**) High-magnification confocal microscopy image reflecting the small white box in **a1**. Note the small round- or oval-shaped ND-GFP-expressing cells near the bulge area of the hair follicle (small red box). (**a3**) High-magnification fluorescence microscopy image showing two individual ND-GFP-expressing stem cells reflecting the red box in **a2**. Note the unique morphology of the hair follicle stem cells and multiple dendrite-like structures of each cell. Red arrows indicate the cell body, and red arrowheads show the multiple dendritic structure of each cell (Original magnifications: **a1** × 100; **a2** × 400; **a3** × 1,600.) (SG, sebaceous gland; EP, epidermis)

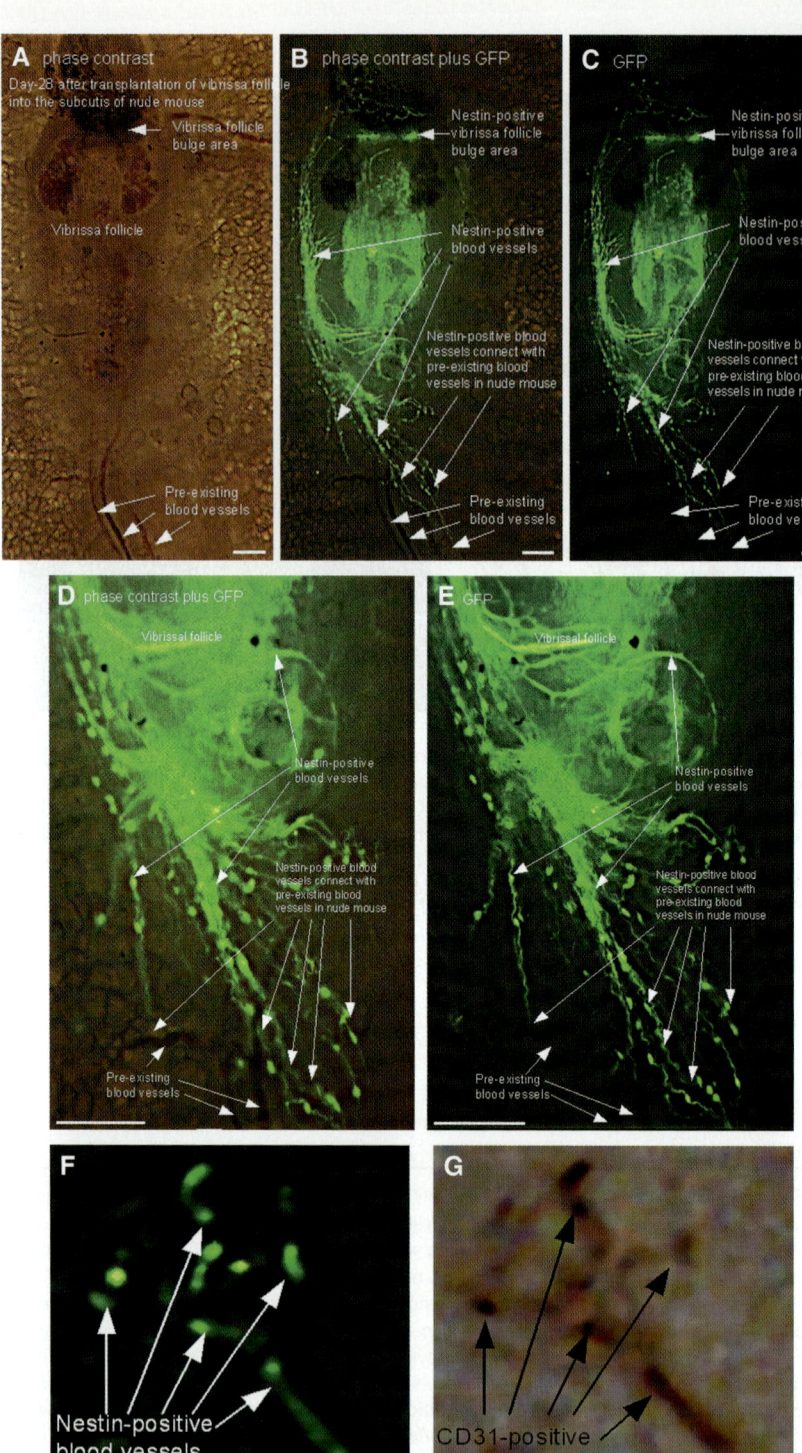

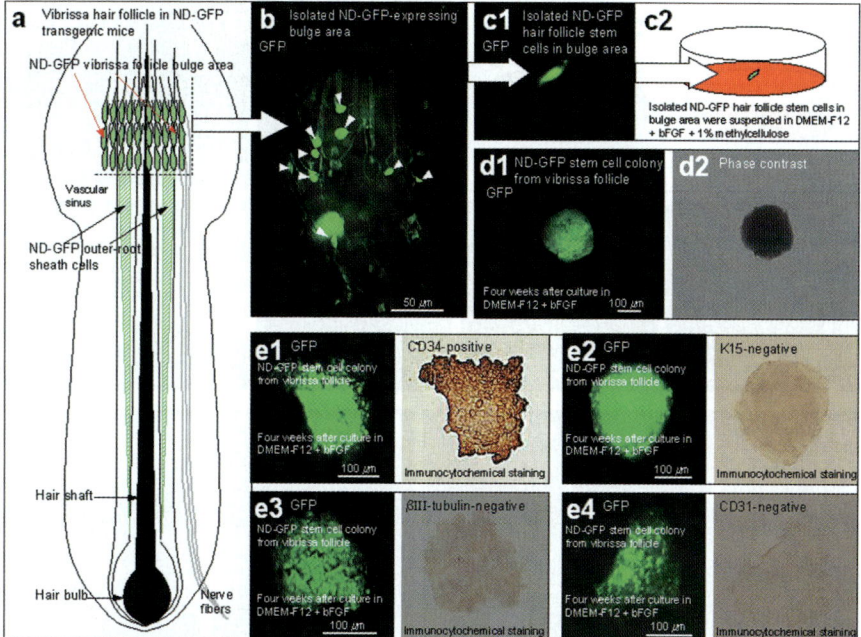

Fig. 15.5 Isolation, culture, and characterization of ND-GFP hair follicle stem cells [20]. (**a**) Schematic representation of a vibrissa hair follicle in ND-GFP transgenic mice showing the position of the ND-GFP-expressing vibrissa follicular stem cells (red arrows) and ND-GFP-expressing outer-root sheath cells (black arrows). (**b**) Isolated ND-GFP-expressing vibrissa follicular stem cells (white arrow heads). (**c1** and **c2**) The ND-GFP-expressing hair-follicle stem cells in the vibrissa were isolated and suspended in DMEM-F12 containing B-27 and 1% methylcellulose supplemented with bFGF every 2 days. (**d1** and **d2**) After 4 weeks, ND-GFP-expressing hair-follicle stem cells from the vibrissa area formed the ND-GFP-expressing cell colony. (**e**) ND-GFP-expressing cells within the colony were CD34-positive (**e1**), and the ND-GFP-expressing cells within the colony were K15- (**e2**), III β-tubulin- (**e3**), and CD31-negative (**e4**)

Fig. 15.4 Transplantation of an ND-GFP vibrissa follicle into the subcutis of a nude mouse [19]. (**a**) Phase-contrast micrograph of follicle 28 days after transplantation. (**b**) Phase-contrast micrograph plus GFP fluorescence. (**c**) GFP fluorescence. In **b** and **c**, ND-GFP blood vessels (arrows) are seen growing from the transplanted ND-GFP hair follicle and associating with preexisting blood vessels in the nude-mouse skin. (**d** and **e**) Higher magnification of the ND-GFP vessels of **b** and **c**, respectively. (**f** and **g**) Colocalization of GFP and the endothelial cell marker CD31 (arrows). **f** is a fluorescent image, and **g** shows the same field air-dried and immunohistochemically stained with CD31 (Scale bars, 100 μm)

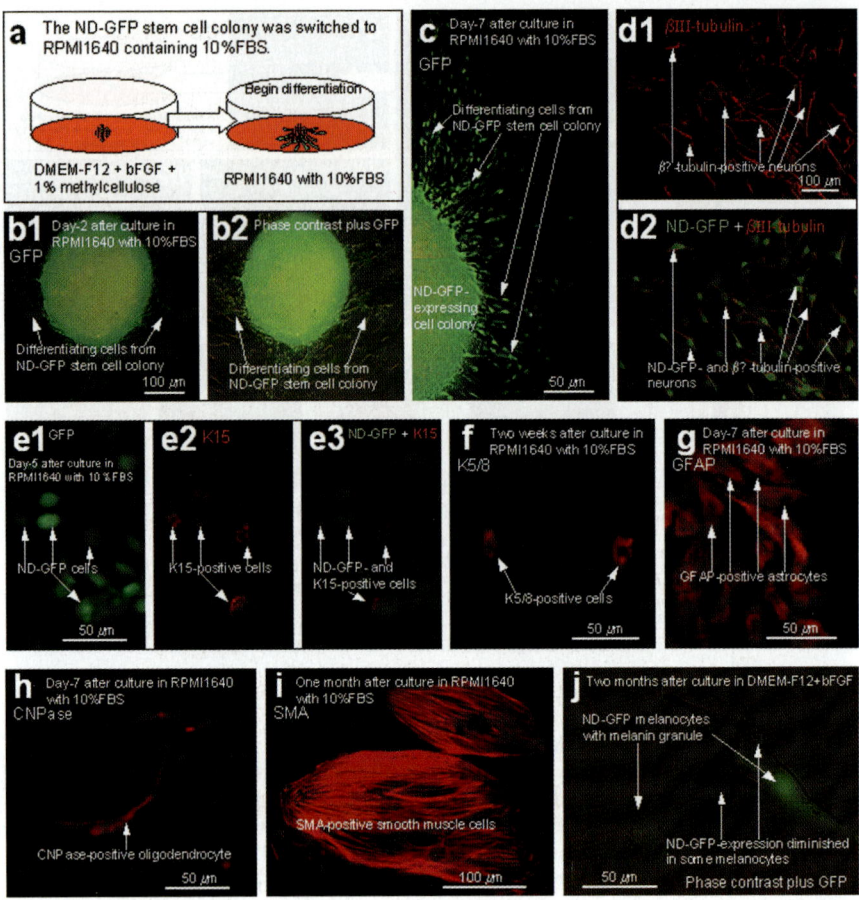

Fig. 15.6 Differentiation of ND-GFP hair follicle stem cells *in vitro* [20]. (**a**) The ND-GFP-expressing cell colony was switched to RPMI medium 1640 containing 10% FBS from DMEM-F12 containing B-27 and 1% methylcellulose supplemented with bFGF every 2 days. (**b1** and **b2**) At 2 days after switching into RPMI medium 1640 containing 10% FBS, differentiating cells migrated out of the ND-GFP-expressing cell colony. (**c**) At 7 days after switching to RPMI medium 1640, many differentiating cells migrated out of the ND-GFP-expressing cell colony. (**d1** and **d2**) ND-GFP-expressing cells differentiated to III β-tubulin-positive neurons which maintain ND-GFP-expression. (**e1–e3**) At 5 days after switching to RPMI medium 1640, ND-GFP-expressing cells differentiated to K15-positive cells (red fluorescence, arrows) (**e2**). The K15-positive cells still expressed ND-GFP. (**f**) ND-GFP-expressing cells differentiated to K5/8-positive cells 2 weeks after switching to RPMI medium 1640. (**g**) At 7 days after switching to RPMI medium 1640, ND-GFP-expressing cells differentiated to GFAP-positive astrocytes. (**h**) At 7 days after switching to RPMI medium 1640, ND-GFP-expressing cells differentiated to 2`,3`-cyclic nucleotide 3′-phosphodiesterase (CNPase)-positive oligodendrocytes. (**i**) At 1 month after culture in RPMI medium 1640 containing 10% FBS, ND-GFP-expressing cells differentiated to SMA-positive smooth muscle cells. (**j**) At 2 months after culture in DMEM-F12 containing B-27 and 1% methylcellulose supplemented with bFGF every 2 days, ND-GFP-expressing cells differentiated to melanocytes containing melanin. Some melanocytes still expressed ND-GFP

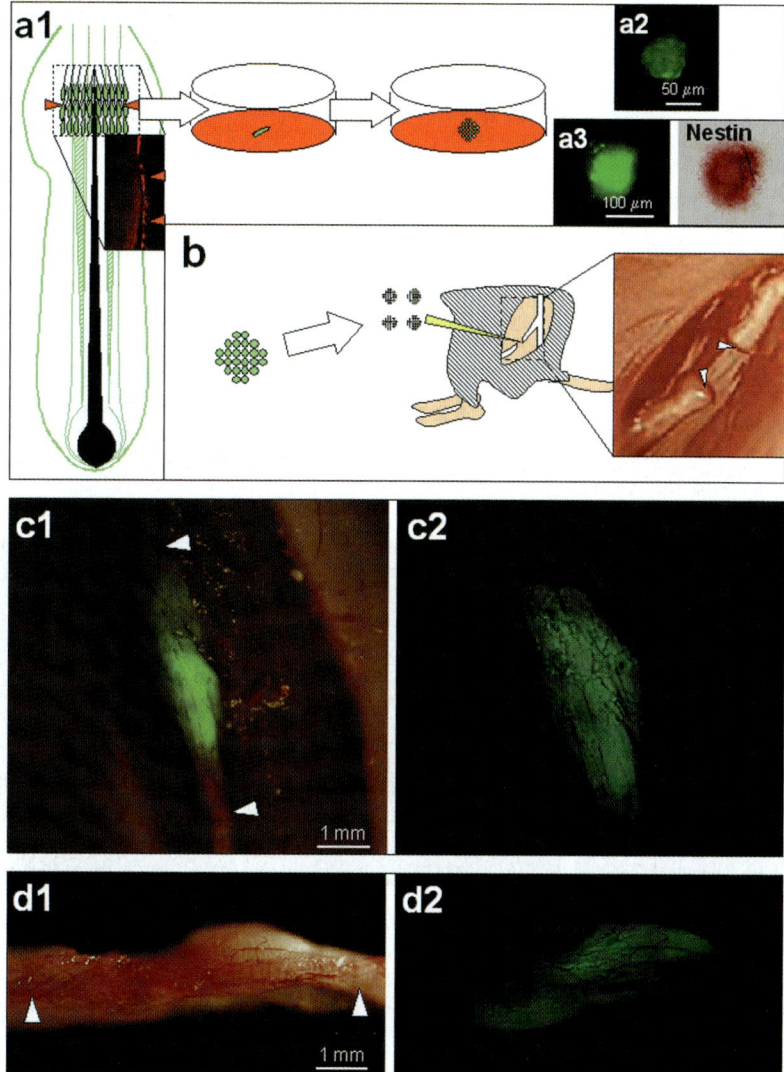

Fig. 15.7 Rejoining severed sciatic nerve with hair follicle stem cells [21]. (**a1**) Schematic of vibrissa follicle of GFP transgenic mice showing the position of GFP- and nestin-expressing vibrissa follicle stem cells (red arrowheads). (**a2**) Colony formed from GFP-expressing hair follicle stem cells from the vibrissa after 2 months in culture. (**a3**) GFP-expressing cells within the colony were nestin-positive. (**b**) GFP-expressing hair follicle stem cells grown for 2 months in DMEM-F12 containing B-27, 1% methylcellulose, and basic FGF were transplanted between the severed sciatic nerve fragments in C57BL/6 immunocompetent mice (white arrowheads). (**c1** and **c2**) Fluorescence images from a live mouse. Two months after transplantation between the severed sciatic nerve, the GFP-expressing cells joined the severed sciatic nerve. **c2** shows higher magnification of *c1*. (**d1** and **d2**) Brightfield (**d1**) and fluorescence (**d2**) images of an excised sciatic nerve. The preexisting sciatic nerve is denoted by white arrowheads

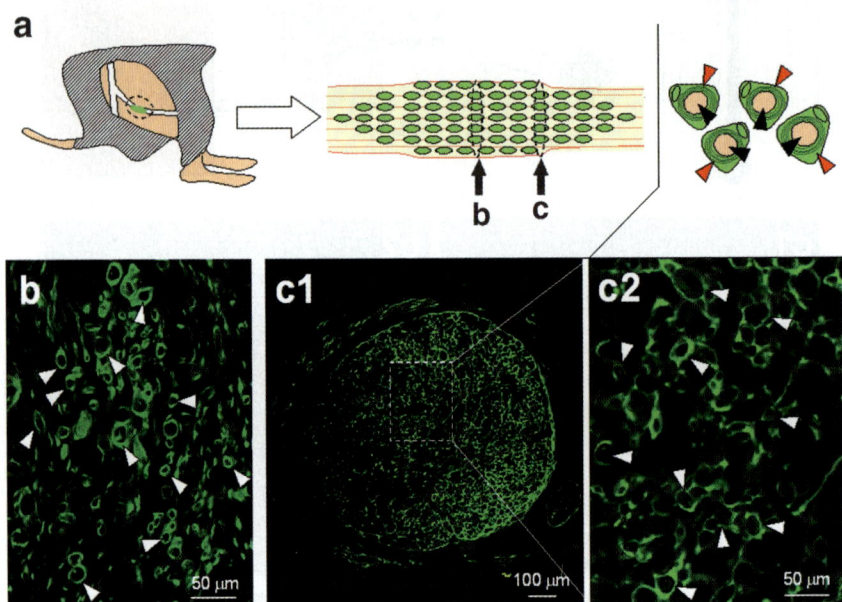

Fig. 15.8 Cell types growing in area of sciatic nerve joined by hair follicle stem cells [21]. (**a**) GFP-expressing vibrissa hair follicle stem cells were growing in the joined sciatic nerve. Most of the GFP-expressing vibrissa hair follicle stem cells differentiated to Schwann cells and formed myelin sheaths surrounding axons (red arrowheads). The axons are denoted by black arrowheads. (**b**) Transverse section of joined nerve. In the central area of the joined nerve, GFP-expressing cells formed many small myelin sheaths (white arrowheads). (**c1**) In the marginal area of the joined nerve, GFP-expressing cells formed many myelin sheaths (white arrowheads). (**c2**) Higher magnification of area of **c1** indicated by the white dashed box